Challenging Pain Syndromes

Editor

ADAM L. SCHREIBER

PHYSICAL MEDICINE AND REHABILITATION CLINICS OF NORTH AMERICA

www.pmr.theclinics.com

Consulting Editor
GREGORY T. CARTER

May 2014 • Volume 25 • Number 2

ELSEVIER

1600 John F. Kennedy Boulevard • Suite 1800 • Philadelphia, Pennsylvania, 19103-2899

http://www.theclinics.com

PHYSICAL MEDICINE AND REHABILITATION CLINICS OF NORTH AMERICA Volume 25, Number 2
May 2014 ISSN 1047-9651, ISBN 978-0-323-29723-3

Editor: Jennifer Flynn-briggs
Developmental Editor: Don Mumford

Reprints. For copies of 100 or more of articles in this publication, please contact the Commercial Reprints Department, Elsevier Inc., 360 Park Avenue South, New York, NY 10010-1710. Tel.: 212-633-3874; Fax: 212-633-3820; E-mail: reprints@elsevier.com.

Physical Medicine and Rehabilitation Clinics of North America (ISSN 1047-9651) is published quarterly by Elsevier Inc., 360 Park Avenue South, New York, NY 10010-1710. Months of issue are February, May, August, and November. Business and Editorial Offices: 1600 John F. Kennedy Blvd., Suite 1800, Philadelphia, PA 19103-2899. Customer Service Office: 3251 Riverport Lane, Maryland Heights, MO 63043. Periodicals postage paid at New York, NY and additional mailing offices. Subscription price per year is $275.00 (US individuals), $486.00 (US institutions), $145.00 (US students), $335.00 (Canadian individuals), $640.00 (Canadian institutions), $210.00 (Canadian students), $415.00 (foreign individuals), $640.00 (foreign institutions), and $210.00 (foreign students). Foreign air speed delivery is included in all *Clinics* subscription prices. All prices are subject to change without notice. **POSTMASTER:** Send address changes to *Physical Medicine and Rehabilitation Clinics of North America,* Customer Service Office: Elsevier Health Sciences Division, Subscription Customer Service, 3251 Riverport Lane, Maryland Heights, MO 63043. **Customer Service: 1-800-654-2452 (US). From outside of the United States, call 314-447-8871. Fax: 314-447-8029. E-mail:** JournalsCustomerService-usa@elsevier.com **(for print support);** JournalsOnlineSupport-usa@elsevier.com **(for online support).**

Physical Medicine and Rehabilitation Clinics of North America is indexed in *Excerpta Medica, MEDLINE/PubMed (Index Medicus), Cinahl,* and *Cumulative Index to Nursing and Allied Health Literature.*

Contributors

CONSULTING EDITOR

GREGORY T. CARTER, MD, MS
Consulting Medical Editor, Medical Director, St Luke's Rehabilitation Institute, Spokane, Washington; University of Washington, School of Medicine, Seattle, Washington

EDITOR

ADAM L. SCHREIBER, DO
Director of Ambulatory Services, Jefferson Rehabilitation Medicine Associates, Assistant Professor, Department of Rehabilitation Medicine, Jefferson Medical College, Thomas Jefferson University, Philadelphia, Pennsylvania

AUTHORS

ANNA-CHRISTINA BEVELAQUA, MD, FAAPMR
Assistant Professor of Rehabilitation Medicine, Department of Rehabilitation and Regenerative Medicine, Columbia University Medical Center, New York Presbyterian Hospital, New York, New York

JOANNE BORG-STEIN, MD
Associate Professor, Department of Physical Medicine and Rehabilitation, Harvard Medical School, Boston, Massachusetts

BARBARA J. BROWNE, MD
Assistant Professor, Rehabilitation Medicine, Magee Rehabilitation Hospital, Jefferson Medical College, Thomas Jefferson University, Philadelphia, Pennsylvania

GREGORY T. CARTER, MD, MS
Consulting Medical Editor, Medical Director, St. Luke's Rehabilitation Institute, Spokane, Washington; University of Washington, School of Medicine, Seattle, Washington

VICKY DUONG, BS, PharmD(c)
Doctoral Candidate, Department of Pharmacotherapy, Washington State University, Spokane, Washington

KRISTOFER J. FEEKO, DO
Clinical Instructor, Department of Rehabilitation Medicine, Jefferson Medical College, Thomas Jefferson University, Philadelphia, Pennsylvania

MITCHELL FREEDMAN, DO
Associate Professor and Clinical Instructor of Rehabilitation Medicine, Jefferson Medical College, Thomas Jefferson University; Director of Physical Medicine and Rehabilitation, Rothman Institute, Philadelphia, Pennsylvania

ROBERT D. GERWIN, MD, FAAN
Associate Professor of Neurology, Department of Neurology, Johns Hopkins University School of Medicine, Baltimore; Pain and Rehabilitation Medicine, Bethesda, Maryland

DAVID GOLDMANN, MD
Elsevier Clinical Solutions, Evidence-Based Medicine Center, Philadelphia, Pennsylvania

CHRISTOPHER L. GREER, BPharm
St. Luke's Rehabilitation Institute; Faculty, Department of Pharmacotherapy, Washington State University, Spokane, Washington

ARI C. GREIS, DO
Clinical Instructor of Rehabilitation Medicine, Jefferson Medical College, Thomas Jefferson University; Rothman Institute, Philadelphia, Pennsylvania

JEFFREY HENSTENBURG
Rochester Institute of Technology College Student Volunteer, Rothman Institute, Philadelphia, Pennsylvania

STANLEY HO, BS, PharmD(c)
Doctoral Candidate, Department of Pharmacotherapy, Washington State University, Spokane, Washington

MARY ALEXIS IACCARINO, MD
Department of Physical Medicine and Rehabilitation, Harvard Medical School, Boston, Massachusetts

BRIAN KAHAN, DO, FAAPMR, DAOCRM, DABIPP, DABPM, FIPP
Founder, The Kahan Center for Pain Management, Annapolis, Maryland

LEONARD B. KAMEN, DO
Clinical Director, MossRehab Outpatient Center, Albert Einstein Healthcare Network; Associate Professor, Department of Physical Medicine and Rehabilitation, Temple University, Philadelphia, Pennsylvania

MICHAEL MALLOW, MD
Assistant Professor of Rehabilitation Medicine, Department of Rehabilitation Medicine, Jefferson Medical College, Thomas Jefferson University, Philadelphia, Pennsylvania

LISA MARINO, DO
Associate Physician, Rothman Institute, Philadelphia, Pennsylvania

MATTHEW MCAULIFFE, MD
Resident Physician, Department of Rehabilitation Medicine, Thomas Jefferson University Hospital, Philadelphia, Pennsylvania

LEVON N. NAZARIAN, MD, FACR
Professor and Vice Chairman for Education, Department of Radiology, Thomas Jefferson University Hospital, Jefferson Medical College, Thomas Jefferson University, Philadelphia, Pennsylvania

KATHRYN C. NGO, BS, PharmD(c)
Doctoral Candidate, Department of Pharmacotherapy, Washington State University, Spokane, Washington

MEGAN SANDS-LINCOLN, MPH, PhD
Elsevier Clinical Solutions, Evidence-Based Medicine Center, Philadelphia, Pennsylvania

MICHAEL SAULINO, MD, PhD
Physiatrist, MossRehab, Elkins Park; Assistant Professor, Department of Rehabilitation Medicine, Jefferson Medical College, Thomas Jefferson University, Philadelphia, Pennsylvania

ADAM L. SCHREIBER, DO, FAAPMR
Director of Ambulatory Services, Jefferson Rehabilitation Medicine Associates, Assistant Professor, Department of Rehabilitation Medicine, Jefferson Medical College, Thomas Jefferson University, Philadelphia, Pennsylvania

FEHREEN SHAMIM, MD
Resident Physician, Department of Rehabilitation Medicine, Thomas Jefferson University Hospital, Philadelphia, Pennsylvania

TATYANA A. SHAMLIYAN, MD, MS
Elsevier Clinical Solutions, Evidence-Based Medicine Center, Philadelphia, Pennsylvania

CARL M. SHAPIRO, DO, FAOCPMR, FAAPMR
Board Certified in the Sub-Specialty of Pain Medicine, ABPMR, Former Assistant Professor of Physical Medicine and Rehabilitation, University of Cincinnati; Past President American Osteopathic College of Physical Medicine and Rehabilitation; Tri-State Spine and Neuromuscular Associates, Cincinnati, Ohio

JEREMY SIMON, MD
Clinical Instructor, Department of Physical Medicine and Rehabilitation, Rothman Institute, Philadelphia, Pennsylvania

ANUPAM N. SINHA, DO
Associate Physician, Rothman Institute, Philadelphia, Pennsylvania

CLARK C. SMITH, MD, MPH, FAAPMR
Assistant Professor of Rehabilitation Medicine, Department of Rehabilitation and Regenerative Medicine, Columbia University Medical Center, New York Presbyterian Hospital, New York, New York

J. BART STAAL, PhD
Scientific Institute for Quality of Healthcare (IQ Healthcare), Radboud University Nijmegen Medical Centre, Nijmegen, The Netherlands

BENJAMIN M. SUCHER, DO, FAOCPMR, FAAPMR
Medical Director, EMG Labs of Arizona Arthritis & Rheumatology Associates, Phoenix, Arizona

AMIR TAHAEI, MD
Resident Physician, Department of Rehabilitation Medicine, Thomas Jefferson University Hospital, Philadelphia, Pennsylvania

JOHN M. VASUDEVAN, MD
Assistant Professor, Physical Medicine & Rehabilitation, University of Pennsylvania, Philadelphia, Pennsylvania

NANCY VUONG, MD
Resident Physician, Department of Rehabilitation Medicine, Thomas Jefferson University Hospital, Philadelphia, Pennsylvania

DOUGLAS L. WEEKS, PhD
St. Luke's Rehabilitation Institute; Faculty, Department of Pharmacotherapy, Washington State University, Spokane, Washington

Contents

Carpal tunnel syndrome (CTS) is a common median nerve compression syndrome and the most common peripheral mononeuropathy. The clinical syndrome is diagnosed by history and physical examination. Electrodiagnostic testing is the objective method used to measure median nerve dysfunction at the wrist and confirm the clinical diagnosis of CTS. Neuromuscular ultrasound imaging of the carpal tunnel provides supportive diagnostic information by revealing pathologic nerve swelling in CTS, and other anatomic anomalies that compress the median nerve. These tests cannot be used to make the diagnosis in the absence of history that includes CTS symptom criteria and excludes other causes.

 Videos of a demonstration of an opponens roll and a sonographically guided needle puncture of the transverse carpal ligament in real time accompany this article

This article describes 2 nonsurgical approaches to the treatment of carpal tunnel syndrome that are not routinely offered, probably due to a lack of awareness. Osteopathic manipulative treatment (OMT) is commonly used for many medical problems, including musculoskeletal issues. OMT of the carpal tunnel is well described and researched, and can be clinically used by a skilled practitioner. The second treatment strategy is a more recent development. The use of ultrasound for guidance of injection is established, but a newer technique using sonographically guided percutaneous needle release of the transverse carpal ligament has shown promising results.

Parsonage-Turner syndrome (PTS) is a rare disorder typically characterized by an abrupt onset of upper extremity pain followed by progressive neurologic deficits, including weakness, atrophy, and occasionally sensory abnormalities. The exact cause and pathophysiology of PTS are complex and incompletely understood. Autoimmune, genetic, infectious, and mechanical processes have all been implicated. No specific treatments have been proven to reduce neurologic impairment or improve the prognosis of PTS. Most patients with PTS are treated with a multidisciplinary

tender, contracted muscle that is readily identified by palpation. The trigger point has well-described electrophysiologic properties and is associated with a derangement of the local biochemical milieu of the muscle. A proper diagnosis of MPS includes evaluation of muscle as a cause of pain, and assessment of associated conditions that have an impact on MPS.

Myofascial pain syndrome (MPS) is a regional pain disorder caused by taut bands of muscle fibers in skeletal muscles called myofascial trigger points. MPS is a common disorder, often diagnosed and treated by physiatrists. Treatment strategies for MPS include exercises, patient education, and trigger point injection. Pharmacologic interventions are also common, and a variety of analgesics, antiinflammatories, antidepressants, and other medications are used in clinical practice. This review explores the various treatment options for MPS, including those therapies that target myofascial trigger points and common secondary symptoms.

Treatment of chronic noncancer pain (CNCP) with high-dose opioids (HDOs) has burgeoned over the past 2 decades in the United States. Characteristic domains and features of the failed CNCP management patient using long-term HDOs are described herein as the/an opioid syndrome (Schreiber AL, personal communication. 2013). Reversing or even modulating HDO use in patients with CNCP requires a paradigm shift on the part of physician, patient, and the societal "quick fix" medical culture. This review offers measures, agents, and strategies to consider in management of this pervasive, erosive medical and societal challenge.

Chronic pain associated with traumatic spinal cord injury (SCI) can be quite challenging to the physiatrist. This highly prevalent condition within the SCI population requires an appropriate evaluative approach including a thorough history, a targeted physical examination, and appropriate use of diagnostic testing. The International Spinal Cord Injury Pain Classification allows for a reasonable categorization of the various pain syndromes and may assist in selecting a reasoned treatment strategy. A multitude of management approaches exist including nonpharmacologic, pharmacologic, and interventional approaches. This article provides an overview of the epidemiology, classification, evaluation, and management of SCI-associated pain.

Stroke is a significant source of mortality and long-term disability in the United States. Of persons who survive a stroke, approximately 50% will have hemiplegia, half of whom will live with a nonfunctional arm. Hemiplegic shoulder pain (HSP), which occurs in most patients with hemiplegia, reduces participation and worsens outcomes in rehabilitation. Management of HSP is challenging because its causes are multifactorial and there is limited, conflicting, or nonspecific evidence in support of most treatments. This article develops an effective approach for diagnosis and treatment using the best available evidence to aid practitioners in obtaining optimal results.

This article discusses current trends in managing cancer pain, with specific regard to opioid transmission, descending pathway inhibation, and ways to facilitate the endogenous antinociceptive chemicals in the human body. Various techniques for opioid and nonopioid control of potential pain situations of patients with cancer are discussed. The benefits of using pharmacogenetics to assess the appropriate medications are addressed. Finally, specific treatment of abdominal cancer pain using radiofrequency lesioning is discussed.

Analgesics, including opioids, steroidal and nonsteroidal anti-inflammatory drugs, aspirin, acetaminophen, antiepileptics, and serotonin-norepinephrine reuptake inhibitors, are medications commonly used to treat many forms of pain. However, all of these agents may have significant adverse side effects. Adverse effects may occasionally be inseparable from desired effects. Side effects are often dose dependent and time dependent. It is critical that the prescribing practitioner and the dispensing pharmacist provide a thorough, understandable review of the potential side effects to all patients before these drugs are administered. Proper monitoring and follow-up during therapy are crucial.

Special Article

Most clinical guidelines do not recommend routine use of epidural steroid injections for the management of chronic low back pain. However, many clinicians do not adhere to these guidelines. This comprehensive evidence overview concluded that off-label epidural steroid injections provide small short-term but not long-term leg-pain relief and improvement in function; injection of steroids is no more effective than injection of local anesthetics alone; post-procedural complications are uncommon, but the risk of contamination and serious infections is very high. The evidence does not support routine use of off-label epidural steroid injections in adults with benign radicular lumbosacral pain.

PHYSICAL MEDICINE & REHABILITATION CLINICS OF NORTH AMERICA

RELATED INTEREST

Medical Clinics of North America, November 2013 (Vol. 97, Issue 6, Pages 1201–1215)
Patients with Chronic Pain
Joseph Salama-Hanna and Grace Chen, *Editors*

VISIT THE CLINICS ONLINE!
Access your subscription at:
www.theclinics.com

NOW AVAILABLE FOR YOUR iPhone and iPad

Foreword

Challenging Pain Syndromes

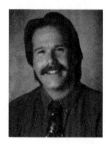

Gregory T. Carter, MD, MS
Consulting Editor

This volume is guest-edited by Dr Adam Schreiber. What you have in your hands now is the result of tremendous efforts by Dr Schreiber, and I believe he has produced an amazingly useful and pertinent issue of *Physical Medicine and Rehabilitation Clinics of North America*. Taking on the topic of challenging pain syndromes is much like taking on the heart and soul of many physiatry practices, including my own, frankly. I applaud Dr Schreiber's efforts in assembling a very qualified, renowned group of authors to create this issue of the *Physical Medicine and Rehabilitation Clinics of North America*.

This is also the first volume of the Clinics where we are adding, in response to our readers' requests, an additional component of evidence-based medicine. An article is featured in this issue on "Discogenic Low Back Pain," arguing that there isn't much evidence that steroid epidurals have shown convincing benefit for this entity. In turn, Elsevier Clinical Solutions, Evidence-Based Medicine Center elected to include an article on "Epidural Steroid Injections for Radicular Lumbosacral Pain – A Systematic Review," to also show that the evidence is insufficient.

Among the other esteemed authors is Dr Sucher, Director of the EMG Labs of Arizona Arthritis & Rheumatology Associates, who has done excellent work in the area of grading the severity of carpal tunnel syndrome (CTS) and developing methods for doing so. While most of us tend to use latencies as a guide, this can be misleading, and using other criteria, such as low amplitudes or conduction block and denervation, may be very useful. Drs Sucher, Nazarian, and Schreiber then give us a treatise on emerging, novel treatment strategies for CTS.

Dr Kamen, of the MossRehab Outpatient Center, and Dr Feeko, give us a comprehensive guide of opioid therapy, taking into consideration all available evidence from preclinical and clinical work. This includes excellent review of the safety and tolerability profile of opioids, pointing out that the adverse event profile varies greatly between opioids. Methods of using these agents to optimize the tolerability profile, especially regarding central nervous system and gastrointestinal effects, are provided.

Phys Med Rehabil Clin N Am 25 (2014) xiii–xiv
http://dx.doi.org/10.1016/j.pmr.2014.03.001
1047-9651/14/$ – see front matter © 2014 Elsevier Inc. All rights reserved.

pmr.theclinics.com

Drs C. Smith and Bevelaqua give an excellent review of Parsonage-Turner syndrome in the context of neuropathic pain and Dr Saulino provides us with a thorough review of the challenges in treating spinal cord injury pain, which can often be refractory to conventional treatment and presents particular challenges to physicians and patients. This article reviews chronic spinal pain pathophysiology and the mechanisms whereby spinally administered analgesics may modify chronic pain as well as guidelines on the use of agents for nociceptive, neuropathic, and mixed pain.

Drs Greis, Marino, and Freedman review the management of complex regional pain syndrome, one of our biggest clinical challenges. They offer directly usable, clinically practical treatment paradigms.

The latter portion of this volume is rounded out with a thorough article by Drs Mallow and Nazarian on greater trochanteric pain syndrome, followed by a comprehensive review of hemiplegic shoulder pain by Drs Vasudevan and Browne. Dr Gerwin reviews the challenging topic of assessing myofascial pain syndrome, followed by a discussion from Drs Borg-Stein and Iaccarino on management strategies. Dr Kahan provides us with an excellent overview of cancer pain; the volume concludes with two articles discussing various aspects of low back pain. This includes an outstanding treatise on failed back surgery syndrome by Dr Shapiro, followed by a comprehensive discussion of the role of epidural steroid injections for radicular lumbosacral pain by Drs Shamliyan, Stall, Goldmann, and San-Lincoln.

I also want to thank each and every one of these distinguished authors, most especially Dr Schreiber, for their hard work and outstanding contributions to this issue of the *Physical Medicine and Rehabilitation Clinics of North America*. I believe this is a very comprehensive presentation of the management of a most challenging population of patients. This issue of *Physical Medicine and Rehabilitation Clinics of North America* gives us directly applicable and useful advice on how to treat these patients, making a sublime addition to the series.

Gregory T. Carter, MD, MS
St Luke's Rehabilitation Institute
711 South Cowley Street
Spokane, WA 99202, USA

E-mail address:
gtcarter@uw.edu

Preface

Challenging Pain Syndromes

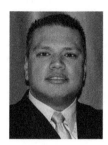

Adam L. Schreiber, DO
Editor

No matter whether a general or subspecialized physiatrist, we all encounter pain syndromes; therefore, when Dr Greg Carter invited me to edit an issue of *Physical Medicine and Rehabilitation Clinics of North America*, the topic appealed to my desire to produce an issue that spans the breadth of the specialty. Another focus of this issue is to serve as a guide to clinical medicine, which entails the best evidence with the experience of our authors to produce practical recommendations.

As I edited the work of the authors, I found common themes that I would like to emphasize. In regard to ordering testing, "care must be exerted with regard to interpretation so as not to 'over-read' the importance of particular abnormality," wrote Dr Michael Saulino. This applies to all aspects of medicine, but by the nature of a syndrome, testing is never pathognomonic. How many of our patients marry the finding of L5 disc bulge? Many times this does not explain any or all of their symptoms, yet 10 years later they remain devout to the beloved bulge, which may have even reabsorbed. Prior to ordering tests, I try to counsel patients that tests will likely have abnormalities; it only matters if the the findings correlate with what "you share with me." An example is Dr Gerry Herbison has been preaching for decades that EMG is confirmation of our clinical impression; to a degree that notion should apply to all testing, especially in regard to pain syndromes.

Another common theme was medication use. There are several medication utilized with pain syndromes. The rationale for use may differ for the clinical syndrome but the side-effect profile remains the same. Therefore, we added an addendum in this issue for side effects to keep the syndrome articles focused on the topic and also as a handy compiled reference for side-effect risk profiles.

I am confident the issue will be of interest to our entire field and serve as a strong reference of clinical information that will help you teach others and treat your patients.

Thanks to this issue authors for their time, expertise, and efforts. Thanks to Dr Greg Carter for the opportunity to give back to our specialty. In addition, a special thanks to

Phys Med Rehabil Clin N Am 25 (2014) xv–xvi
http://dx.doi.org/10.1016/j.pmr.2014.02.002
1047-9651/14/$ – see front matter © 2014 Elsevier Inc. All rights reserved.

pmr.theclinics.com

my wife, Jeanne, and sons, Noah and Leo, for providing the support to take on such an endeavor.

Adam L. Schreiber, DO
Department of Rehabilitation Medicine
Jefferson Medical College of Thomas Jefferson University
Jefferson Rehabilitation Medicine Associates
25 South 9th Street
Philadelphia, PA 19107, USA

E-mail address:
adam.schreiber@jefferson.edu

Carpal Tunnel Syndrome Diagnosis

Benjamin M. Sucher, DO[a],*, Adam L. Schreiber, DO[b]

KEYWORDS

- Carpal tunnel • Median nerve • Nerve compression • Neuropathy • Ultrasound

KEY POINTS

- Symptoms include numbness, tingling, and/or pain in the ventral-lateral hand, possibly thenar atrophy and weakness, which typically worsens at night.
- Positive provocative testing includes Tinel, Phalen, and carpal compression.
- Positive electrical testing includes nerve conduction studies revealing initially prolonged median peak sensory latencies (slowing across the wrist), with normal ulnar and radial latencies.
- Ultrasound imaging reveals median nerve enlargement at the proximal wrist, median nerve compression during stress testing, and muscle intrusion during hand motion (digit flexion or extension) that compresses the median nerve.

INTRODUCTION

Carpal tunnel syndrome (CTS) is a very common nerve compression syndrome, generally not considered difficult to diagnose.[1–4] However, the method of diagnosis may vary among clinicians. Although diagnosis is important, determination of the degree or severity is useful because it may influence the treatment approach.[5] For example, during the early stages and milder forms of CTS, there may be ample time to begin a trial of conservative treatment without risk of significant denervation. However, in more advanced cases with axon loss, delayed interventional treatment increases the risk of irreversible progressive median nerve (MN) injury. In addition, neuromuscular ultrasound (NMUS) can demonstrate contributing factors that often injure the MN, and once identified, these factors can be addressed in the treatment plan for improved outcomes.[6,7]

Definition

CTS refers to a constellation or aggregate of hand symptoms that are linked to the median neuropathy at the wrist.[1–4] There are many various causes, some

---

[a] EMG Labs of Arizona Arthritis & Rheumatology Associates, 4550 East Bell Road, #170, Phoenix, AZ 85032, USA; [b] Jefferson Rehabilitation Medicine Associates, Jefferson Medical College of Thomas Jefferson University, 25 South 9th Street, 1st Floor, Philadelphia, PA 19107, USA
* Corresponding author.
E-mail address: DrSucher@msn.com

Phys Med Rehabil Clin N Am 25 (2014) 229–247
http://dx.doi.org/10.1016/j.pmr.2014.01.004
1047-9651/14/$ – see front matter © 2014 Elsevier Inc. All rights reserved.

beyond the scope of this article; however, it is usually considered to be multifactorial[6,7]:

- Increased intracarpal pressure
- Decreased MN mobility (from fibrous fixation)
- Median nerve deformation (ie, compression, stretching, traction)
- Increased stiffness of the synovium and flexor retinaculum (ie, transverse carpal ligament [TCL])
- Relative thenar muscle hypertrophy or increased thenar muscle mass with intrusion into the carpal tunnel
- Flexor tendon thickening and tightening during activity

Symptom Criteria

The following are typical symptoms that accompany CTS. It is important to keep in mind that these symptoms may be quite variable, thus requiring clinical examination and electrodiagnostic (EDX) testing to confirm.[1–4]

- Numbness: thumb and first 2 to 3 fingers (and lateral aspect of the fourth digit), primarily ventral
- Tingling: same distribution as numbness
- Weakness: thumb abduction and opposition (dropping or problems holding objects)
- Pain: ventral wrist and hand
- Autonomic features (temperature or color changes, dry skin, swelling)
- Provocative factors: nocturnal worsening; aggravated by sustained wrist flexion or extension, repetitive hand activity

CLINICAL FINDINGS
Physical Examination

Sensory examination is often normal in CTS, despite patient complaints and other diagnostic findings.[1] The pattern of sensory loss may not follow the classic MN distribution in the hand (which includes the ventral thumb, index, middle, and lateral half of the ring finger) due to anatomic variations.[1] Examination for pin sensation is quite subjective, but monofilament testing adds some degree of objectivity and can be used to map out sensory loss within the MN distribution.[8] Abnormal 2-point discrimination (and vibratory loss) is a later manifestation due to more severe nerve injury.[1,8]

Positive provocative Tinel and Phalen (**Fig. 1**) tests are not considered reliable or confirmatory, but may be helpful by adding to the clinical impression.[1–3] The problem is that they are not objective tests, and the precise method of application is highly variable among clinicians. **Fig. 1A** illustrates the proper and commonly used improper method of performing the Phalen test. Carpal compression may also be useful and can be applied simultaneously with the Phalen test as the operator grasps the patient's wrist and maintains flexion dorsally while providing focal pressure over the MN ventrally (see **Fig. 1B**).

Palpation of the wrist for mechanical restriction over the carpal canal can assist in diagnosis[9] and has been demonstrated to have a sensitivity of greater than 90%,[10] using EDX as the gold standard. The most reliable motion testing involves transverse extension and thenar extension/abduction (**Fig. 2**).[9] Palpatory diagnosis also correlates well with EDX.[9–11]

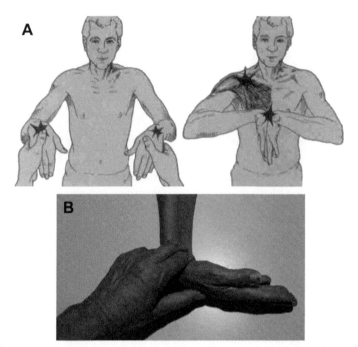

Fig. 1. Phalen test (*A*) performed properly (*left*) and improperly (*right*). The left image illustrates independent testing of each carpal tunnel. The right image illustrates a common shortcut examination technique, which is a good general screening for nerve compression, but not specific to the carpal tunnel because it also challenges the thoracic outlet (therefore misleading if it evokes symptoms). (*B*) The Phalen test combined with carpal compression test—examiner maintains wrist flexion while simultaneously applying firm digital pressure directly over the carpal canal. This maneuver is typically held for up to 30 seconds and less than 1 minute.

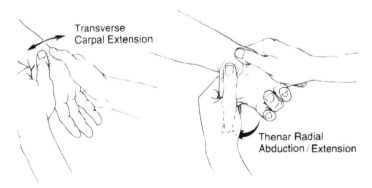

Fig. 2. Palpatory examination of the wrist and carpal canal during transverse carpal extension (*left*) and radial abduction with extension of the thumb (*right*). (*From* Sucher BM. Palpatory diagnosis and manipulative management of carpal tunnel syndrome. J Am Osteopath Assoc 1994;94:648. Figure 2; with permission.)

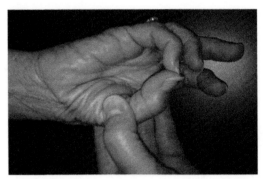

Fig. 3. Strength testing of the thenar muscles. Opposition and abduction of the shorter muscles are tested simultaneously by applying resistance along the first metacarpal or at the first metacarpophalangeal joint.

Strength testing can identify thenar muscle weakness if applied correctly—the examiner being aware that resistance must be applied along the first metacarpal or at the number 1 metacarpal-phalangeal joint, and toward the radial side of the index to avoid testing the radial innervated abductor pollicis longus (**Fig. 3**).[1,2] The median innervated thumb muscles should never be tested by pulling a digit through the patient's flexed index and thumb, because that tests the thumb adductor and long thumb and finger flexors, which receive ulnar innervation for the former, while the flexor pollicis longus and index finger flexors receive their median innervation proximal to the tunnel.[1,2] It is also important to exclude contribution from the abductor pollicis longus, which would not be affected by CTS either, because it is radial nerve innervated. It may seem that the patient has normal strength if the distal abductor pollicis brevis and opponens pollicis muscles are not properly isolated and challenged.

One sign that may be apparent with advanced MN injury is the observation of thenar atrophy. Indentation or hollowing of the thenar mound is a late sign accompanying weakness and implies severe CTS. In fact, some authors have determined that it may be too late to operate once the nerve damage has reached this state.[12] Bland[12] discovered that patients with absent sensory or motor responses (degeneration of many MN fibers) had the worst outcomes.

Differential Diagnosis

Neuromusculoskeletal and vascular differential diagnoses of carpal tunnel symptoms include, but are not limited to: brain, cervical spine, musculoskeletal system, and neurologic diseases other than CTS (**Box 1**).[1,13] It may be helpful to consider the history and physical examination in any attempt to clarify the perspective from central to distal. There are many predisposing factors including, but not limited to: alcoholism, endocrine diseases (diabetes and thyroid), rheumatologic disease, amyloidosis, trauma, infections, uremia, and obesity.[1]

Objective Diagnostic Studies

Diagnostic studies that produce measurable changes to document nerve injury help confirm the diagnosis of CTS. The most commonly used tests include EDX[1–4,13–17] and NMUS.[6,7,18–23] Quantitative sensory testing will not be discussed here.

Box 1
Differential diagnosis of CTS

Brain

Cerebral insult (including tumors, thalamic lesions, lacunar strokes)

Demyelinating diseases

Cervical spine

Cervical disc disease, spondylosis, stenosis, and associated radiculopathy

Spinal cord injury (including syringomyelia, tumors)

Musculoskeletal (peripheral)

Myofascial pain syndrome

Osteoarthritis, inflammatory arthropathies (including Raynaud's)

Tendonitis, tendinosis, epicondylitis

Compartment syndrome

Ganglions and hand tumors

Neurologic

Brachial plexopathy (including Parsonage Turner syndrome and thoracic outlet syndrome)

Complex regional pain syndrome

Compression neuropathy proximal to the wrist

Ischemic monomelic neuropathy

Polyneuropathy (including diabetic, mononeuropathy multiplex)

Motor neuron disease

Demyelinating diseases

Infections (Lyme disease, tabes dorsalis, leprosy)

Data from Rosenbaum RB, Ochoa JL. Carpal tunnel syndrome and other disorders of the median nerve. 2nd edition. Amsterdam: Butterworth Heinemann; 2002; and Ashworth NL. Carpal tunnel syndrome. Available at: http://emedicine.medscape.com/article/316715-overview. Accessed February 4, 2014. [Updated and republished March 5, 2013].

ELECTRODIAGNOSIS

The electrodiagnostic approach to CTS is not simply looking at latencies and other waveform parameters. It includes the use of this information while taking into account the clinical acumen to decide

- If there are electrodiagnostic abnormalities, are they meaningful and do they support the clinical impression of CTS, or does one reject the clinical impression based on the electrodiagnostic findings for management purposes?
- If there are no electrodiagnostic abnormalities, is the suspected diagnosis of CTS still likely for purposes of treatment strategies?

These queries are 2 ends of the diagnostic spectrum with which the electrodiagnostician must struggle. The area in between poses much less challenge.

The spectrum of peripheral nerve injury includes axon and/or myelin disruption and tends to be simplified because effects are measured rather than underlying pathophysiology. Myelin injury may occur in isolation or with secondary axonal death. Axonal death is also referred to as axonopathy, denervation, and Wallerian degeneration (WD). WD includes both axon death and myelin digestion. CTS typically involves myelin disruption initially, followed by axonal death. Macrophages and Schwann cells clear the myelin debris associated with WD. However, if there is a loss of Schwann cells and other growth-supporting molecules, reinnervation becomes less likely.[24] Muscle wasting is a sign of long-standing WD and heralds a poor prognosis for resolution of the atrophy, regardless of any intervention.

Initially, CTS symptoms are transient because of vascular compromise with resultant ischemia caused by overwork or wrist flexion during sleep. Eventually "symptom-producing conduction block" (sCB) may ensue when there is a loss of myelin of 2 successive internodes between nodes of Ranvier.[25] Depending on how many axons are involved, there will be varying degrees (intensity and frequency) of paresthesias, dyesthesias, and eventually weakness. Recovery of conduction block by remyelination promotes recovery of sensation and strength. The remyelinated segment may conduct slower; however, slowing does not cause weakness.[26] A classic example of slowing unrelated to the presence of clinical symptomology is early Charcot-Marie-Tooth disease.[27,28] In addition, there may be axons suffering from slowing and others with sCB.[26]

Dysmyelination or Myelinopathy

All types and severities of myelin injury were traditionally referred to as "demyelination," but this oversimplification implies a lack of myelin, which occurs infrequently. If this were true, symptoms would be constant, and the periodic symptoms associated with activity or nocturnally would not exist. Dysmyelination or myelinopathy and sCB better describe the physiologic states of CTS, as follows[29,30]:

1. Varying degrees of myelin damage
   a. Partial thickness (thinning) of internode(s)
   b. Total thickness of one internode
   c. Total thickness of internodes but not consecutively
   d. Total thickness of consecutive internodes (sCB)
2. Extent of remyelination following myelin injury
3. Extent of remyelination following axonal injury regrowth/reinnervation and sprouting

Patterns of myelin damage may have both electrodiagnostic and clinical manifestations. The thinning of myelin along an axon or loss of myelin at nonconsecutive internodes each cause slowing of conduction that lacks clinical manifestations, whereas the loss of myelin at 2 consecutive internodes would result in sCB.[25] Summation of the axon conducting properties in the MN will express varying degrees of these patterns—slowing with no clinical manifestations, or partial to complete block that manifests in sensory and eventually motor symptoms.[26,31] Remyelinated segments will conduct slowly due to suboptimal myelin.

Axonopathy

The compound muscle action potential (CMAP) attenuates both proximally and distally if acute injury outpaces reinnervation by axonal regrowth or peripheral sprouting from neighboring axon nerve terminals. The CMAP amplitude may return to normal, but residual slowing (prolonged latencies) is likely from either poorly myelinated (dysmyelinated) regenerating parent axons or sprouts from neighboring axons. These axons will never conduct as fast as the original uncompromised axon. Therefore, denervation may be present, or there could be only minor electrical changes such as mild slowing. When a large amount of motor denervation occurs and exceeds reinnervation, then there is detectable clinical weakness.

In chronic repeated compression, the MN is often thinned and flattened at the site of compression, yet may be enlarged both proximal and distal to the compression.[32] With repeated compression, WD occurs gradually, and over a longer period of time there may be collapse of the endoneurial tubes, thus preventing axonal regrowth (a time-sensitive process).[33] CTS has an advantage compared with other nerve injuries, as the reinnervation distance is relatively short, requiring less time to complete the nerve repair before there is a loss of all supporting molecules.

Technique

Multiple electrophysiologic techniques have been described for use in confirming a diagnosis of CTS. However, there is a lack of consensus as to a single best approach. For a broad description of the various EDXs used to evaluate CTS, the reader is encouraged to review several recent articles.[14–16,23] There are also joint organization practice publications that break down recommendations by standards, guidelines, and options.[17]

More focus is usually given to the measurement of sensory fiber conduction because large-diameter myelinated sensory axons are affected before smaller diameter motor axons. Ipsilateral studies should include measurement of sensory and motor conduction in the MN across the wrist, including comparison with nearby nerves (radial and/or ulnar) that do not traverse the carpal tunnel, to minimize the effects of temperature, polyneuropathy, or other factors that may lead to misinterpretation of abnormal MN findings. It is essential to perform sensory conductions from the wrist to the second or third digit, and if there is an abnormality, then from the palm to the digit. Proximal segment conduction attenuation relative to the distal palmar response theoretically will establish if sCB is present, with a significantly larger sensory nerve action potential at the palm than the wrist, suggesting focal compression of the MN at the wrist.[34] However, caution must be exercised using motor comparisons because of volume conduction from ulnar innervated muscles, which might not cause an initial downward deflection due to phase cancellation from the multiple muscles activated by dual stimulation of the median and ulnar nerves.[35]

Motor nerve conduction velocity measured in the forearm is also often slowed. Some attribute this to degeneration of motor fibers proximal to the site of entrapment. However, recording electrodes over the abductor pollicis brevis may pick up slower motor fibers, while faster fibers are blocked at the wrist and not recorded at the end organ. When such slowing is detected between the elbow and the wrist, there is a tendency to attribute it to MN dysfunction at the wrist, but further conduction studies should be considered to demonstrate that the slowed conduction between the wrist and the elbow (mixed conduction) is due to blockage of the fastest conducting fibers:

- A lack of conduction with this technique may be due to retrograde degeneration of the MN axons and would mitigate against recovery with decompression of the MN at the wrist.
- If there is slowing of conduction between the elbow and the wrist, evaluation of forearm muscles should be done to rule out electrodiagnostic abnormalities proximal to the level of the wrist, which would impact the interpretation of a slowing across the wrist.

Needle electromyography (EMG) can confirm denervation if there is motor involvement. Fibrillations and positive sharp waves identify axonal injury and assist in determining chronicity, but are poor indicators of the degree of denervation. Volitional potential abnormalities can assist chronicity determination. If there is a low CMAP from stimulation at the wrist (with pickup at the abductor pollicis brevis muscle and without a reliable palmar study), the EMG will clarify if this is due to sCB or denervation and whether there is any reinnervation. Needle EMG should also be performed if a radiculopathy is a possible cause of symptoms.

SUMMARY

Werner and Andary[14] state that a diagnosis of CTS can usually be made on the basis of clinical symptoms and signs because CTS is a clinical syndrome. If the patient has electrical abnormalities in the absence of any clinical symptoms or signs, they should be reported as "electrodiagnostic evidence of median neuropathy at the wrist with no clinical symptoms or signs," which is a frequent electrical finding, best understood in the light of the wide variation in normal values for latencies and amplitudes in the literature.[36] If the patient has clinical symptoms and signs of CTS in the absence of electrodiagnostic abnormalities, they should be reported as "there is no electrodiagnostic evidence of median neuropathy at the wrist. Given the history and physical, there is clinical evidence of carpal tunnel syndrome." The theoretical reasons for a negative study in a patient with CTS include (1) the condition being too mild, affecting too few nerve fibers; (2) symptoms due to intermittent ischemia, which is fully reversible[37]; (3) testing occurring after reinnervation of sensory nerve action potential.

A predominant amount of the EDX literature is devoted to slowing of conduction, yet Kimura[38] writes, "Slowing of conduction by itself leads to little, if any, clinical symptoms, as long as all impulses arrive at the target organ." The value of slowed nerve conduction parameters is to localize nerve injury. Electrical (and ultrasound) abnormalities may be used to support a clinical impression of CTS but are not used to make a diagnosis of CTS. The practical value of EDX is to confirm that the patient does not have another condition and to demonstrate whether there is a conduction block and/or axonal death, which impacts management of the patient as well as the prognosis.

NMUS

NMUS not only helps confirm the diagnosis but also adds vital information that no other evaluation method can provide.[18–23] It opens a clinical window to look inside the tunnel and observe the structure and behavior of the MN during various activities or hand/wrist positions, providing the clinician with a unique opportunity to study the behavior of the nerve and surrounding structures.

The most reliable ultrasonographic measurement is to obtain the cross-sectional area (CSA) of the MN on transverse imaging at the wrist and distal forearm (**Fig. 4**), typically measured at the level of the pisiform (see **Fig. 4**A and B).[6,7,18–23] The maximum CSA is preferred, which is near the pisiform—the goal is to locate and measure the MN where most swelling has occurred—by tracing along the inner edge of the hyperechoic (brighter) rim that surrounds the nerve (epineurium).[18–23] The upper limit of normal size is generally approximately 11 mm^2, but each laboratory may want to establish normal value limits based on experience.[6,7,18–23] Enlarged nerve size is considered an objective sign of nerve edema, causing the nerve to look darker (more hypoechoic), usually accompanied by loss of definition of the nerve fascicles (tiny hypoechoic dots, surrounded by hyperechoic connective tissue, perineurium), often termed "loss of fascicular echotexture."[18,19,22] **Fig. 5** illustrates an abnormally enlarged MN at 15 mm^2 in a CTS patient (see **Fig. 5**B).

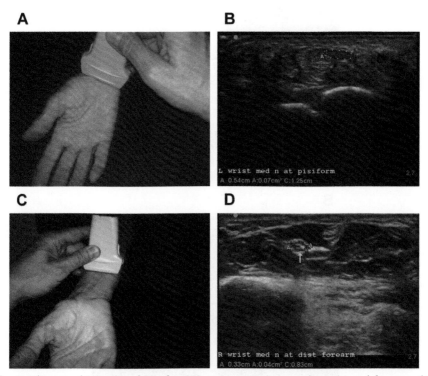

Fig. 4. Ultrasound imaging of MN for CTS: transverse views at the wrist and forearm. (*A*) Transducer placement technique for imaging at the proximal tunnel, at the level of the pisiform, for CSA measurement. (*B*) Ultrasound image of a normal MN. The MN is the darker (hypoechoic) ellipsoid structure in the upper right central portion of the image: dotted outline surrounds the MN ("A" marker on left edge of nerve) just along the inner edge of the brighter (hyperechoic) rim of epineurium that encompasses the nerve; CSA measures 7 mm² (0.07 cm²). (*C*) Transverse imaging in distal forearm, for wrist-forearm ratio determination. (*D*) Ultrasound image from the forearm, white vertical arrow identifies MN (surrounded by dotted outline of "A" markers), which is relatively bright (hyperechoic) at this level due to the darker (hypoechoic) adjacent forearm muscles.

If the CSA is not clearly abnormal, but borderline or near the high end of normal, then obtaining a CSA in the distal forearm allows calculation of the wrist-forearm ratio (see **Fig. 4**C and D), which is a sensitive method of determining abnormal enlargement of the nerve.[39] The wrist-forearm ratio upper limit of normal is approximately 1.5.[39] This work was subsequently confirmed by others[40] and it was determined that the distal forearm measurement could be obtained at 4 or 12 cm proximal to the distal radius. In fact, the 4-cm measurement was considered easier to obtain and is thus preferred.[40] However, some authors have found that absolute numbers may be better than the ratio and have determined if the CSA difference between forearm and wrist is 2 mm² or greater, that it has a 99% sensitivity and 100% specificity for CTS.[41]

Motion studies allow the examiner to evaluate the dynamic behavior of the nerve in response to tendon and muscle movement.[19,23] The most common muscle intrusion into the carpal canal involves the lumbrical muscles (see **Fig. 5**), because they are attached to the long flexor tendons and are often carried into the tunnel during digit flexion (grasp maneuver). In addition, the flexor digitorum superficialis muscle can be pulled into the tunnel from the distal forearm during wrist and digit extension (**Fig. 6**).

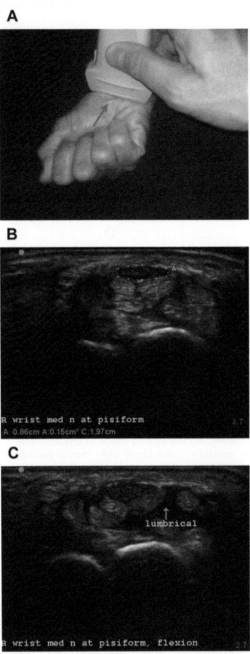

Fig. 5. Ultrasound imaging of the carpal tunnel–motion study for digit flexion. (*A*) Transducer position for transverse imaging with digit flexion to evaluate for lumbrical muscle intrusion into the tunnel during hand activity (grasp). (*B*) Ultrasound image with digits relaxed and extended in a neutral position; MN is the darker (hypoechoic) ellipsoid structure in the upper right central portion of the image (dotted outline surrounds the MN, with "A" marker on the right side of the nerve); nerve is enlarged at 15 mm² in this patient with CTS, and there is partial loss of fascicular echotexture (compare with the normal nerve in **Fig. 4**B). (*C*) Ultrasound image in the same patient with digits flexed (grasp), revealing a mild-moderate amount of lumbrical muscle intrusion and altered shape of the MN (compressive effect, no longer ellipsoid).

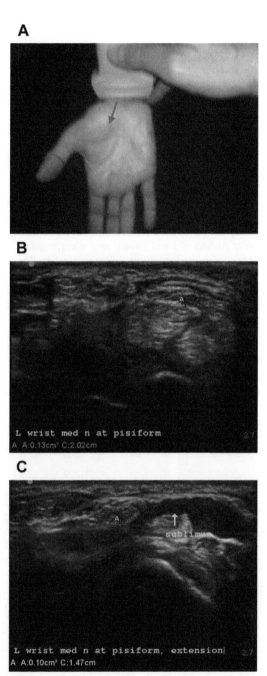

Fig. 6. Ultrasound imaging of the carpal tunnel in a patient with CTS, motion study for combined wrist and digit extension. (*A*) Transducer position for transverse imaging with wrist and digit extension to evaluate for flexor digitorum superficialis muscle intrusion. (*B*) Ultrasound image with wrist and digits in neutral position (dotted outline surrounds the MN, note the "A" marker; also note that this is an abnormal enlarged nerve, CSA measures 13 mm²). (*C*) Ultrasound image in the same patient with wrist and digits extended, revealing a marked amount of superficialis muscle intrusion (dark, hypoechoic structure in the upper right section of the image, labeled with *arrow* as "sublimus") into the tunnel and altered shape of the MN (compressive effect) as revealed by the dotted outline ("A" marker) just to the left of the superficialis ("sublimus") muscle.

Longitudinal imaging views (**Fig. 7**A) can be used to study the MN further for compression (see **Fig. 7**B). This nerve compression is typically accompanied by proximal swelling, optimally measured on transverse imaging at the level of the pisiform (see **Fig. 7**C), and occasionally distal flattening of can be identified (see **Fig. 7**D).

Finally, a dynamic stress test has been developed that challenges the nerve in the mid-distal carpal canal, where most compression typically occurs.[6,7] The dynamic stress test was developed to increase sensitivity of detecting contour changes or "notching" of the nerve on longitudinal imaging that is usually seen only in severe cases of CTS.[22,23] The stress simply involves the application of normal prehensile hand activity while observing how the MN responds.[6,7] The examiner measures the MN diameter before and during stress to look for objective evidence of nerve compression. One study demonstrated an average 40% decrease in diameter during stress, whereas normal nerves did not reveal any compression.[7] The initial resting (prestress) view is obtained in the longitudinal plane (see **Fig. 7**A). The "thenar digital flexion stress test" is applied while maintaining the same view—the patient holds a semirigid rubber ball between the thumb and digits 2 and 3 (**Fig. 8**A), requiring only a gentle isometric contraction of the thumb and fingers against the ball. Firm pressure is not required and actually may interfere with optimal imaging if the patient squeezes too hard. The most consistent location where MN compression occurs is at the level of the third carpometacarpal joint, where the capitate bone articulates with the third metacarpal head (**Fig. 9**). At this site, the flexor tendons to the second and third digits can be seen to tighten under the nerve as the thenar fibromuscular attachment to the TCL contracts or tightens and bulges into the nerve (it moves dorsally). There are 5

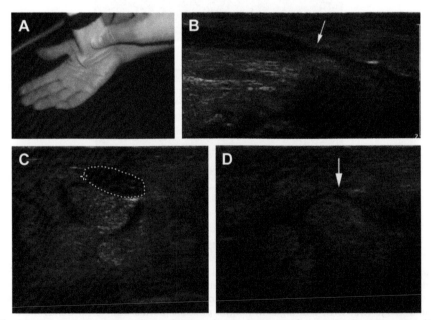

Fig. 7. Ultrasound imaging of CTS. (*A*) Tranducer placement for longitudinal imaging. (*B*) Longitudinal image in a CTS patient shows an enlarged MN proximally (*left side of image*), which narrows abruptly (*arrow*) as it passes under the TCL. (*C*) The first transverse image, just proximal to the tunnel, shows cursors tracing the perimeter of the large (23 mm²), hypoechoic MN. (*D*) The second transverse image, within the tunnel, shows the markedly flattened nerve (*arrow*).

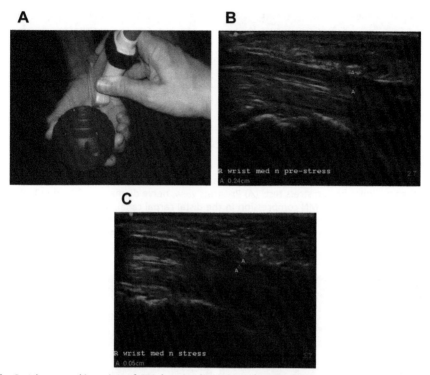

Fig. 8. Ultrasound imaging of CTS, longitudinal views for MN diameter measurement during the thenar digital flexion stress test. (*A*) Transducer placement and position of stress ball for patient to contract the thenar muscles and digits 2 and 3 flexors. (*B*) Ultrasound image, longitudinal view for diameter measurement in relaxed prestress position (as demonstrated in **Fig. 7**A). Caliper markers (A-A) measure the nerve diameter as 2.4 mm (0.24 cm). (*C*) Same patient as in (*B*), but during the stress test as demonstrated in (*A*). Notice the MN diameter has decreased from 2.4 to 0.5 mm at a prominent focal region, due to the thenar muscle intrusion, and the nerve appears uncompromised both proximal and distal to the site of constriction (at the A-A markers). Also, note that the site of compression is in the distal carpal canal and aligns with the digit 3 CMC joint (also see **Fig. 9**), at the level where the capitate articulates with the third metacarpal bone (bright-edged hyperechoic structures near bottom of image and directly in line with the "A" markers).

variations in the pattern of compression as the nerve is "sandwiched" between the thenar muscle and tendon:

1. Focal bulging of the thenar attachment dorsally into the nerve (see **Fig. 8**)
2. Very focal or more pointed bulging of the thenar attachment dorsally into the nerve (**Fig. 10**)
3. Regional bulging (over a longer segment) of the thenar attachment dorsally into the nerve (**Fig. 11**)
4. Flexor tendons bulge or tether up ventrally into the nerve (**Fig. 12**)
5. Combinations of the above, most commonly digits 1 and 4 (**Fig. 13**)

   The quantity of thenar muscle mass present at this location also varies, with some patients having a moderate amount of muscle and others having very little, such that in the latter case there is almost no hypoechoic muscle mass but just the hyperechoic fibromuscular attachment as it anchors into the TCL.

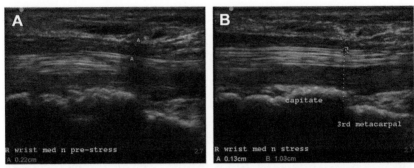

Fig. 9. Ultrasound imaging of CTS, longitudinal views for MN diameter measurement during the thenar digital flexion stress test. (*A*) Prestress view, nerve diameter is 2.2 mm (0.22 cm). (*B*) Stress view, showing MN compression in the distal carpal canal, at the level of the third carpometacarpal joint, where maximum narrowing of nerve diameter is measured at 1.3 mm (0.13 cm), which is a 41% decrease from the prestress diameter.

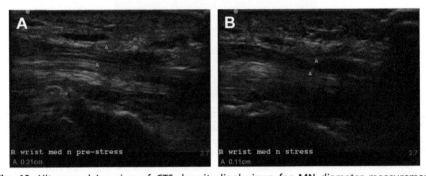

Fig. 10. Ultrasound imaging of CTS, longitudinal views for MN diameter measurement during the thenar digital flexion stress test. (*A*) Prestress view, nerve diameter is 2.1 mm (0.21 cm). (*B*) Stress view demonstrates very focal thenar bulging into the MN, where diameter narrows to 1.1 mm (0.11 cm).

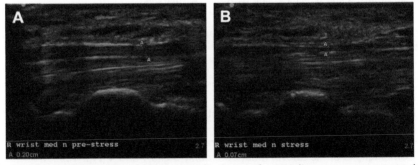

Fig. 11. Ultrasound imaging of CTS, longitudinal views for MN diameter measurement during the thenar digital flexion stress test. (*A*) Prestress view, nerve diameter is 2.0 mm (0.20 cm). (*B*) Stress view demonstrates regional type of the thenar muscle bulging into the MN, with narrowing across a relatively long segment of the nerve, diameter measured at 0.7 mm (0.07 cm).

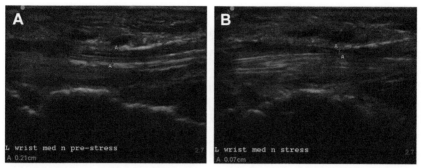

Fig. 12. Ultrasound imaging of CTS, longitudinal views for MN diameter measurement during the thenar digital flexion stress test. (*A*) Prestress view, nerve diameter is 2.1 mm (0.21 cm). (*B*) Stress view demonstrates flexor tendon bulging up or tethered (dorsally) into the nerve, diameter measured at 0.7 mm (0.07 cm).

Key ultrasound imaging views of the median nerve for carpal tunnel syndrome include the following:

- Transverse view at the wrist, at the level of the pisiform (see **Fig. 4**A)
- Transverse view at the wrist with digit flexion, for lumbrical muscle intrusion into the carpal tunnel (see **Fig. 5**)
- Transverse view at the wrist with wrist and digit extension, for superficialis muscle intrusion into the carpal tunnel (see **Fig. 6**)
- Longitudinal view across the carpal tunnel in neutral relaxed position (see **Fig. 7**A), for baseline prestress diameter measurement of the MN (see **Fig. 8**B)
- Longitudinal view across the carpal tunnel during thenar digital flexion stress test (see **Fig. 8**A), for diameter measurement of the MN (see **Fig. 8**C) to assess for compression

Other (Optional) Ultrasound Views

- Transverse "open-mouth" view, looking "down the throat" of the carpal tunnel (**Fig. 14**)[7]
- Video-clip stress testing in transverse and longitudinal views[6]

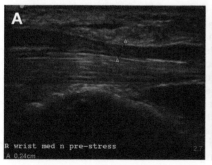
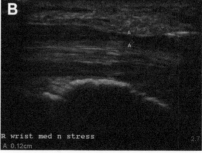

Fig. 13. Ultrasound imaging of CTS, longitudinal views for MN diameter measurement during the thenar digital flexion stress test. (*A*) Prestress view, nerve diameter is 2.4 mm (0.24 cm). (*B*) Stress view demonstrates a combination of focal muscle bulging (at the upper A marker) and tendon bulging up (dorsally, lower A marker) into the MN, diameter measured at 1.2 mm (0.12 cm).

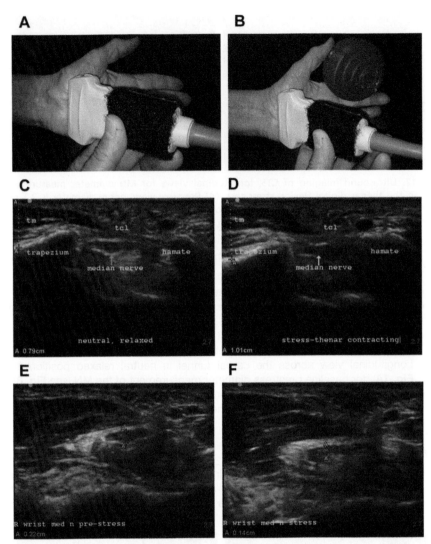

Fig. 14. Ultrasound technique for the carpal tunnel, "open mouth" view. (A) At rest, demonstrating proper transducer position. (B) Same as (A) during stress with thenar muscle contraction using a hard rubber ball to provide resistance (isometric). (C) Ultrasound image in a normal subject using the technique demonstrated in (A) at rest. tcl, transverse carpal ligament; tm, thenar muscle. Notice the thickness of the ligament, especially as it attaches to the trapezium just below the thenar muscle and to the left of the nerve. (D) Ultrasound image of same subject as in (C), using the technique demonstrated in (B), during stress. Notice that the width (thickness) of the thenar muscle has increased (from 0.79 to 1.01 cm), confirming muscle activation; this is a normal subject, and there is no appreciable change in the MN. (E, F) Ultrasound images of a patient with CTS, demonstrating compressive narrowing of the MN during stress, noting the thickness of the nerve decreases from 2.2 mm (0.22 cm) prestress (E) to 1.4 mm (0.14 cm) during stress (F), a 36% "flattening" compression.

These supplemental imaging views can provide more information. The open-mouth view allows better imaging of the thenar musculature, and its impact dynamically on the carpal tunnel and the MN. Video clips allow detailed review and study of the biomechanics during hand activity, because the examiner can replay the motion study repeatedly and observe the impact on the nerve.

IMAGING STUDIES (OTHER)

Plain film imaging of the wrist and carpal tunnel are not considered routine or helpful.[1,13] Magnetic resonance imaging may be useful if a structural or space-occupying lesion is suspected, but there is no specific correlation with the median neuropathy, and the expense usually outweighs the value of this type of testing.[1,3,13]

SUMMARY

CTS is a clinical diagnosis. EDX and NMUS are the most useful objective studies to assist the clinician in determining the neurophysiologic involvement of motor and sensory nerves and their type of injury (myelinopathy and/or axonopathy), and the anatomic causes of CTS, respectively. This data can be used to serve the clinician better with the treatment plan.

ACKNOWLEDGMENTS

We are indebted to Dr Levon Nazarian for generous support and helpful suggestions, as well as allowing the use of the ultrasound images for **Fig. 7**B–D.

We are indebted to Dr Gerald J. Herbison for his thoughtful mentoring, generous support, and helpful suggestions.

REFERENCES

1. Rosenbaum RB, Ochoa JL. Carpal tunnel syndrome and other disorders of the median nerve. 2nd edition. Amsterdam: Butterworth Heinemann; 2002.
2. Hennessey WJ, Kuhlman KA. The anatomy, symptoms, and signs of carpal tunnel syndrome. In: Johnson EW, editor. Physical medicine & rehabilitation clinics of NA: carpal tunnel syndrome, vol. 8. Philadelphia: W.B. Saunders Company; 1997. p. 439–57.
3. American Academy of Neurology, Quality Standards Review Subcommittee: practice parameter for carpal tunnel syndrome (Summary statement). Neurology 1993;43:2406–9.
4. Jablecki CK, Andary MT, Floeter MK, et al. Second AAEM literature review of the usefulness of nerve conduction studies and needle electromyography for the evaluation of patients with carpal tunnel syndrome. Muscle Nerve 2002;10: 924–78.
5. Sucher BM. Grading severity of carpal tunnel syndrome in electrodiagnostic reports: why grading is recommended. Muscle Nerve 2013;48:331–3.
6. Sucher BM. Carpal tunnel syndrome: ultrasonographic imaging and pathologic mechanisms of median nerve compression. J Am Osteopath Assoc 2009;109: 641–7.
7. Sucher BM. Ultrasound imaging of the carpal tunnel during median nerve compression. Curr Rev Musculoskelet Med 2009;2:134–46.
8. Kozakiewicz RT, Bowyer BL. Quantitative testing and thermography in carpal tunnel syndrome. In: Johnson EW, editor. Physical medicine & rehabilitation clinics of

NA: carpal tunnel syndrome, vol. 8. Philadelphia: W.B. Saunders Company; 1997. p. 503–11.

9. Sucher BM. Palpatory diagnosis and manipulative management of carpal tunnel syndrome. J Am Osteopath Assoc 1994;94:647–63.

10. Sucher BM, Glassman JH. Upper extremity syndromes. In: Stanton D, Mein E, editors. Phys Med Rehabil Clin N Am: manual medicine. Philadelphia: WB Saunders; 1996.

11. Sucher BM. Palpatory diagnosis and manipulative management of carpal tunnel syndrome: part 2. 'Double crush' and thoracic outlet syndrome. J Am Osteopath Assoc 1995;95:471–9.

12. Bland JD. Do nerve conduction studies predict outcome of carpal tunnel decompression. Muscle Nerve 2001;24:935–40.

13. Ashworth NL. Carpal tunnel syndrome. Available at: http://emedicine.medscape.com/article/316715-overview. Accessed February 4, 2014 [updated and republished: March 5, 2013].

14. Werner RA, Andary M. Electrodiagnostic evaluation of carpal tunnel syndrome. Muscle Nerve 2011;44:597–607.

15. Robinson LR. Electrodiagnosis of carpal tunnel syndrome. Phys Med Rehabil Clin N Am 2007;18:733–46.

16. American Association of Electrodiagnostic Medicine (AAEM). Literature review of the usefulness of nerve conduction studies in needle electromyography for the evaluation of patients with carpal tunnel syndrome. Muscle Nerve 1999; 22(Suppl 8):S145–67.

17. American Association of Electrodiagnostic Medicine, American Academy of Neurology, American Academy of Physical Medicine and Rehabiliation. Practice parameter for electrodiagnostic studies in carpal tunnel syndrome: summary statement. Muscle Nerve 2002;25:918–22.

18. Peer S, Bodner G. High-resolution sonography of the peripheral nervous system. 2nd edition. Berlin: Springer; 2008.

19. Cartwright MS. Ultrasound of focal neuropathies. In: Walker FO, Cartwright MS, editors. Neuromuscular ultrasound. Philadelphia: Elsevier Saunders; 2011. p. 72–90.

20. Leep Hunderfund AN, Boon AJ, Mandrekar JN, et al. Songorophy in carpal tunnel syndrome. Muscle Nerve 2011;44:485–91.

21. Cartwright MS, Hobson-Webb LD, Boon AJ, et al. Evidenced-based guideline: neuromuscular ultrasound for the diagnosis of carpal tunnel syndrome. Muscle Nerve 2012;46:287–93.

22. Beekman R, Visser LH. Sonography in the diagnosis of carpal tunnel syndrome: a critical review of the literature. Muscle Nerve 2003;27:26–33.

23. Strakowski JA. Ultrasound evaluation of focal neuropathies: correlation with electrodiagnosis. New York: Demos Medical; 2014.

24. Zochodne DW. Reversing neuropathic deficits. J Peripher Nerv Syst 2012; 17(Suppl 2):4–9.

25. LaFontaine S, Rasminsky M, Saida T, et al. Conduction block in rat myelinated fibers following exposure to anti-galactocerebroside serum. J Physiol 1982;323: 287–306.

26. Kimura J. Consequence of peripheral nerve demyelination: basic and clinical aspects. Can J Neurol Sci 1993;20:263–70.

27. Garcia CA, Malamut RE, England JD, et al. Clinical variability in two pairs of identical twins with the Charcot-Marie-Tooth disease type 1A duplication. Neurology 1995;45:2090.

28. Birouk N, Gouider R, Le Guern E, et al. Charcot–Marie–Tooth disease type 1A with 17p11.2 duplication. Brain 1997;120:813.
29. Schreiber AL, Herbison GJ. Nerve conduction. 38th Annual Jefferson Medical College Electrodiagnostic Medicine. Philadelphia, March 2, 2010.
30. Schreiber AL, Herbison GJ. A functional approach to nerve conduction studies. American Osteopathic College of Physical Medicine & Rehabilitation Mid-year meeting. Phoenix, April 16, 2011.
31. Schrijver HM, Gerritsen AA, Strijers RL, et al. Correlating nerve conduction studies and clinical outcome measures on carpal tunnel syndrome: lessons from a randomized controlled trial. J Clin Neurophysiol 2005;22:216–21.
32. Brown WF, Furguson GG, Joses MW, et al. The location of conduction abnormalities in human entrapment neuropathies. Can J Neurol Sci 1976;3:111–22.
33. Selzer ME. Regeneration of peripheral nerve. In: Sumner AJ, editor. The physiology of peripheral nerve disease. Philadelphia: W.B. Saunders; 1979. p. 359.
34. Lesser EA, Venkatesh S, Preston DC, et al. Stimulation distal to the lesion in patients with carpal tunnel syndrome. Muscle Nerve 1995;18:503–7.
35. Park TA, Welshofer JA, Dzwierzynski WW, et al. Median "pseudoneurapraxia" at the wrist: reassessment of palmar stimulation of the recurrent median nerve. Arch Phys Med Rehabil 2001;82:190–7.
36. Buschbacher RM, Prahlow ND, editors. Manual of nerve conduction studies. 2nd edition. New York: Demos; 2006.
37. Dawson DD, Hallet M, Wilbourn AJ, editors. Chapter 3: carpal tunnel syndrome in entrapment neuropathies. 3rd edition. Philadelphia: Lippincott-Raven; 1999.
38. Kimura J. Facts, fallacies, and fancies of nerve conduction studies: twenty-first annual Edward H. Lambert lecture. Muscle Nerve 1997;20:777–87.
39. Hobson-Webb L, Paduca L. Median nerve ultrasonography in carpal tunnel syndrome: findings from two laboratories. Muscle Nerve 2009;40:94–7.
40. Ulasli AM, Duymus M, Nacir B, et al. Reasons for using swelling ratio in sonographic diagnosis of carpal tunnel syndrome and a reliable method for its calculation. Muscle Nerve 2013;47:396–402.
41. Klauser AS, Halpern EJ, DeZordo T, et al. Carpal tunnel syndrome assessment with US: value of additional cross-sectional area measurements of the median nerve in patients versus healthy volunteers. Radiology 2009;250(1):171–7.

Two Novel Nonsurgical Treatments of Carpal Tunnel Syndrome

Adam L. Schreiber, DO[a],*, Benjamin M. Sucher, DO[b],
Levon N. Nazarian, MD[c]

KEYWORDS

- Carpal tunnel syndrome • Treatment • Osteopathic manipulative treatment
- Ultrasound

KEY POINTS

- There is a wide range of treatment strategies for carpal tunnel syndrome (CTS), from conservative to surgical, with varying degrees of supportive evidence that must be considered. The choice of treatment is complicated by clinical severity, chronicity, and patient preference.
- Osteopathic manipulative treatment of the carpal tunnel is well described and researched, and can be clinically used by a skilled practitioner.
- Sonographically guided percutaneous needle release of the transverse carpal ligament has shown promising results.

 Videos of a demonstration of an opponens roll and a sonographically guided needle puncture of the transverse carpal ligament in real time accompany this article at http://www.pmr.theclinics.com/

INTRODUCTION

Of the challenging pain syndromes discussed in this issue, carpal tunnel syndrome (CTS) will be the most commonly encountered by the physiatrist. After a clinical diagnosis is made and, if necessary, electrodiagnostic or ultrasonographic testing is performed (see the article entitled "Carpal Tunnel Syndrome Diagnosis" by Sucher and Schreiber elsewhere in this issue), treatments to consider include conservative and

[a] Department of Rehabilitation Medicine, Jefferson Rehabilitation Medicine Associates, Jefferson Medical College, Thomas Jefferson University, 25 South 9th Street, 1st Floor, Philadelphia, PA 19107, USA; [b] EMG Labs of Arizona Arthritis & Rheumatology Associates, 4550 East Bell Road, #170, Phoenix, AZ 85032, USA; [c] Department of Radiology, Thomas Jefferson University Hospital, Room 763E Main Building, 132 South 10th Street, Philadelphia, PA 19107-5244, USA
* Corresponding author.
E-mail address: Adam.Schreiber@Jefferson.edu

Phys Med Rehabil Clin N Am 25 (2014) 249–264
http://dx.doi.org/10.1016/j.pmr.2014.01.008
1047-9651/14/$ – see front matter © 2014 Elsevier Inc. All rights reserved.

surgical strategies, with varying degrees of supportive evidence. The choice of treatment is complicated by clinical severity and chronicity of the disease, and patient preference.[1] Typical treatment options include, but are not limited to, splinting, occupational and/or physical therapy, nutritional support, anti-inflammatory regimens (including injection), and ergonomic modifications, all of which should be considered in carefully selected patients.[2] This article highlights 2 nonsurgical approaches to treatment that are not commonly used, probably because of a lack of awareness. Osteopathic manipulative treatment (OMT) is often used for many different medical problems, including musculoskeletal issues that practitioners tend to link to spine care. In fact, OMT for CTS is well described and researched, and can be clinically used by a skilled practitioner. The second treatment strategy has been more recently developed with the increased use of ultrasonography as a therapeutic imaging tool, and application of its diagnostic capabilities described in the article entitled "Carpal Tunnel Syndrome Diagnosis" by Sucher and Schreiber in this issue. The use of ultrasound for the guidance of injection is established, but a newer technique using sonographically guided percutaneous needle release of the transverse carpal ligament (TCL) has promising results. OMT of the carpal tunnel and sonographically guided percutaneous needle release of the TCL are described herein.

OSTEOPATHIC MANIPULATIVE TREATMENT OF CTS

OMT is an essential component of the conservative management regime for CTS. Various manual techniques have been proved to be effective.[3–10] Training to develop proficiency in OMT for CTS is not difficult for clinicians; especially those skilled in manual medicine. Sucher and colleagues[8,10] have determined the most effective techniques to elongate the TCL, thereby increasing volume within the carpal tunnel (CT) and decreasing pressure on the median nerve (MN). The OMT described is a powerful and effective form of nonsurgical decompression of the MN at the CT.[3–7]

Indications

Patients may be considered for this treatment if they fulfill the following criteria:

1. Clinical diagnosis of CTS. It is not required that the patient have electrodiagnostic testing before the procedure, although the authors recommend testing whenever possible to confirm diagnosis and rule out other causes. The finding of mechanical restriction over the carpal canal by palpatory diagnosis is the primary indication for applying OMT at this site (see the article by Sucher and Schreiber elsewhere in this issue).
2. Osteopathic principles guide physicians to evaluate the entire musculoskeletal system, then apply treatment to all areas of somatic dysfunction[d,11] diagnosed by appreciation of tissue-texture change, asymmetry, restriction, and tenderness (TART findings). Therefore, exclusive focus on the CT could ignore other important areas of restriction that affect wrist and hand function. Proximal dysfunction will affect biomechanical behavior distally, and should be addressed (but is beyond the scope of this article).

---

[d] Somatic dysfunction is defined as the impaired or altered function of related components of the somatic (bodywork) system including: the skeletal, arthrodial, and myofascial structures, and their related vascular, lymphatic, and neural elements.

Contraindications and Precautions

- Focused OMT can be administered vigorously without concern of injuring the MN by specifically avoiding direct pressure over the CT[3,5,7,9]; this is not a problem if the manipulating fingers work along the edges of the CT.
- Arthritic changes in the first carpometacarpal joint can limit the degree of range of motion necessary to create sufficient traction along the TCL, thus preventing adequate stretch or elongation of the ligament.
- Fragile skin can cause ecchymosis, especially on the dorsal hand. Inadvertent counterforce applied on the dorsal aspect of the hand by the operator's manipulating fingers can injure the skin and lead to bruising. Vigorous force is required to successfully elongate the TCL.
- Any increased pressure on a badly damaged nerve could lead to more axon loss. However, severe cases of CTS do not respond well to conservative treatment[11,12] or surgery.[13] There is the distinct possibility that vigorous application of manipulative forces, even for brief periods of time, could further injure a fragile nerve that has already sustained axon loss. The caveat is that severe CTS may not improve with surgery, and not all patients want surgery. Severe CTS is a relative contraindication, and requires clinical judgment combined with patient participation (informed consent).

Techniques

Anatomy

Descriptive terminology used to identify movement through the anatomic planes can vary somewhat in the literature. The terms applied for the techniques described herein are consistent with the specific literature referenced for application of OMT in CTS.

Osteopathic manipulative treatments

1. Transverse extension (TE): **Fig. 1**[3,7,9,10]
2. Thenar extension and abduction (ThEA): **Fig. 1**[3,7,9]
3. Hyperextension (wrist and digits): **Fig. 1**[3,7,9]
4. Opponens roll (thenar): **Figs. 2** and **3**[5,7,9]
5. Guy-wire (GW): **Fig. 4**[5,8–10]
6. Combination maneuvers: Figs. **1**, **4**B and **5**[3,7–10]

Transverse extension Carefully targeting of the edges of the carpal bones facilitates the practitioner in elongating the TCL by direct TE with 3-point bending (1 central contact point dorsally in the hand and 2 contact points ventrally along the canal edges, **Fig. 1**).[3,7,9,10] This technique is a good initial approach and is very effective, but can be challenging to apply to large wrists or if the practitioner's hands are small (or not very strong).

Thenar extension and abduction The thumb can be used as a lever arm to create a fulcrum effect to apply traction along the TCL, by placing the thumb into abduction and extension (see **Fig. 1**), again avoiding direct pressure on the MN. This maneuver is fairly easy to perform in isolation or in combination with TE (see **Fig. 1**).

Hyperextension Hyperextension of the wrist and digits pulls the thicker myotendinous junctions distally and creates a bougienage effect by dilating the tunnel from within, as well as generally stretching the fascia over the ventral wrist and CT (see **Fig. 1**B). In addition, this maneuver mobilizes the MN by reducing adhesions or fibrous fixation of the nerve to the TCL, flexor tendons, or the walls of the tunnel.[5,14]

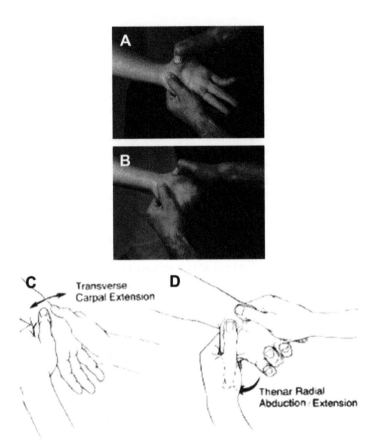

Fig. 1. Manipulation for carpal tunnel syndrome (CTS): transverse extension (TE) of the carpal tunnel and thenar abduction/extension. (*A*) Operator's fingers (not visible beneath patient's hand) press upward on the dorsal part of the patient's wrist (centrally). Operator's thumbs apply pressure along the attachment edges of the transverse carpal ligament (TCL) at the medial and lateral borders of the carpal bones. In addition, the patient's thumb is grasped firmly by the operator's right hand and pulled into radial abduction with extension. (*B*) Same technique as in *A*, except the patient's wrist and digits are hyperextended, further opening or extending the canal, and the operator's thumbs have progressed away from midline, stripping the ligamentous and myofascial attachments back. (*C*) TE. Action-line arrows demonstrate movement of thumbs apart to widen the carpal tunnel. (*D*) Graphic of thenar radial abduction with extension. Action-line arrow demonstrates the movement of the thumb required to release the abductor pollicis brevis and opponens pollicis muscle attachments at the TCL. ([*A, B*] *From* Sucher BM. Myofascial release of carpal tunnel syndrome. J Am Osteopath Assoc 1993;93:92–4. © 1993 American Osteopathic Association. Reprinted with the consent of the American Osteopathic Association; and [*C, D*] *From* Sucher BM. Palpatory diagnosis and manipulative management of carpal tunnel syndrome. J Am Osteopath Assoc 1994;94: 647–63. © 1994 American Osteopathic Association. Reprinted with the consent of the American Osteopathic Association.)

Opponens roll The opponens roll maneuver is a progression of the thenar technique by adding lateral axial rotation (see **Fig. 2**), which elevates the edge of the TCL off the MN as it is being stretched (see **Fig. 3**, Video 1).

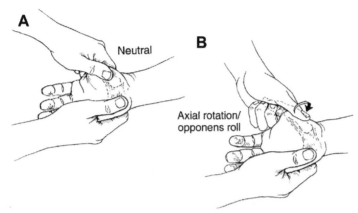

Fig. 2. Manipulation for CTS: opponens roll maneuver. (*A*) Relaxed or neutral position. (*B*) Thenar abduction with extension and lateral axial rotation (retroposition). (*From* Sucher BM. Palpatory diagnosis and manipulative management of carpal tunnel syndrome. J Am Osteopath Assoc 1994;94:649. © 1994 American Osteopathic Association. Reprinted with the consent of the American Osteopathic Association.)

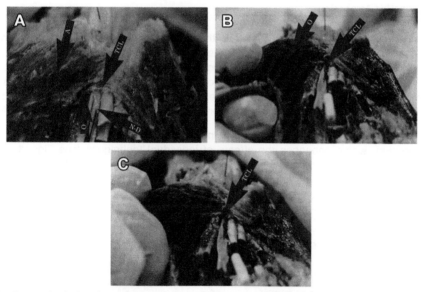

Fig. 3. Manipulation for CTS: opponens roll maneuver of the carpal tunnel in a cadaver; view of distal aspect of carpal canal. (*A*) Stretch position for the abductor pollicis muscle into radial abduction and extension pulls TCL taut, up against the median nerve (MN), identified by *arrow* marked N-D, and electromyogram electrode. Notice pressure effect just distal to edge of ligament (identified by *arrow* marked TCL). (*B*) The more superficial abductor has been dissected away. Thumb is pulled back into radial abduction with extension, and lateral axial rotation has just been initiated. Opponens pollicis muscle (identified by *arrow* marked O) and its ligamentous attachment are pulled taut, slightly contacting the MN. (*C*) Opponens roll. Maximum axial rotation is introduced, rotating thumb laterally (notice change in position of operator's fingers around thumb). Observe how the still taut ligament is now elevated up off the MN with slight "gapping" even as ligament is being stretched. (*From* Sucher BM. Palpatory diagnosis and manipulative management of carpal tunnel syndrome. J Am Osteopath Assoc 1994;94:649. © 1994 American Osteopathic Association. Reprinted with the consent of the American Osteopathic Association.)

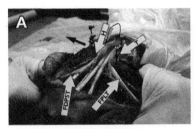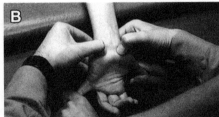

Fig. 4. Manipulation for CTS: guy-wire (GW) maneuver and TE. (*A*) GW technique applied to cadaver limb, dissected with ligament cut away, to illustrate the flexor pollicis longus tendon (FPLT) deflected around the inner edge of the trapezium (T) and flexor digitorum porfundus-5 tendon (FDP5T) deflected around the inner edge of the hamate (H), creating a fulcrum effect, tending to pull apart the carpal arch (*thin black arrows*). The electromyogram electrode (needle) identifies the MN centrally. (*B*) Combination TE with the GW manipulation technique. The GW maneuver is performed by an assistant holding the thumb and little finger while the physician applies distal-row TE. (*From* Sucher BM, Hinrichs RN. Manipulative treatment of carpal tunnel syndrome: biomechanical and osteopathic intervention to increase the length of the transverse carpal ligament. J Am Osteopath Assoc 1998;98: 685. © 1998 American Osteopathic Association. Reprinted with the consent of the American Osteopathic Association.)

Guy-wire The GW maneuver builds on the hyperextension technique by using the tendons of the flexor pollicis longus and flexor digitorum profundus to widen the CT from within. Force vectors are generated from the tendons as they are tethered vigorously at their deflection points where they contact against the inside edges of the distal row of carpal bones (trapezium and hamate, respectively), creating a fulcrum effect to literally pry apart the carpal bones, thus widening the transverse carpal arch (see **Fig. 4**A).

Combination maneuvers Finally, combinations of some of these maneuvers can be applied, which enhances the effects of individual techniques (see Figs. **1**, **4**B and **5**).[3,7–10] In addition, the use of an assistant more readily allows the operator(s)

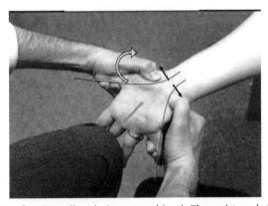

Fig. 5. Manipulation for CTS: all techniques combined. The wrist and digits are hyperextended (*central palmar green arrow*) against the operator's knee, transverse extension is applied by the operator's thumbs (*short transverse blue arrows* on either side of the wrist), opponens roll lateral axial rotation is applied by the operator's left hand (*short curved yellow arrow* on the left), and the GW maneuver is applied by both of the operator's hands extending and abducting the patient's thumb and little finger (*long thin red arrows* crossing over the patient's thumb and little finger).

to combine maneuvers and generate more vigorous application of the techniques, which is useful for larger wrists and patients with marked palpatory restriction about the CT (**Fig. 6**).[7]

Stretching exercises for CTS
Exercises performed by the patient complement OMT by extending and building on the manipulative efforts to alleviate symptoms of CTS. Stretching works best following manipulative priming of the TCL.[10] The techniques are easy to teach to patients and are based on the manipulative maneuvers (**Figs. 7–9**). These exercises should initially be performed several times daily to effectively lengthen the TCL, and gradually tapered to a maintenance level as symptoms subside.

Splinting
The most well-known treatment of CTS is a neutral positioned wrist splint, but a modified thumb spica has been developed based on the neuromuscular ultrasonography (NMUS) findings that thenar muscle intrusion into the CT compresses the MN.[15,16] This type of orthosis (**Fig. 10**) creates a thenar block that inhibits muscle contraction, thereby sparing the MN.

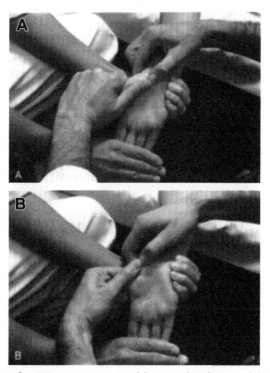

Fig. 6. Manipulation for CTS: operator-assisted (2-person) technique. (*A*) Starting or neutral position; operator uses both hands to firmly secure the patient's thenar muscle mass and first metacarpal while the assistant stabilizes the palm medially and digits distally. (*B*) Same as *A* except the operator's hands have moved laterally after slowly and vigorously rotating the patient's first metacarpal to the tolerable limit of range of motion. (*From* Sucher BM, Glassman JH. Upper extremity syndromes. Phys Med Rehabil Clinics N Am 1996;7(4):791; with permission.)

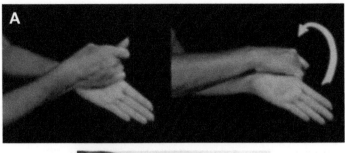

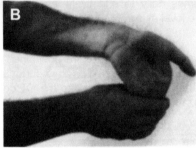

Fig. 7. Basic self-stretching exercises for CTS. (*A*) Thenar, carpal ligament stretch. Left frame shows initiation of stretch. Patient hooks hypothenar region of opposite hand (in this case, right hand) into thenar area of hand to be stretched (in this case, left hand), pulling laterally while simultaneously grasping thumb itself and extending. Right frame shows progressive phase of stretch into further extension and abduction. (*B*) Extension stretch of wrist and carpal canal. (*From* Sucher BM. Myofascial release of carpal tunnel syndrome. J Am Osteopath Assoc 1993;93:92–4. © 1993 American Osteopathic Association. Reprinted with the consent of the American Osteopathic Association.)

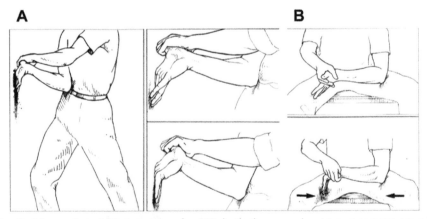

Fig. 8. Advanced stretching exercises for CTS: both thenar and wrist components are addressed. (*A*) While standing, use of a wall frees the other hand to control the thumb. The focused views on the right show the elbow tucked into the iliac crest, so that as the patient leans forward (see enlargement on the left), the body weight assists the stretch. (*B*) While seated, placing the forearm between the thighs allows control of the wrist and digit component of the stretch, and frees the other hand for the thenar portion. Slowly squeezing the thighs together extends the wrist and digits. (*From* Sucher BM. Myofascial manipulative release of carpal tunnel syndrome: documentation with magnetic resonance imaging. J Am Osteopath Assoc 1993;93:1274, 1275. © 1993 American Osteopathic Association. Reprinted with the consent of the American Osteopathic Association.)

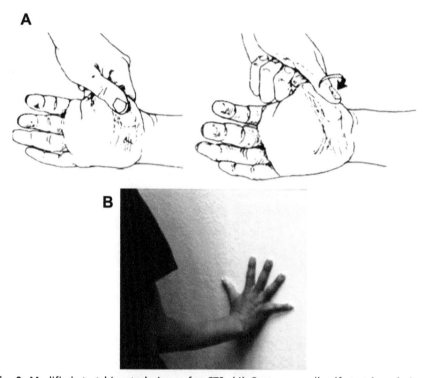

Fig. 9. Modified stretching techniques for CTS. (*A*) Opponens roll self-stretch technique. Lateral axial rotation stretches the opponens pollicis muscle. Left frame shows relaxed position. Right frame shows maximum stretch position. (*B*) GW self-stretch technique. Patient maximally spreads apart the digits and places hand against wall with wrist and digits hyperextended. Elbow is tucked into the hip (iliac crest area) for support and counterforce that is induced by leaning forward to use body weight as assistance for maximum stretch. The hand can be placed lower to enhance the stretch effect. The guy-wire effect is created by having the patient contract the thumb and fifth digit into flexion against the wall and holding for several seconds. It can also be achieved with the forearm supinated (palm facing up). (*From* Sucher BM. Palpatory diagnosis and manipulative management of carpal tunnel syndrome: part 2. "Double crush" and thoracic outlet syndrome. J Am Osteopath Assoc 1995; 95:472. © 1995 American Osteopathic Association. Reprinted with the consent of the American Osteopathic Association.)

Clinical Implications

Research in cadavers[8,10] demonstrated that the TE + GW maneuvers were most effective at elongating the TCL. However, subsequent dynamic studies in live subjects[15,16] with NMUS revealed that thenar muscle intrusion ventrally into the CT combines with tightening of the flexor tendons dorsally to create a sandwich-like compression of the MN. Thus, application of the following maneuvers can be used to specifically address these more recently discovered contributing causes of CTS:

- ThEA addresses to thenar muscle tightness, shortening, mounding, and/or trigger-point formation
- Hyperextension addresses shortening and tightness of the flexor tendons

In addition, since manipulative priming was discovered,[10] support has grown for vigorous manipulation with TE + GW, followed by self-stretching. The research

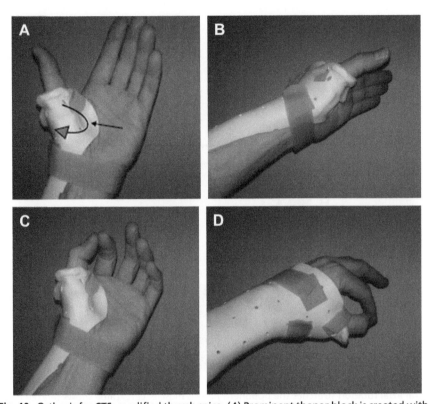

Fig. 10. Orthosis for CTS: modified thumb spica. (*A*) Prominent thenar block is created with a molded indentation (*straight arrow*) that maintains retroposition (opposite of opposition–*curved arrow*) and prevents vigorous contraction of the opponens pollicis and abductor pollicis brevis muscles. (*B*) Side view of orthosis shows thumb maintained in retroposition. (*C*) Weak opposition pinch is allowed for light activity. (*D*) Side view of weak pinch in the orthosis.

findings mimic the typical clinical situation whereby the manipulative maneuvers can provide the priming in the office setting, with a subsequent home program of self-stretching more readily addressing the thenar and tendon component (patients cannot as easily simulate the TE or GW components on themselves).

Use of the opponens roll maneuver is a good initial choice in more advanced cases of CTS, because it elevates the TCL off the MN.[5] It may also be helpful to provide a steroid injection or topical nonsteroidal anti-inflammatory medication before manipulation, to decrease inflammation and edema of the nerve, which should improve the tolerance and response to manipulation.

Electrodiagnostic evaluation may be used to monitor the effects of manipulation objectively by observing distal latency reductions after successful OMT.[4,5] Typically, electrical changes by nerve conduction studies (NCS) lag behind clinical changes, by weeks or months, yet can still be used to follow the physiologic status of the MN and assist with management of the patient's progress.[5]

Palpatory restriction over the carpal canal can be diminished rapidly with OMT, and often precedes clinical and electrophysiologic improvement.[5] The observation of decreased restriction into the normal range can be used as a predictive tool to encourage the patient, and may enhance compliance with the home exercise program.[5]

Outcomes

Sucher[3–6] has published extensively about documenting the effects of OMT. The primary goal and result of treatment is to reduce symptoms. In addition, concomitant improvement in the NCS abnormalities (less slowing, less conduction block, increased amplitudes) may be recorded. Sucher also demonstrated an increase in the size of the CT as measured objectively by magnetic resonance imaging, revealing that the anterior-posterior and transverse dimensions of the tunnel increased as symptoms decreased and NCS values improved.[4] Subsequent work revealed that the TCL can be elongated as the width of the transverse carpal arch increased after application of OMT and stretching.[8,10]

NUMS is another method used to confirm that OMT alters the biomechanics of the CT and alleviates MN compression in CTS. Dynamic stress testing in CTS demonstrates that MN compression occurs between the thenar muscles and flexor tendons.[15,16] Furthermore, it can be objectively demonstrated by repeat stress testing imaged with NMUS after manipulation that the MN compression is less pronounced (**Fig. 11**).

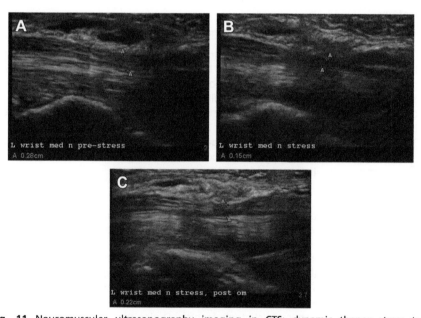

Fig. 11. Neuromuscular ultrasonography imaging in CTS: dynamic thenar stress test sequence before and after manipulation. The median nerve (MN) is the hypoechoic (*dark*), tubular structure that is oriented transversely across middle of the images; the flexor tendons are relatively hyperechoic (*white*), with a fibrillar pattern, and located just below (dorsal) the MN; the thenar fibromuscular attachment (along the TCL) can be seen just above (ventral) the MN, and is relatively hyperechoic with some hypoechoic muscular patches interspersed. (*A*) Resting position without stress, before manipulation. MN diameter measures 0.28 cm (between the 2 "A" markers). (*B*) Stress test before manipulation reveals MN compression as the diameter decreases to 0.15 cm; note that the fibromuscular thenar attachment above the MN protrudes downward (dorsally) into the nerve as the flexor tendons are pulled up (ventrally) into the nerve, which is sandwiched in between. (*C*) Stress test after manipulation reveals that the nerve diameter is only compressed to 0.22 cm (compression is reduced by more than 50%).

SONOGRAPHICALLY GUIDED PERCUTANEOUS NEEDLE RELEASE OF THE TRANSVERSE CARPAL LIGAMENT

Local corticosteroid injections have been widely used for the short-term treatment of CTS. A systematic review of 12 studies with 671 participants concluded that corticosteroid injections give better clinical improvement then placebo injection for 1 month after injection, and greater improvement than oral corticosteroids for 3 months after injection.[17] High-resolution sonographic imaging of the CT allows for real-time sonographic guidance with accurate placement of the needle and injectate.[18] Smith and colleagues[18] suggest sonographically guided CT injections for patients who have failed nonguided injection, have persistent symptoms after CT release, or are anticoagulated.

Real-time sonography has opened up new possibilities for percutaneous treatments beyond traditional corticosteroid injections when conservative management has failed. Several investigators have explored the use of sonography to guide percutaneous surgical release of the transverse carpal ligament.[19–21] An option now available to minimize the potential morbidity of traditional surgery, described by McShane and colleagues,[22] is an office procedure called sonographically guided percutaneous needle release of the TCL.

Indications

Patients may be considered for this treatment if they fulfill the following criteria:

1. Clinical diagnosis of CTS. It is not required that the patient have electrodiagnostic testing before the procedure, although the authors recommend testing whenever possible to confirm diagnosis and rule out other causes.
2. Sonography reveals findings that fulfill the measurement criteria for CTS as described by Klauser and colleagues,[23] and mass effect on the MN is identified by a thickened TCL within the CT.
3. Treatment of CTS has not responded adequately to conservative approaches such as splinting, exercise/therapy, and/or corticosteroid injections, and the patient is considered a potential surgical candidate.

Technique

- Patient positioning. The patient is seated with the dorsal aspect of the hand and wrist lying on a Mayo tray with a rolled towel beneath to place the wrist into extension.
- Preparation. The site of maximal thickening of the TCL within the CT is localized in the longitudinal plane using a high-frequency linear ultrasound transducer, typically 12 to 15 MHz (**Figs. 12** and **13**). Standard ultrasound gel is layered on the transducer, over which a sterile probe cover is placed. The patient is prepped and draped in usual sterile fashion. During the procedure either sterile ultrasound gel or povidone-iodine solution is used as an acoustic coupling agent.
- Procedure. Using continuous sonographic guidance, a 25-gauge hypodermic needle is advanced into the subcutaneous tissues and the TCL, and 1% lidocaine is infiltrated for local anesthetic. Next an 18-gauge needle is advanced into the ligament from a proximal to distal approach (**Fig. 14**). The tip of the needle is used to puncture the TCL repeatedly until it palpably softens (Video 2). When the needle no longer meets significant resistance and/or a fluid plane can be created between the MN and the ligament, 0.5 mL betamethasone (40 mg/mL) or equivalent is injected into the ligament. The needle is then removed and hemostasis maintained. Often a decreased mass effect on the

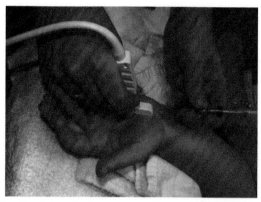

Fig. 12. Position of patient's hand, ultrasound probe, and needle for percutaneous needle release of the carpal tunnel.

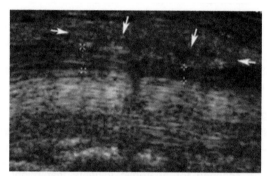

Fig. 13. Longitudinal ultrasonography image of the carpal tunnel. Proximal to the carpal tunnel the median nerve is thickened (× *cursors*) and is narrowed within the tunnel (+ *cursors*) as it passes under the thickened TCL (*arrows*).

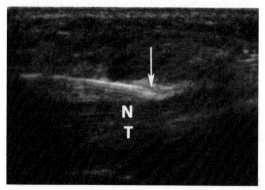

Fig. 14. Longitudinal ultrasonography image showing the needle (*arrow*) within the TCL. N, median nerve; T, flexor digitorum superficialis tendon.

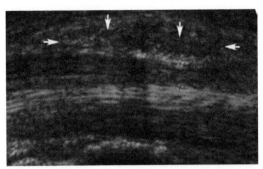

Fig. 15. Immediate postprocedure longitudinal ultrasonography image of the carpal tunnel. The narrowing of the nerve has markedly improved (*cursors*). Arrows indicate the TCL.

nerve (less compression) is detectable immediately after the procedure (**Fig. 15**).

Postfenestration/Postinjection Care

- A small adhesive bandage is placed over the needle entry site, and the patient is sent home with instructions to apply ice to the treated area for 20 minutes per hour on the day of the procedure, and take oral acetaminophen (if there are no contraindications) as needed.
- Although McShane and colleagues[22] recommend therapy starting the next day, it has not been established whether therapy is necessary.

Technical Challenges and Contraindications

- Because of the proximity of the needle to the MN, the operator needs to have adequate training and expertise in musculoskeletal sonography and sonographically guided procedures so as to avoid nerve injury. Before the procedure the CT should also be scanned for anatomic variants that might alter the needle approach, such as bifid MN and persistent median artery.
- The patient is consented for potential risks of bleeding, infection, and nerve injury. A coagulation profile is not routinely checked unless the patient has a known coagulopathy. If so, to minimize the risk of bleeding an international normalized ratio of less than 1.5 is preferred. Warfarin, dabigatran, or clopidogrel is held for 3 days before the procedure if deemed safe by the patient's primary care provider. Patients do not need to hold aspirin or nonsteroidal anti-inflammatory medicines before the procedure.
- Severe CTS is not a contraindication, but the patient should be counseled that outcomes may not be as favorable if there is significant preexisting MN damage.

Outcomes

A preliminary study demonstrated MN decompression and substantial clinical improvement in 17 patients who were reevaluated at a mean of 25 months after the procedure. The MN had significantly smaller cross-sectional area when compared with pretreatment measurement. In addition, patients had significantly fewer symptoms, less functional impairment, and an improved hand diagram score.[22] Among the patients, 84.6% had negative clinical diagnostic test results for CTS (Tinel test, Phalen test, and carpal compression test), and 86% said they were satisfied with the procedure. There were no procedure-related infections or nerve injuries.[22]

SUMMARY

The 2 treatment techniques described herein are novel nonsurgical treatments that should be considered by clinicians for their CTS treatment paradigm. OMT of the CT is a safe technique that can be applied in the office and reinforced at home with vigorous self-stretching exercises and modified splinting. Several studies have shown the efficacy of this type of OMT. Larger randomized controlled studies are needed to validate these techniques in comparison with other treatments. Sonographically guided percutaneous release of the TCL has multiple advantages over the traditional surgical treatment of CTS. The procedure is much less invasive than surgery, can be performed in an office setting, and uses local anesthetic. Because it only involves puncture with an 18-gauge needle or smaller (anecdotally it appears that similar results can be obtained with 20–22-gauge needles), there is little concern for scarring or pain after the procedure. The nerve is continuously visualized throughout the procedure, allowing for accurate fenestration of the ligament while minimizing the possibility of nerve injury. Moreover, the flexor retinaculum is not completely sectioned, so the attachments of the thenar muscles remain functionally intact and the flexor tendons remain in place. Finally, after the procedure there is rapid healing and no restrictions on patient activity. Future randomized controlled studies are needed to validate this technique and to compare its outcomes with those after surgery. Both OMT and sonographically guided percutaneous release of the TCL are safe, effective treatments for CTS.

SUPPLEMENTARY DATA

Videos related to this article can be found online at http://dx.doi.org/10.1016/j.pmr.2014.01.008.

REFERENCES

1. Caliandro P, Giannini F, Pazzaglia C, et al. A new clinical scale to grade the impairment of median nerve in carpal tunnel syndrome. Clin Neurophysiol 2010;121:1066–71.
2. Tortland PD. Nonsurgical management of carpal tunnel syndrome. Tech Orthop 2003;18:23–9.
3. Sucher BM. Myofascial release of carpal tunnel syndrome. J Am Osteopath Assoc 1993;93:91–101.
4. Sucher BM. Myofascial manipulative release of carpal tunnel syndrome: documentation with magnetic resonance imaging. J Am Osteopath Assoc 1993;93:1273–8.
5. Sucher BM. Palpatory diagnosis and manipulative management of carpal tunnel syndrome. J Am Osteopath Assoc 1994;94:647–63.
6. Sucher BM. Palpatory diagnosis and manipulative management of carpal tunnel syndrome: part 2. "Double crush" and thoracic outlet syndrome. J Am Osteopath Assoc 1995;95:471–9.
7. Sucher BM, Glassman JH. Upper extremity syndromes. In: Stanton D, Mein E, editors. Phys Med Rehabil Clin N Am: manual medicine, vol. 7. Philadelphia: WB Saunders; 1996. p. 787–810.
8. Sucher BM, Hinrichs RN. Manipulative treatment of carpal tunnel syndrome: biomechanical and osteopathic intervention to increase the length of the transverse carpal ligament. J Am Osteopath Assoc 1998;98:679–86.
9. Sucher BM. Carpal tunnel syndrome. In: Rakel D, editor. Integrative medicine. Philadelphia: Saunders; 2003. p. 455–561.

10. Sucher BM, Hinrichs RN, Welcher RL, et al. Manipulative treatment of carpal tunnel syndrome: biomechanical and osteopathic intervention to increase the length of the transverse carpal ligament: part 2. Effect of sex differences and manipulative "priming". J Am Osteopath Assoc 2005;105:135–43.

11. Chila A, editor. Foundations of osteopathic medicine. 3rd edition. Philadelphia: Lippincott Williams and Wilkins; 2010.

12. Rosenbaum RB, Ochoa JL. Carpal tunnel syndrome and other disorders of the median nerve. 2nd edition. Amsterdam: Butterworth Heinemann; 2002.

13. Bland JD. Do nerve conduction studies predict the outcome of carpal tunnel decompression? Muscle Nerve 2001;24:935–40.

14. Hunter JM. Recurrent carpal tunnel syndrome, epineural fibrous fixation, and traction neuropathy. Hand Clin 1991;7:491–504.

15. Sucher BM. Ultrasound imaging of the carpal tunnel during median nerve compression. Curr Rev Musculoskelet Med 2009;2:134–46.

16. Sucher BM. Carpal tunnel syndrome: ultrasonographic imaging and pathologic mechanisms of median nerve compression. J Am Osteopath Assoc 2009;109: 641–7.

17. Marshall SC, Tardif G, Ashworth NL. Local corticosteroid injection for carpal tunnel syndrome. Cochrane Database Syst Rev 2007;(2):CD001554.

18. Smith J, Wisniewski SJ, Finnoff JT, et al. Sonographically guided carpal tunnel injections: the ulnar approach. J Ultrasound Med 2008;27:1485–90.

19. Rojo-Manaute JM, Capa-Grasa A, Rodriguez-Maruri GE, et al. Ultra-minimally invasive sonographically guided carpal tunnel release: anatomic study of a new technique. J Ultrasound Med 2013;32:131–42.

20. Nakamichi K, Tachibana S, Yamamoto S, et al. Percutaneous carpal tunnel release compared with mini-open release using ultrasonographic guidance for both techniques. J Hand Surg Am 2010;35:437–45.

21. Buncke G, McCormack B, Bodor M. Ultrasound-guided carpal tunnel release using the Manos CTR system. Microsurgery 2013;33:362–6.

22. McShane JM, Slaff S, Gold JE, et al. Sonographically guided percutaneous needle release of the carpal tunnel for the treatment of carpal tunnel syndrome: a preliminary report. J Ultrasound Med 2012;31:1341–9.

23. Klauser AS, Halpern EJ, De Zordo T, et al. Carpal tunnel assessment with US: value of additional cross-sectional area measurements of the median nerve in patients versus healthy volunteers. Radiology 2009;250:171–7.

Challenging Pain Syndromes
Parsonage-Turner Syndrome

Clark C. Smith, MD, MPH*, Anna-Christina Bevelaqua, MD

KEYWORDS

- Parsonage-Turner syndrome • Neuralgic amyotrophy • Brachial plexus
- Acute brachial plexitis

KEY POINTS

- The current best approach to Parsonage-Turner syndrome (PTS) is a multidisciplinary approach that includes both physical therapy and pharmacologic treatment, often with multiple agents.
- Corticosteroid treatment may improve pain and hasten recovery.
- Surgical options are available for patients who fail conservative treatment.
- Due to the relatively low incidence of this disorder, further research is needed.

DEFINITION

Parsonage-Turner syndrome (PTS) is a rare disorder typically characterized by an abrupt onset of upper extremity pain followed by progressive neurologic deficits, including weakness, atrophy, and occasionally sensory abnormalities. The cause is unknown. The distribution of the nerves involved as well as the extent of involvement is variable. Any peripheral nerve may be affected but most commonly the upper trunk of the brachial plexus is involved.[1,2] Recovery is often prolonged and incomplete. A hereditary form of the syndrome, hereditary neuralgic amyotrophy, has also been studied, although it occurs much less frequently. Clinically it presents similarly to PTS, but often at a younger age and has a higher incidence of recurrent attacks.[3–5]

Although this clinical condition is most commonly referred to as Parsonage-Turner syndrome, neuralgic amyotrophy, or brachial neuritis, it can be found described in literature under many other names (**Box 1**).[4–6]

HISTORY

One of the first descriptions of PTS dates back to 1887 when Julius Dreschfeld described 2 cases of recurrent episodes of nontraumatic brachial plexopathy.[5,6]

Disclosures: The authors have no relevant disclosures.
Department of Rehabilitation and Regenerative Medicine, Columbia University Medical Center, New York Presbyterian Hospital, 180 Fort Washington Avenue, New York, NY 10032, USA
* Corresponding author.
E-mail address: cs3028@columbia.edu

Phys Med Rehabil Clin N Am 25 (2014) 265–277
http://dx.doi.org/10.1016/j.pmr.2014.01.001

> **Box 1**
> **Alternative names for PTS**
>
> Acute brachial neuropathy
>
> Acute brachial plexitis
>
> Acute multiple brachial neuropathy
>
> Brachial neuritis
>
> Brachial plexus neuropathy
>
> Cryptogenic brachial plexus neuropathy
>
> Idiopathic brachial neuritis
>
> Idiopathic brachial plexopathy
>
> Kiloh-Nevin syndrome
>
> Localized neuritis of the shoulder girdle
>
> Multiple neuritis of the shoulder girdle
>
> Neuralgic amyotrophy
>
> Paralytic brachial neuritis
>
> Shoulder girdle neuritis
>
> Shoulder girdle syndrome

Over the next 60 years, there were several case reports describing similar clinical presentations, but it was not until 1943 that Spillane gave the first full description of the condition in his article, "Localised neuritis of the shoulder girdle."[7–9] Spillane described 46 patients with an "acute onset of pain in the shoulder, arm, and side of the neck, over the scapula and down the affected arm" persisting for 7 to 10 days. Several days later, usually after the pain subsided, the patients developed paralysis around the shoulder girdle.[10] In 1948, M.J. Parsonage and John W. Alden Turner published an article titled, "Neuralgic amyotrophy: the shoulder girdle syndrome," which more firmly established and detailed the clinical aspects of the syndrome.[11] This article described a case series of 136 patients who experienced a sudden onset of pain across the shoulder blade lasting from a few hours to 2 weeks, followed by paralysis involving muscles of the shoulder girdle and in some cases patchy numbness along the lateral aspect of the upper arm. In 98 of the cases there was thought to be some precipitating factor, such as surgery, trauma, infection, lumbar puncture, air encephalogram, or antisyphilitic treatment.[11]

CAUSE AND PATHOPHYSIOLOGY

The exact cause and pathophysiology of PTS are complex and incompletely understood. Autoimmune, genetic, infectious, and mechanical processes have all been implicated.[12] Of the many proposed causes, an infectious or immune-mediated process seems to be the most supported due to the high incidence of preceding infections and immunizations.[2,5,6] An antecedent event has been identified in 30% to 70% of PTS cases.[1,11,13,14] It is theorized that an event may trigger an immune-mediated response that incites the development of PTS. In 20% to 52% of cases, infection precedes the development of PTS.[1,11,14] Approximately 15% of cases occur after immunization.[11,14]

PTS has been associated with several surgical procedures, including coronary artery bypass surgery, oral surgery, hysterectomy, and a variety of orthopedic surgeries.[2,15] Although in surgeries involving the chest or upper extremity, plexopathy may develop from a traction injury because of improper positioning or prolonged pressure over the nerve. However, PTS has been observed following surgical procedures that involve little to no traction on the brachial plexus or surrounding nerves. It may be difficult to distinguish a traction injury from PTS. What distinguishes PTS is nerve involvement without common innervation root, brachial plexus trunk, or cord distribution and muscles with common innervation may be unaffected.[2] Other less frequently observed antecedent events are listed in **Box 2**.[1,2,8,9,11,14–16]

Histologic studies have demonstrated evidence of an immune-mediated process. Suarez and colleagues[17] showed the presence of inflammatory cells, particularly T-lymphocytes, within the brachial plexus of a small sample of patients with PTS. In addition, complement fixing antibodies to peripheral nerve myelin have been found elevated in the acute phase of PTS, and levels tended to decrease during the recovery phase.[18]

van Alfen[12] suggests that the pathophysiology of the condition involves an interaction between a genetic predisposition, mechanical vulnerability, and an autoimmune trigger. No mutations have been found in patients with idiopathic neuralgic amyotrophy but studies have shown mutations of the septin gene in some families with the hereditary autosomal-dominant form. The septin family of genes is highly expressed in glial cells in neuronal tissue.[4] In some cases PTS is preceded by increased physical exertion, suggesting that biomechanical factors may also play a role in triggering the attack.[14]

EPIDEMIOLOGY

One study suggests that the annual incidence of PTS is 1.64 per 100,000 in the United States.[19] The actual incidence may be higher given the difficulty of recognition. It is described in patients ranging from age 3 months[14] to 81 years[16] but occurs most frequently between the third and seventh decades.[14] PTS occurs more frequently in men than women. Studies have shown the ratio of male-to-female involvement ranges from 1.75:1 to 11.5:1.[13] The hereditary form is thought to occur 10 times less frequently than the idiopathic form and typically occurs in the second decade of life.[1,3]

Box 2
Reported antecedent events and associated illnesses

Viral infection—upper respiratory tract infection, flulike syndrome, hepatitis, mononucleosis, malaria, pneumonia, abscess, Typhus, small pox, rheumatic fever, typhoid, poliomyelitis

Immunizations—tetanus toxoid, influenza, horse tetanus antitoxin, DPT

Strenuous exercise

Trauma—fall on shoulder, gunshot wound

Peri-partum

Perioperative—orthopedic, hernia surgery, appendectomy, pilonidal cyst excision, varicocele repair, coronary artery bypass surgery, hysterectomy, tonsillectomy

Medical procedures—lumbar puncture, encephalogram, antisyphilitic treatment

Autoimmune—rheumatoid arthritis, polyarteritis, temporal arteritis

Psychological stress

Data from Refs.[1,2,8,9,11,14–16]

PATIENT EVALUATION OVERVIEW

The classic presentation of PTS begins with acute onset of severe pain lasting for several days to weeks, followed by the development of weakness and muscle atrophy. The presentation is highly variable and may present with a wide range of symptoms, including pain, paresthesias, and sensory disturbances. Patients typically do not have constitutional symptoms such as fever or malaise.[11]

Pain is the predominant presenting symptom in 90% to 95% of patients.[1,14] The pain is usually worse at night and frequently awakens patients from sleep. It is often described as "constant," "sharp," "stabbing," "throbbing," or "aching" and in some cases is associated with muscle tenderness.[14] Characteristically the pain is located in the shoulder and often radiates into the arm or neck. The pain is commonly aggravated by movement of the shoulder but not typically by movement of the neck or Valsalva maneuvers.[20,21] In rare cases, symptoms are localized outside the brachial plexus and in some cases in the lower extremity. The pain is usually unilateral, on the same side in which the weakness develops. Some patients experience bilateral pain followed by unilateral motor symptoms.[4,14] Although the pain on average, lasts 1 to 2 weeks and then subsides,[2] the duration of pain is highly variable, ranging from several hours to months.[1,14] After the acute episode, a portion of patients develops a lingering neuropathic pain in the distribution of the affected nerve and or musculoskeletal pain in the affected muscles or compensating muscles.[12]

Muscle weakness typically begins to develop days to weeks after the onset of pain and often worsens as the pain subsides.[1,14] In a study of 99 patients, weakness began within the first 2 weeks after the onset of pain in 70% of the cases.[14] The location of the initial pain does not necessarily correlate to the distribution of muscle weakness.[21] It may be difficult to ascertain the exact onset of weakness because pain may limit the patient's use of the extremity. In addition, weakness may be hard to recognize if the muscles involved are hard to isolate manually and test.[2] Atrophy of the involved muscles usually occurs relatively quickly.[21]

A characteristic feature of PTS is the patchy distribution of motor and sensory symptoms. Muscles innervated by one peripheral nerve, multiple peripheral nerves, one or more trunks of the plexus, or a combination of peripheral nerves and trunks may be affected.[13,21] The most common pattern of weakness involves muscles supplied by the upper part of the brachial plexus, especially the long thoracic nerve. Muscles most commonly affected include the deltoid, supraspinatus, infraspinatus, serratus anterior, biceps, and triceps.[5] Muscles that have been reported to be affected are listed in **Box 3**.

Individual nerves in isolation or in multiple nerve distributions may be affected. Isolated involvement of the radial, long thoracic, suprascapular, axillary, median, and anterior interosseous nerves are most commonly described.[5] Less frequently, nerves remote from the brachial plexus are involved, including the lumbosacral plexus, phrenic nerve, lower cranial nerves, and recurrent laryngeal nerve.[1,6] Involvement of nerves outside the brachial plexus is seen more frequently in the hereditary form of the syndrome, hereditary neuralgic amyotrophy.[23] Nerves that have been reported to be affected are listed in **Box 4**.

Bilateral brachial plexus involvement occurs approximately 30% of the time. In most cases, one side is more affected than the other.[1,6] In bilateral cases pain and weakness may begin on both sides at the same time or weeks may elapse before involvement of the second side.[13] Involvement of the clinically unaffected side may be found more often on needle electromyography (EMG) than on clinical examination.[5]

> **Box 3**
> **Muscles reported affected in PTS**
>
> *Commonly affected muscles*
>
> Infraspinatus
>
> Supraspinatus
>
> Deltoid
>
> Serratus anterior
>
> Biceps
>
> Triceps
>
> Rhomboids
>
> *Less commonly affected muscles*
>
> Extensor carpi radialis and ulnaris
>
> Pronator teres
>
> Brachioradialis
>
> Trapezius (lower)
>
> Latissiumus dorsi
>
> Pectoralis
>
> Flexor carpi radialis and ulnaris
>
> Teres major
>
> Finger extensors
>
> Pronator quadratus
>
> Flexor digitorum profundus
>
> Dorsal interosseus
>
> Adductor pollicis
>
> Extensor pollicis longus
>
> Supinator
>
> Sternocleidomastoid
>
> Paraspinal neck extensors
>
> *Data from* Refs.[1,11,13,14,22]

Sensory symptoms are variable and occur in anywhere from 42% to 78% of cases.[1,11,13,14] Hypoesthesia and paraesthesias are the most commonly described sensory symptoms.[1] As with weakness, the sensory loss is often patchy in distribution and often corresponds to the sites of plexus or nerve involvement.[5,21] Most frequently, the sensory loss is incomplete and occurs over the lateral shoulder and upper arm or the radial surface of the forearm.[5,20,21]

Autonomic symptoms have also been described, although less frequently. These changes include trophic skin changes, edema in the involved extremity, temperature dysregulation, changes in nail or hair growth, and increased sweating. Autonomic findings occur more commonly in patients with involvement of the posterior cord and lower trunk of the brachial plexus than those with upper trunk involvement.[1,6]

Box 4
Nerves reported to be affected in PTS

Commonly affected nerves

Axillary nerve

Suprascapular nerve

Long thoracic nerve

Musculocutaneous nerve

Radial nerve

Anterior interosseous nerve

Less commonly affected nerves

Median nerve

Subscapular nerve

Phrenic nerve

Recurrent laryngeal nerve

Spinal accessory nerve

Glossophargyneal

Hypoglossal nerve

Lateral antebrachial cutaneous

Data from Refs.[1,2,5,6,16]

DIFFERENTIAL DIAGNOSIS

The diagnosis of PTS is difficult to make, especially in the early stages. PTS may present similarly to other, more common, neurologic and musculoskeletal conditions that cause pain and weakness around the shoulder (**Box 5**). Acute cervical radiculopathies and PTS may both present with a sudden onset of severe pain, although unlike PTS, pain secondary to a cervical radiculopathy may be exacerbated by extension of the neck. In addition, in a cervical radiculopathy, sensory and motor symptoms are usually distributed along a single nerve root. Differentiating between a cervical radiculopathy and PTS may be complicated by the fact that the referred radicular pattern of pain from a cervical radiculopathy, the dynatome, is often different than the traditional dermatomal map.[24] Peripheral nerve entrapments may present similarly to PTS; however, the onset of symptoms is generally more insidious and the pain is less severe. Similarly, mononeuritis multiplex has a more progressive onset and typically involves the distal arm and leg, unlike PTS.[23] Many patients with PTS are initially misdiagnosed with shoulder joint pathologic abnormality. In the acute stage, patients with PTS usually have full passive shoulder range of motion, making intrinsic shoulder joint pathology less likely.[4] Testing passive shoulder range of motion may be difficult in patients with PTS secondary to guarding. To make an accurate diagnosis, it is critical to complete a thorough neurologic and musculoskeletal examination of both the symptomatic and the asymptomatic extremities, including testing manual muscle strength, range of motion, sensation, and reflexes as well as evaluating the shoulder for signs of impingement, adhesive capsulitis, rotator cuff injury, and scapular dyskinesis. It may be challenging to manually test individual muscles surrounding the shoulder. When the scapula is not stabilized, rotator cuff muscles may appear weak even

---

Box 5
Differential diagnosis for PTS

Neurologic disorders

Cervical radiculopathy

Mononeuritis multiplex

Multifocal motor neuropathy

Motor neuron disease

Entrapment neuropathies

Transverse myelitis

Complex regional pain syndrome

Brachial plexopathy secondary to trauma, traction, infiltration (ie, Pancoast tumor)

Tumors of the spinal cord or brachial plexus

Herpes zoster

Hereditary neuropathy with liability to pressure palsies

Neurogenic thoracic outlet syndrome

Musculoskeletal disorders

Rotator cuff injury

Calcific tendinitis

Adhesive capsulitis

Bursitis

Shoulder impingement

Myofascial pain syndrome

Neck disorders, such as osteoarthritis, stenosis, facet

---

when there is no intrinsic weakness. Proper positioning during physical examination helps prevent misdiagnosing rotator cuff weakness.[25] Many of the conditions in the differential diagnosis can be eliminated with the classic history of acute severe pain that decreases spontaneously with the onset of weakness.

DIAGNOSTIC STUDIES
EMG/Nerve Conduction Study

PTS is a clinical diagnosis; however, further diagnostic studies can confirm clinical suspicion and help exclude other causes. Electrodiagnostic studies are particularly useful in localizing the lesion, confirming the diagnosis, and determining the extent of injury. Early EMG testing may be nondiagnostic and therefore should not be performed before 4 to 6 weeks after the onset of symptoms. PTS is thought to be an axonopathy, although findings may vary.[2,14,21] Routinely tested nerve conduction studies are often normal, although delayed distal latencies, decreased compound muscle action potentials, decreased sensory nerve action potentials, and proximal conduction blocks have all been observed.[2,4,20] When sensory abnormalities are present, the lateral antebrachial cutaneous nerve is one of the most frequently affected and should be tested. The diagnosis relies on the needle EMG.[2] Because of the often patchy distribution of involvement, it may be necessary to test a variety of muscles, including muscles that are not routinely tested. EMG performed 3 to 4 weeks after the onset of symptoms shows evidence of acute denervation (fibrillations and positive sharp waves) and often a reduction in motor unit recruitment in a nonmyotomal pattern. There is selective denervation of muscles of different root levels and different peripheral nerves distributions. Typically the paraspinal muscles are not affected.[21] EMG studies 4 to 12 months after the onset of symptoms may show old denervation and reinnervation with polyphasic motor unit potentials.[2] Typical electrodiagnostic findings are summarized in **Table 1**.

Imaging

Radiographic imaging may be useful in excluding other disorders. A chest radiograph can help rule out a Pancoast tumor if there is a clinical suspicion and will detect an elevated hemidiaphragm caused by involvement of the phrenic nerve.[23] A magnetic resonance imaging (MRI) of the cervical spine may reveal cervical disc disease or nerve root compression. An MRI of the shoulder may identify other causes of shoulder pain, including rotator cuff tears, labral tears, shoulder impingement, nerve entrapment, or mass lesions. Abnormalities signifying denervation may be detected on MRI in cases of PTS.[20] MRI findings most characteristic of PTS include diffuse high signal intensity on T2-weighted images, involving one or more muscles innervated by the brachial plexus.[16,26] Later in the subacute phase, T1-weighted images may demonstrate atrophy and fatty infiltration.[16] MRI may not be sensitive enough to detect early (within the first 2–3 weeks) changes in PTS, although magnetic resonance neurography (MRN) may provide better resolution early on, demonstrating hyperintense thickening of the involved areas of the brachial plexus.[27] MRN, however, is currently not readily available at most institutions.

Other Studies

Laboratory studies are generally not helpful in making the diagnosis of PTS. Blood tests are nonspecific and can show elevated liver function levels, mildly elevated creatine kinase, antiganglioside antibodies, and slightly increased cerebrospinal fluid protein and pleocytosis in up to 25% of patients.[1] As mentioned previously, the diagnosis of PTS is ultimately based on clinical history and physical examination.

Pharmacologic Treatment Options

No specific treatments have been proven to reduce neurologic impairment or improve the prognosis of PTS. A *Cochrane Review* concluded that no available studies provided appropriate evidence for a particular form of treatment.[1] There is anecdotal

Table 1 Electrodiagnostic findings	
Nerve conduction studies	May show reduced amplitude, prolonged distal latency, or conduction block Often are normal
Early EMG findings (3–4 wk after symptom onset)	Acute denervation: Fibrillation potentials, positive sharp waves Reduced motor unit recruitment in muscles innervated by different root levels and peripheral nerves
Late EMG findings (3–6 mo after symptom onset)	Old denervation, early reinnervation: Large duration, large amplitude polyphasic motor units, decreased recruitment

evidence that early corticosteroid therapy may improve pain and hasten recovery in some patients.[3] In one study, several patients treated with a 2-week course of oral prednisolone 60 mg in the first week and tapered to 10 mg per day in the second week noted a faster rate of recovery.[1] van Alfen and van Engelen[1] suggests early treatment with oral prednisone 1 mg/kg for the first week and tapering during the second week. Two case reports of PTS showed partial benefit from treatment with intravenous immunoglobulin; however, it has not been reproduced in any larger studies.[28,29]

Severe pain in the acute stage of PTS is often treated with a combination of nonsteroidal anti-inflammatory medications (NSAIDs) and opioids. Antiepileptic medications, such as gabapentin and carbamazepine, and tricyclic antidepressants, such as amytriptyline, are often used to treat the lingering neuropathic pain that often persists after the acute painful attack. Antiepileptic medications are not as effective at treating the acute severe pain of PTS because of their delayed onset.[4] Patients with a history of viral infection or when post-herpetic neuralgia is suspected should be treated with antivirals.[2,4] Strategies used to treat PTS may mimic those used to treat other neuropathic pain conditions such as post-herpetic neuralgia. The American Academy of Neurology recommends gabapentin, lidocaine patch 5%, pregabalin, tricyclic antidepressants, controlled release oxycodone, and morphine sulfate as first-line therapy for the neuropathic pain of post-herpetic neuralgia.[30] A recent review of randomized clinical trials on neuropathic pain outlined an evidence-based algorithm for the treatment of peripheral neuropathic pain. The algorithm suggests that tricylic antidepressants (amitriptyline, nortriptyline, desipramine, imipramine), opioids (CR oxycodone, methadone, morphine), tramadol, gabapentin, and pregabalin are all beneficial in providing pain relief.[31]

Nonpharmacologic Treatment Options

Because PTS is a relatively underrecognized disorder, extensive studies on treatment options have not been performed. In fact, the best treatment of PTS is unknown.[6] Options for nonpharmacologic treatment are mostly based on small, nonrandomized, nonblinded studies and anecdotal evidence. Currently, nonpharmacologic treatments used in the treatment of PTS include physical therapy, osteopathic manipulation, therapeutic modalities, and acupuncture. Despite a proposed role of physical therapy for preventing loss of range of motion and further disability, physical therapy does not seem to speed up recovery.[3]

Goals of physical therapy should include maintenance of range of motion and prevention of loss of function. Depending on the level of pain, range-of-motion exercises for the shoulder may be started immediately. The goal of range-of-motion exercises includes preventing secondary loss of function due to conditions such as contractures or adhesive capsulitis.[2,5] Physical therapy may have a role in pain control. Desensitization exercises may improve allodynia if present. There may also be strategies to reduce traction on involved nerves.[4]

The timing of strengthening exercises depends on several key factors, including level of pain, amount of weakness, and degree of denervation.[22] Most authors advise a cautious approach toward strengthening exercises in physical therapy because an overly aggressive approach can overload muscles that are weak or in the early reinnervated stage.[2] For this reason, authors advise patients to avoid strength training outside of physical therapy sessions during their recovery. Treatment of this condition in high-level athletes should follow the same basic principles. Intensive sport-specific biomechanic training is important before returning high-level athletes to sport. This principle is particularly true in sports that involve throwing, overhead movements (such as basketball, baseball, or tennis), or sports that otherwise involve the shoulder.[2]

The timing of starting biomechanic training depends on the patient's recovery of motor function. Strength training should not be started until significant weakness has recovered.[2]

Although the mainstays of therapy include stretching, range-of-motion, and therapeutic exercise, there may be a role for other therapeutic modalities. Transcutaneous electrical nerve stimulation may play a role in pain control. The role of electrical stimulation as a modality to promote recovery is controversial.[2] There may be a role for acupuncture, particularly in pain control.[2]

The role of interventional procedures has also not been established. In one study, several patients treated with a corticosteroid shoulder injection reported pain relief.[1] In cases where there is coexisting cervical spine pathologic abnormality, cervical epidural steroid injection may be an important diagnostic and therapeutic modality to distinguish between PTS and cervical radiculopathy.[2]

Combination Therapies

Most patients with PTS are treated with a multidisciplinary approach that includes both physical therapy and pharmacologic treatment, often with multiple agents.

From anecdotal evidence, combination pharmacologic therapy may be most effective for pain control. To the extent that oral corticosteroids may help improve symptoms but often provide incomplete pain relief, it is reasonable to begin with oral opioids with the oral corticosteroid taper.[6] As discussed in an earlier section, the recommended dose of oral corticosteroids is a 2-week course of oral prednisolone, 60 mg daily in the first week and tapering to 10 mg per day in the second week.[3] After the initial corticosteroid taper, van Alfen and van Engelen[1] recommend that a combination of NSAID with a short-acting or slow-release opioid may be best.

Surgical Treatment Options

In cases that are refractory to conservative pharmacologic and nonpharmacologic treatments, surgery is often considered. Surgical procedures for PTS include neurolysis, nerve grafts, and nerve transfers. Timing of surgical intervention is challenging. Penkert and colleagues[32] suggest that delay of treatments beyond 2 to 6 months

---

Box 6
Complications of PTS

Potential complications

- Shoulder dysfunction
  - Adhesive capsulitis
  - Shoulder subluxation/dislocation due to weakness
- Chronic pain
- Loss of function
  - Weakness in proximal more than distal arm
  - Loss of function due to pain
- Shoulder subluxation/dislocation due to weakness
- Loss of work/disability
  - Need for workplace modification
  - Long-term disability

Box 7
Factors associated with prognosis in PTS
Good prognosis
• Predominantly upper trunk involvement[4]
• Primarily sensory symptoms[34]
Poor prognosis
• Prolonged pain
• Prolonged weakness[4]

may result in worse outcomes. Kretschmer and colleagues[33] have reported 60% favorable outcomes after surgical treatment. Surgery is often considered when there are secondary complications. Tendon and muscle transfers are often used to facilitate function in the setting of significant weakness. Surgical intervention is also sometimes performed in the setting of secondary shoulder complications, such as recurrent dislocation.[4,32,33]

Evaluation of Outcome and Long-Term Recommendations

The disease course of PTS is variable.[4] In the best possible outcome, pain and weakness can resolve spontaneously in about 1 month[22] with conservative treatment alone. Unfortunately, many patients develop long-term complications such as shoulder dysfunction (adhesive capsulitis, shoulder subluxation), chronic pain, loss of function, loss of work, and disability (**Box 6**).

With respect to disease course, 66% of patients begin to show motor function recovery within 1 month of onset of weakness.[4] A study by Tsairis and colleagues[14] observed the full recovery may follow a more protracted course. The percentage of patients with PTS who reported "excellent" recovery was 36% at 1 year, 75% by 2 years, and 89% by 3 years. A 2006 study by van Alfen and van Engelen[1] observed that although many patients do achieve timely and complete resolutions of symptoms, one-third of patients continue to experience chronic pain and persistent functional deficits (after an average follow-up of greater than 6 years). In patients with greater than 3-years follow-up, mild, moderate, and severe paralysis were seen in 69%, 14%, and 3% of patients, respectively. Factors associated with a good prognosis include predominantly upper trunk involvement and primarily sensory symptoms (**Box 7**).[4,34] Prolonged pain and weakness are associated with a poor prognosis.[4] There is no established relationship between prognosis and age.[4]

Another issue that PTS patients face is recurrence of symptoms. Although rare repeat attacks are sometimes severe, subsequent attacks are usually less severe than the first episode.[4]

SUMMARY

PTS is an underrecognized condition. High-quality evidence for the treatment of PTS is lacking. PTS should be considered as a diagnosis in the setting of an abrupt onset of upper extremity pain followed by progressive neurologic deficits including weakness, atrophy, and occasionally sensory abnormalities. Although there are many proposed theories, a common unifying cause has not been established. No specific treatments have been proven to reduce neurologic impairment or improve the prognosis of PTS, although there is anecdotal evidence that early corticosteroid therapy may improve pain and hasten recovery in some patients. Most patients with PTS syndrome are treated with a multidisciplinary approach that includes both physical therapy and pharmacologic treatment, often with multiple agents. The goals of physical therapy should include maintenance of range of motion and prevention of loss of function. Most authors advise a cautious approach toward strengthening exercises in physical therapy as an overly aggressive approach can overload muscles that are weak or in early reinnervated stages. In cases that are refractory to conservative pharmacologic and nonpharmacologic treatments, surgery is often considered. Further research in treatments to hasten recovery and reduce long-term neurologic impairment is needed.

REFERENCES

1. van Alfen N, van Engelen BG. The clinical spectrum of neuralgic amyotrophy in 246 cases. Brain 2006;129(2):438–50.
2. Feinberg JH, Radecki J. Parsonage Turner syndrome. HSS J 2010;6:199–205.
3. van Alfen N, van Engelen BG, Hughes RA. Treatment for idiopathic and hereditary neuralgic amyotrophy (brachial neuritis). Cochrane Database Syst Rev 2009;(3):CD006976.
4. Tjoumakaris FP, Anakwenze O, Kancherla V, et al. Neuralgic amyotrophy (Parsonage-Turner syndrome). J Am Acad Orthop Surg 2012;20:443–9.
5. Rubin DI. Neuralgic amyotrophy: clinical features and diagnostic evaluation. Neurologist 2001;7:350–6.
6. Stutz CM. Neuralgic amyotrophy: Parsonage Turner syndrome. J Hand Surg Am 2010;35(12):2104–6.
7. Dixon GJ, Dick TB. Acute brachial radiculitis. Lancet 1945;1:707–8.
8. Turner J. Acute brachial radiculitis. Br Med J 1944;2:992–4.
9. Fibuch EE, Mertz J, Geller B. Postoperative onset of idiopathic brachial neuritis. Anesthesiology 1996;84:455–8.
10. Spillane JD. Localised neuritis of the shoulder girdle: a report of 46 cases in the MEF. Lancet 1943;2:532–5.
11. Parsonage MJ, Turner JW. Neuralgic amyotrophy: shoulder girdle syndrome. Lancet 1948;1:973–8.
12. Van Alfen N. Reviews: clinical and pathophysiologic concepts of neuralgic amyotrophy. Nat Rev Neurol 2011;7:315–21.
13. Magee KR, DeJong RN. Paralytic brachial neuritis: discussion of clinical features with review of 23 cases. JAMA 1960;174:1258–62.
14. Tsairis P, Dyck PJ, Milder DW. Natural history of brachial plexus neuropathy: report on 99 patients. Arch Neurol 1972;27(2):109–17.
15. Malmut RI, Marques W, England JD, et al. Postsurgical idiopathic brachial neuritis. Muscle Nerve 1994;17:320–4.
16. Gaskin CM, Helms CA. Parsonage Turner syndrome: MR imaging findings and clinical information of 27 patients. Radiology 2006;240:501–7.
17. Suarez GA, Giannini C, Bosch EP, et al. Immune brachial plexus neuropathy: suggestive evidence of an inflammatory-immune pathogenesis. Neurology 1996; 46(2):559–61.
18. Vriesendrop FJ, Dmytrenko GS, Dietrich T, et al. Anti-peripheral nerve myelin antibodies and terminal activation products of complement in serum of patients with acute brachial plexus neuropathy. Arch Neurol 1993;50:1301–3.
19. Beghi F, Kurland LT, Mudler DW, et al. Brachial plexus neuropathy in the population of Rochester, Minnesota, 1970–1981. Ann Neurol 1985;18:320–3.

20. Sathasivam S, Lecky B, Manohar R, et al. Neuralgic amyotrophy. J Bone Joint Surg Br 2008;90(5):550–3.
21. McCarty E, Tsairis P, Warren R. Brachial neuritis. Clinic Orthop Relat Res 1996; 368:37–42.
22. Misamore GW, Lehman DE. Parsonage-Turner syndrome (acute brachial neuritis). J Bone Joint Surg Am 1996;78(9):1405–8.
23. Van Alfen N. The neuralgic amyotrophy consultation. J Neurol 2007;254:695–704.
24. Slipman CW, Plastaras CT, Palmitier RA, et al. Symptom provocation of fluoro-scopically guided cervical nerve root stimulation. Are dynatomal maps identical to dermatomal maps? Spine 1998;23(20):2235–42.
25. Schreiber A, Abramov R, Fried G, et al. Expanding the differential of shoulder pain: Parsonage Turner syndrome. J Am Osteopath Assoc 2009;109(8):415–22.
26. Sureka J, Cherian RA, Alexander M, et al. Pictorial review: MRI of brachial plexo-pathies. Clin Radiol 2009;64:208–18.
27. Duman I, Guvenc I, Kalyon TA. Neuralgic amyotrophy, diagnosed with magnetic resonance neurography in acute stage: a case report and review of the literature. Neurologist 2007;13(4):219–21.
28. Johnson NE, Petraglia AL, Huang JH, et al. Rapid resolution of severe neuralgic amyotrophy after treatment with corticosteroids and intravenous immunoglobulin. Muscle Nerve 2011;44(2):304–5.
29. Nakajima M, Fujioka S, Ohno H, et al. Partial but rapid recovery from paralysis after immunomodulation during early stage of neuralgic amyotrophy. Eur Neurol 2006;55:227–9.
30. de Leon-Casasola O. Opioids for chronic pain: new evidence, new strategies, safe prescribing. Am J Med 2013;126:3–11.
31. Finnerup NB, Otto M, McQuay HJ, et al. Algorithm for neuropathic pain treatment: an evidence based proposal. Pain 2005;118:289–305.
32. Penkert G, Carvalho GA, Nikkhah G, et al. Diagnosis and surgery of brachial plexus injuries. J Reconstr Microsurg 1999;15:3.
33. Kretschmer T, Ihle S, Antoniadis G, et al. Patient satisfaction and disability after brachial plexus surgery. Neurosurgery 2009;65:A189.
34. Seror P. Isolated sensory manifestation in neuralgic amyotrophy: report of eight cases. Muscle Nerve 2004;29(1):134–8.

Greater Trochanteric Pain Syndrome Diagnosis and Treatment

Michael Mallow, MD[a],*, Levon N. Nazarian, MD[b]

KEYWORDS

- Great trochanteric pain syndrome • Greater trochanteric bursitis
- Ultrasound-guided injection

KEY POINTS

- Greater trochanteric pain syndrome (GTPS) is a relatively common condition causing lateral lower limb pain in a diverse group of patients.
- GTPS can be effectively evaluated by ultrasound, and this can also provide guidance for treatment options.
- There are many treatment options for GTPS; however, comparative effectiveness research is needed.

 Video of an injection of the greater trochanteric bursa accompanies this article at http://www.pmr.theclinics.com/

INTRODUCTION

The term *greater trochanteric pain syndrome* (GTPS) refers to pain originating from various structures in the lateral hip, including tendon and bursa. The latter structure is now thought to play a smaller role in this entity than previously thought, and the term *trochanteric bursitis* is somewhat of a misnomer because inflammation is not commonly found. Other implicated structures and entities include gluteal tears and snapping hip.[1] This article reviews the epidemiology, anatomy, diagnosis, and treatment of GTPS with special attention in imaging and image-guided interventions.

Funding Sources: None.
Conflict of Interest: Dr M. Mallow: None; Dr L.N. Nazarian: Editor-in-Chief, *Journal of Ultrasound in Medicine*.
[a] Department of Rehabilitation Medicine, Jefferson Medical College of Thomas Jefferson University, 25 South 9th Street, Philadelphia, PA 19107, USA; [b] Department of Radiology, Jefferson Medical College of Thomas Jefferson University, 132 South 10th Street, Philadelphia, PA 19107, USA
* Corresponding author.
E-mail address: michael.mallow@jefferson.edu

EPIDEMIOLOGY

Hip pain is a common complaint prompting visitation to a primary care provider or musculoskeletal medicine specialist. In a large national survey, 14.3% of individuals more than 60 years of age reported frequent hip pain.[2] In the survey, women reported pain more frequently than men; in men, age was not a predictor of hip pain. In a large observational study by Segal and colleagues,[3] unilateral GTPS was noted to have a prevalence of 8.5% in women and 6.6% in men. In patients referred to a spine practice for a complaint of back pain, the prevalence of GTPS was 20.2% and again more frequent in women.[4] Noted in this study, greater that 50% of patients had already undergone magnetic resonance imaging (MRI) of the lumbar spine.

Based on the aforementioned data, GTPS is a common clinical entity in patients presenting with both hip pain and low back pain. Attention to the differential of GTPS in any patient with hip and back pain is essential.

ASSOCIATED CONDITIONS AND FACTORS

Because the buttock and hip can be a common site of referred pain from the spine and other structures, as well as the biomechanical loads placed on structures in this region, there are a host of conditions that may coexist with GTPS. Iliotibial band (ITB) tenderness, knee osteoarthritis, and low back pain were positively related to the occurrence of GTPS in an observational study.[3] Body mass index was not found to be associated with GTPS. In a prospective study, GTPS was found in 18% to 45% of patients with chronic low back pain.[5]

ANATOMY

Several muscles insert on or near the greater trochanter of the femur, the gluteus medius and minimus, piriformis, obturator externus, and obturator internus. The most superficial gluteal muscle, the gluteus maximus, has a broad origin including fibers from the ilium and sacrum and inserts onto the gluteal tuberosity of the femur and the iliotibial tract. Deep to this muscle lies the gluteus medius, a smaller muscle in surface area, which originates from the ilium and inserts onto the greater trochanter of the femur. Deep to the gluteus medius, the gluteus minimus is found and takes origin from the ilium and also inserts onto the greater trochanter.

The tensor fascia lata originates from the iliac crest and inserts onto the iliotibial tract in the lower limb. This fibrous band of tissue inserts distally onto the lateral condyle of the tibia. As mentioned earlier, the gluteus maximus muscle inserts onto the iliotibial tract and the femur.

The greater trochanter is associated with bursae that provide protection for the surrounding tendons, namely, the gluteus medius and minimus, ITB, and tensor fascia lata. The most superior bursa, the subgluteus medius bursa, sits superior to the greater trochanter under the gluteus medius tendon. The subgluteus maximus bursa sits between the tendons of the gluteus medius and maximus and lateral to the greater trochanter. The deep subgluteus maximus bursa is a division sometimes revered to as the *trochanteric bursa*. In some individuals, a superficial bursa exists within the gluteus maximus muscle. Dissection study supports the idea that bursa may be acquired as a result of friction between the greater trochanter and gluteus maximus.[6] Bursal tissue from patients with GTPS undergoing total hip arthroplasty showed no signs of acute or chronic inflammation. This finding supports the understanding that inflammation, or bursitis, plays a limited role in GTPS.[7]

PRESENTATION

Patients with GTPS will present with hip pain, but this verbal symptom must be carefully discussed and a full history taken. Patients should be asked about the associated presence of low back pain, groin pain, as well as more distal complaints of knee or ankle pain. Recent increases or decreases in activity should be discussed as well as questions about recent or past trauma. Groin pain often points one in the direction of hip osteoarthritis or perhaps lumbar spine disorders, whereas pain felt laterally, just distal to the waistline, prompts further consideration of GTPS.

Acutely, patients with GTPS will complain of lateral hip pain that is worse with pressure on that side of the body, such as while lying down. They often complain of pain with walking and may admit that pain is worse while standing on the affected leg. There may be associated lateral thigh pain radiation but rarely below the knee. A dermatomal distribution of pain should prompt investigation of alternative causes, such as lumbar radiculopathy. This evaluation, however, can be challenging as the two conditions may coexist.

Some patients with advanced cases can demonstrate tears of the gluteus medius or minimus on ultrasound or MRI. These tears maybe analogous to rotator cuff tears,[8] usually present similarly to GTPS and benefit from a period of conservative treatment, covered later.[1]

External snapping hip syndrome is caused by tightness of the ITB as it overlies the greater trochanter. When the hip is flexed, the ITB may snap over the greater trochanter and can be painful at times in younger, active patients. This syndrome can also be treated with conservative measures.[9]

DIFFERENTIAL DIAGNOSIS

Various disorders and clinical entities can cause lateral hip pain. A comprehensive differential diagnosis is presented here[10]:

- GTPS
  - Gluteus medius dysfunction, gluteus medius or gluteus minimus tendinopathy
  - Piriformis tendinopathy
  - Iliotibial tract friction syndrome
  - Trochanteric bursitis
- Traction enthesopathy
- Piriformis syndrome
- Other snapping hip syndrome
- Meralgia paresthetica
- Other peripheral compressive neuropathy
- Hip (femoroacetabular) osteoarthrosis
- Slipped capital femoral epiphysis
- Femoroacetabular impingement
- Acetabular labral tear
- Femoral head avascular necrosis
- Femoral neck fracture
- Femoral neck stress fracture
- Iliopsoas tendinopathy
- Sports hernia
- Fibromyalgia
- Myofascial trigger points
- Complex regional pain syndrome

- Lumbosacral spine disorders
  - Intervertebral disk disease
  - Facet joint arthropathy
  - Lumbosacral radiculopathy
  - Lumbosacral spine sprain or strain
  - Lumbosacral spondylolisthesis
  - Pars interarticularis injury
  - Sacroiliac joint injury or dysfunction
- Referred pain from intra-abdominal processes
  - Endometriosis
  - Prostate disease
  - Gastroenteritis
  - Inflammatory bowel disease
  - Irritable bowel syndrome
  - Inguinal hernia
  - Ovarian cysts
  - Ureteral stone or dysfunction

EXAMINATION

A complete neuromusculoskeletal examination should be performed, including observation of swelling or skin breakdown and gait observation. Proper manual muscle testing cannot be overemphasized because neurologic conditions, such as lumbar radiculopathy, can present as lateral hip pain. It is important to identify any weakness, sensory loss, and or diminished reflexes because these findings may direct the clinician to an alternative workup. Gluteus medius weakness, however, is often present with GTPS.

Pain in GTPS may be reproduced by direct palpation and often by resisted abduction and external rotation. In a series of 24 patients, Bird and colleagues[11] showed that the Trendelenburg sign was most sensitive for the detection of gluteus medius tears confirmed by MRI. It should be noted that evidence of bursitis was rare in these patients versus the finding of gluteus medius tendinopathy.

IMAGING
Radiography

Plain radiography can depict greater trochanteric enthesopathy as manifested by surface irregularities of the greater trochanter and/or tendon calcifications.[12] Radiography can also identify other causes of hip pain, such as osteoarthritis or fractures. The limitation of radiography is the inadequate imaging of soft tissue.

MRI

MRI is considered by many to be the imaging gold standard for GTPS because it can depict both osseous and soft tissue pathology. Blankenbaker and colleagues[13] reported that all patients with GTPS had a combination of peritrochanteric edema and gluteus minimus or medius pathology, generally tendinosis rather than tear. Tendinosis was the only finding that was significantly more common in patients than in normal subjects. MRI can also detect calcifications in the gluteus medius and minimus.[14] Although fluid is often seen in the local bursas, namely, the greater trochanteric bursa (also known as *the subgluteus maximus bursa*), subgluteus minimus bursa, and subgluteus medius bursa,[15] it is rare that bursal fluid is the dominant or only finding.[13]

Sonographic Imaging

Sonography can be helpful in establishing the cause of GTPS.[16,17] The advantages over MRI include lower cost, greater accessibility, and the ability to compare imaging findings with tenderness at the time of the examination. High-resolution images can be obtained of the gluteus medius (**Figs. 1** and **2**) and gluteus minimus tendons (**Fig. 3**) and ITB (**Fig. 4**). The local bursas can also be visualized.

The pain at the greater trochanter is usually not secondary to bursitis, although reactive bursal fluid can be present. Instead, sonography most often reveals pathology involving the gluteus medius and minimus tendons as well as the ITB. The most common pathology is tendinosis, whereby any combination of these structures may be thickened and heterogeneous with a loss of the normal fibrillar pattern. Calcifications are commonly seen within the gluteus medius and gluteus minimus tendons (**Figs. 5** and **6**), and there is often bony irregularity on the greater trochanter indicating enthesopathy.[16] Tendon tears (**Fig. 7**) can also be seen with high accuracy.[17]

The real-time nature of ultrasound also allows for the evaluation of patients who have painful snapping at the greater trochanter. The examiner places the ultrasound probe over the greater trochanter and asks patients to perform the maneuver that reproduces the snapping. Dynamic imaging usually shows that either the ITB or the gluteus maximus muscle is responsible for the symptoms (**Fig. 8**).[18]

CONSERVATIVE TREATMENT

Patients should be initially managed with relative rest, ice, and antiinflammatory medication if deemed necessary for pain control and/or in acute cases. Most patients improve with conservative measures.[19] As noted earlier, most GTPS cases are unlikely to be the result of inflammation; therefore, nonsteroidal antiinflammatory drugs may not be beneficial beyond their analgesic effects. Activity modification is important to avoid potentially injurious hip motions, such as lying on that hip or repetitive motions.

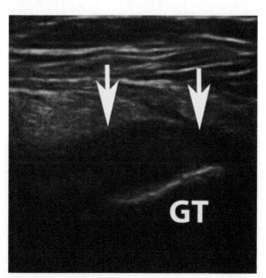

Fig. 1. Gluteus medius tendinosis: Longitudinal sonogram at the level of the greater trochanter in a patient with GTPS shows a thickened, hypoechoic gluteus medius tendon (*arrows*) consistent with tendinosis.

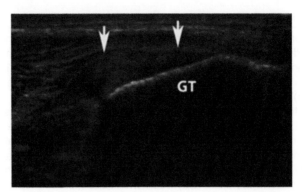

Fig. 2. Gluteus medius normal: Longitudinal sonogram at the level of the greater trochanter (GT) in an asymptomatic subject shows a normal insertion site of the gluteus medius tendon (*arrows*).

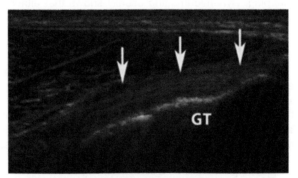

Fig. 3. Gluteus minimus normal: Longitudinal sonogram at the level of the greater trochanter (GT) in an asymptomatic subject shows a normal insertion site of the gluteus minimus tendon (*arrows*).

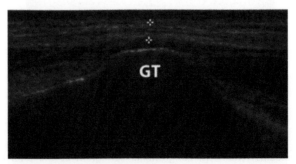

Fig. 4. ITB normal: Longitudinal sonogram at the level of the greater trochanter (GT) in an asymptomatic subject shows a normal ITB (*cursors*).

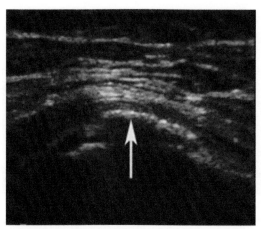

Fig. 5. Calcific tendinosis: Longitudinal sonogram at the level of the greater trochanter in a patient with GTPS shows a calcification (*arrow*) within the gluteus medius tendon.

Given that the hip abductors are active during ambulation to stabilize the pelvis, it is logical to postulate that correcting weakness of hip abduction would improve the ability of this musculature to function correctly and improve pain. There is, however, a lack of data in the literature to support home exercise regimens or formal physical therapy strategies to treat GTPS. Rompe and colleagues[20] assigned patients sequentially to home training, single steroid injection, or 3 sessions of shock wave treatment. The home program consisted of piriformis stretching, ITB stretching, straight leg raises, wall squats, and gluteal strengthening. Participants in this group participated in 6 instructional sessions of 20 minutes duration and were instructed to perform this program twice daily for 12 weeks. Although corticosteroid injection was superior to the other treatments at 1 month, at 15 months from baseline, home training (80% success rate) was superior to shock wave treatment (74% success rate) and single steroid injection (48% success rate). A treatment plan that corrects other kinetic chain

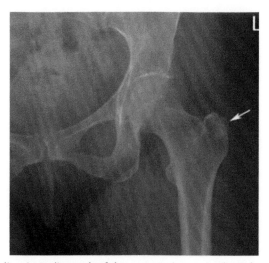

Fig. 6. Calcific tendinosis: Radiograph of the same patient as in **Fig. 5** shows the calcification (*arrow*) superficial to the greater trochanter.

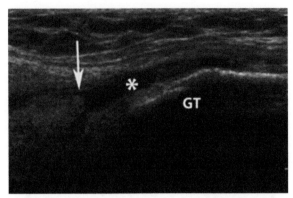

Fig. 7. Gluteus minimus tear: Longitudinal sonogram at the level of the greater trochanter (GT) in a patient with GTPS shows a torn gluteus minimus tendon (*asterisk*) with the retracted edge indicated by the arrow.

abnormalities, such as knee and ankle pathology or weakness, is also reasonable, although not well studied, and could be included in any treatment plans.

Furia and colleagues[21] also evaluated conservative treatment and compared patients treated with extracorporeal shock wave therapy (ESWT) and other nonoperative treatments, including corticosteroid injections, with patients treated with the same nonoperative treatments without ESWT in a case control study. They showed greater efficacy in the group treated with ESWT at 1, 3, and 12 months.

SONOGRAPHICALLY GUIDED TREATMENTS

Although GTPS is not caused by bursitis, most patients feel intermediate-term relief from the injection of corticosteroids and local anesthetic into the greater trochanteric bursa (Video 1).[22]

When symptoms recur, repeat injections can be performed.[23] Greater trochanteric bursal injections are usually done using landmarks and without image guidance. In

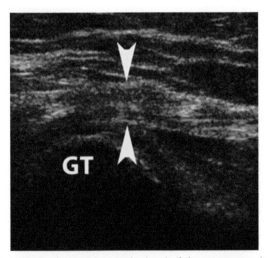

Fig. 8. Thick ITB: Longitudinal sonogram at the level of the greater trochanter (GT) in a patient with GTPS shows a thickened, heterogeneous ITB (*arrowheads*).

patients with a large body habitus or in whom non–image-guided injections were unsuccessful, image guidance can confirm accurate placement of the needle and of the injectate. One study of fluoroscopically guided injections showed that this method increased costs without improving outcomes.[24] Two other studies showed that sonographically guided corticosteroid injections into the greater trochanteric bursa were effective, but these studies did not have control groups who were injected without image guidance.[25,26] Further studies are necessary to document whether sonographically guided corticosteroid injections into the greater trochanteric bursa improve outcomes.

When injections are ineffective or only work for a brief period of time, sonographically guided treatment options that directly target the underlying pathology need to be considered. These treatments include percutaneous needle tenotomy, injection of platelet-rich plasma or whole blood, prolotherapy, and others. At this time, there is only preliminary work describing such treatments for the gluteus medius tendon and only in the context of the treatment of a wide range of tendons.[27] Randomized trials comparing the effectiveness of these various treatments are needed in order to define their role in GTPS.

SURGICAL TREATMENT

GTPS that is refractory to many of the aforementioned measures is, at times, managed surgically with various techniques,[28] including new endoscopic approaches.[29] In certain patients, surgical intervention may be superior to conservative care[19]; however, the results of surgical studies are challenging to evaluate given their small sample size.

SUMMARY

GTPS is a complex clinical entity. Once thought to be primarily caused by bursal inflammation, current evidence and experience points to tendinopathy as the primary cause of pain. Therefore, antiinflammatory medications may be of limited utility. Other treatments, such as exercise, and modalities surely play a role. For cases recalcitrant to initial conservative measures, injection therapy should be considered. More recently, sonographic imaging can provide anatomic abnormalities and/or provide procedural guidance. GTPS can be successfully treated with awareness of diagnosis, understanding of pathology, and utilization of available treatment options.

SUPPLEMENTARY DATA

Video related to this article can be found online at http://dx.doi.org/10.1016/j.pmr.2014.01.009.

REFERENCES

1. Strauss EJ, Nho SJ, Kelly BT. Greater trochanteric pain syndrome. Sports Med Arthrosc 2010;18:113–9.
2. Christmas C, Crespo CJ, Franckowiak SC, et al. How common is hip pain among older adults? Results from the Third National Health and Nutrition Examination Survey. J Fam Pract 2002;51:345–8.
3. Segal NA, Felson DT, Torner JC, et al. Greater trochanteric pain syndrome: epidemiology and associated factors. Arch Phys Med Rehabil 2007;88:988–92.
4. Tortolani PJ, Carbone JJ, Quartararo LG. Greater trochanteric pain syndrome in patients referred to orthopedic spine specialists. Spine J 2002;2:251–4.

5. Collée G, Dijkmans BA, Vandenbroucke JP, et al. Greater trochanteric pain syndrome (trochanteric bursitis) in low back pain. Scand J Rheumatol 1991;20: 262–6.

6. Dunn T, Heller CA, McCarthy SW, et al. Anatomical study of the "trochanteric bursa". Clin Anat 2003;16:233–40.

7. Silva F, Adams T, Feinstein J, et al. Trochanteric bursitis: refuting the myth of inflammation. J Clin Rheumatol 2008;14:82–6.

8. Robertson WJ, Gardner MJ, Barker JU, et al. Anatomy and dimensions of the gluteus medius tendon insertion. Arthroscopy 2008;24:130–6.

9. Reich MS, Shannon C, Tsai E, et al. Hip arthroscopy for extra-articular hip disease. Curr Rev Musculoskelet Med 2013;6:250–7.

10. Ho GW, Howard TM. Greater trochanteric pain syndrome: more than bursitis and iliotibial tract friction. Curr Sports Med Rep 2012;11:232–8.

11. Bird PA, Oakley SP, Shnier R, et al. Prospective evaluation of magnetic resonance imaging and physical examination findings in patients with greater trochanteric pain syndrome. Arthritis Rheum 2001;44:2138–45.

12. Steinert L, Zanetti M, Hodler J, et al. Are radiographic trochanteric surface irregularities associated with abductor tendon abnormalities? Radiology 2010;257: 754–63.

13. Blankenbaker DG, Ullrick SR, Davis KW, et al. Correlation of MRI findings with clinical findings of trochanteric pain syndrome. Skeletal Radiol 2008;37:903–9.

14. Dwek J, Pfirrmann C, Stanley A, et al. MR imaging of the hip abductors: normal anatomy and commonly encountered pathology at the greater trochanter. Magn Reson Imaging Clin N Am 2005;13:691–704, vii.

15. Pfirrmann CW, Chung CB, Theumann NH, et al. Greater trochanter of the hip: attachment of the abductor mechanism and a complex of three bursae–MR imaging and MR bursography in cadavers and MR imaging in asymptomatic volunteers. Radiology 2001;221:469–77.

16. Connell DA, Bass C, Sykes CA, et al. Sonographic evaluation of gluteus medius and minimus tendinopathy. Eur Radiol 2003;13:1339–47.

17. Fearon AM, Scarvell JM, Cook JL, et al. Does ultrasound correlate with surgical or histologic findings in greater trochanteric pain syndrome? A pilot study. Clin Orthop Relat Res 2010;468:1838–44.

18. Bureau NJ. Sonographic evaluation of snapping hip syndrome. J Ultrasound Med 2013;32:895–900.

19. Lustenberger DP, Ng VY, Best TM, et al. Efficacy of treatment of trochanteric bursitis: a systematic review. Clin J Sport Med 2011;21:447–53.

20. Rompe JD, Segal NA, Cacchio A, et al. Home training, local corticosteroid injection, or radial shock wave therapy for greater trochanter pain syndrome. Am J Sports Med 2009;37:1981–90.

21. Furia JP, Rompe JD, Maffulli N. Low-energy extracorporeal shock wave therapy as a treatment for greater trochanteric pain syndrome. Am J Sports Med 2009; 37:1806–13.

22. Williams BS, Cohen SP. Greater trochanteric pain syndrome: a review of anatomy, diagnosis and treatment. Anesth Analg 2009;108:1662–70.

23. Sayegh F, Potoupnis M, Kapetanos G. Greater trochanter bursitis pain syndrome in females with chronic low back pain and sciatica. Acta Orthop Belg 2004;70: 423–8.

24. Cohen SP, Strassels SA, Foster L, et al. Comparison of fluoroscopically guided and blind corticosteroid injections for greater trochanteric pain syndrome: multicentre randomised controlled trial. BMJ 2009;338:b1088.

25. McEvoy JR, Lee KS, Blankenbaker DG, et al. Ultrasound-guided corticosteroid injections for treatment of greater trochanteric pain syndrome: greater trochanter bursa versus subgluteus medius bursa. AJR Am J Roentgenol 2013;201:W313–7.
26. Labrosse JM, Cardinal E, Leduc BE, et al. Effectiveness of ultrasound-guided corticosteroid injection for the treatment of gluteus medius tendinopathy. AJR Am J Roentgenol 2010;194:202–6.
27. Finnoff JT, Fowler SP, Lai JK, et al. Treatment of chronic tendinopathy with ultrasound-guided needle tenotomy and platelet-rich plasma injection. PM R 2011;3:900–11.
28. Baker CL, Massie RV, Hurt WG, et al. Arthroscopic bursectomy for recalcitrant trochanteric bursitis. Arthroscopy 2007;23:827–32.
29. Govaert LH, van Dijk CN, Zeegers AV, et al. Endoscopic bursectomy and iliotibial tract release as a treatment for refractory greater trochanteric pain syndrome: a new endoscopic approach with early results. Arthrosc Tech 2012;1:e161–4.

Complex Regional Pain Syndrome
Diagnosis and Treatment

Mitchell Freedman, DO[a,b,*], Ari C. Greis, DO[a,b], Lisa Marino, DO[b],
Anupam N. Sinha, DO[b], Jeffrey Henstenburg[b]

KEYWORDS

- Complex regional pain syndrome • Neuropathic pain syndromes
- Reflex sympathetic dystrophy sympathetic nerve block • Spinal cord stimulation

KEY POINTS

- Complex regional pain syndrome (CRPS) is characterized by pain out of proportion to the usual time or degree of a specific lesion.
- The diagnosis of CRPS is based on 4 distinct subgroups of signs and symptoms: sensory, vasomotor, sudomotor, and motor/trophic changes.
- Treatment should be multidisciplinary, consisting of medications, physical/occupational therapy, psychotherapy, and sympathetic blocks targeted toward pain relief and functional restoration.
- More aggressive treatment, such as sympathectomy and spinal cord stimulation, have a low level of evidence but may be considered for therapy-resistant CRPS type I.

INTRODUCTION

Complex regional pain syndrome (CRPS) is characterized by pain that is out of proportion to the usual time or degree of a specific lesion. It does not present within the distribution of one peripheral nerve or nerve root, and has a distal predominance of abnormal sensory, motor, sudomotor, vasomotor, and/or trophic findings. Progression is variable.[1] CRPS has been known by many other names including reflex sympathetic dystrophy (RSD) and causalgia. These terms date back to Claude Bernard, who in 1851 referred to a pain syndrome that was accompanied by changes in the sympathetic nervous system. During the American Civil War, Silas Weir Mitchell described cases of soldiers suffering from ongoing burning pain after recovering from gunshot wounds, and coined the term Causalgia.[2,3] Evans first used the term reflex sympathetic dystrophy in the 1940s to emphasize that the sympathetic nervous system

Disclosures: None.
[a] Department of Rehabilitation Medicine, Jefferson Medical College, Thomas Jefferson University, 9th and Chestnut Street, Philadelphia, PA 19107, USA; [b] Rothman Institute, 925 Chestnut Street, Philadelphia, PA 19107, USA
* Corresponding author. Rothman Institute, 925 Chestnut Street, Philadelphia, PA 19107.
E-mail address: mitchell.freedman@rothmaninstitute.com

Phys Med Rehabil Clin N Am 25 (2014) 291–303
http://dx.doi.org/10.1016/j.pmr.2014.01.003

was involved in the pathophysiology of the disease.[4] CRPS replaced the term RSD for several reasons. Sympathetic changes and dystrophy may not be present throughout the disease course.[5,6] Furthermore, there is no specific reflex arc that is responsible for the CRPS; pain is secondary to multisynaptic pathologic changes involving the brain, spinal cord, and peripheral nerves.

EPIDEMIOLOGY

CRPS has a female to male ratio of 2:1 to 4:1, which is more common with increasing age. There are 50,000 new cases of CRPS in the United States annually. The most common initiating events of the syndrome include fractures, sprains, and trauma such as crush injuries and surgery. Immobilization after injury is a contributing factor in more than half of patients.[7,8]

DIAGNOSIS

The Budapest Consensus Workshop introduced criteria to identify patients with CRPS and exclude other neuropathic conditions. More stringent criteria are used for research purposes to eliminate false-positive inclusions. Less stringent criteria are used in the clinical setting to avoid missing the diagnosis. A patient must report symptoms of, and display signs on physical examination, in the following categories: sensory, vasomotor, sudomotor/edema, and motor/trophic (**Figs. 1** and **2**). For both clinical and research purposes, a patient with CRPS should have physical examination evidence of at least 1 sign in 2 or more of the categories. The symptom criteria are different when assessing patients in a clinical rather than a research setting. In a clinical setting, patients must report 1 symptom in 3 out of the 4 categories, whereas in the research setting the patient must report 1 symptom in each of the 4 categories (**Box 1**). This minor adjustment in data collection creates a sensitivity of 0.85 and a specificity of 0.69 for the research group, compared with the clinical criteria that have a sensitivity of 0.94 and a specificity of 0.36.[1,9]

There are 2 subgroupings of CRPS. CRPS I is CRPS without major nerve damage (formerly known as RSD) while CRPS II is CRPS with major nerve damage (formerly known as causalgia). A third subtype is CRPS NOS (not otherwise specified), which captures patients who only partially meet the current criteria but were diagnosed with CRPS under previous criteria.[1,6,9]

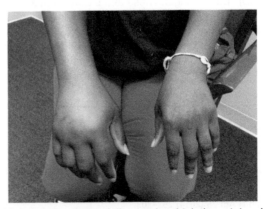

Fig. 1. A patient with 3 months of pain following brachial plexus injury has significant fusiform edema and color changes in the right upper extremity.

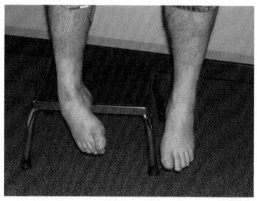

Fig. 2. A patient with chronic complex regional pain syndrome exhibits dystonic posture of the right ankle along with trophic skin changes.

Accurate diagnosis of CRPS is challenging despite the standardization of diagnostic criteria. There is no one definitive objective test that confirms the clinical diagnosis. Physical findings may not be present at all times, but the diagnostic criteria for signs require that the findings be present at the time of the diagnosis. At present, the diagnosis is made primarily on the basis of physical examination, but there are objective tests that may help verify the physical examination findings. Functional imaging, visual

---

Box 1
Budapest clinical diagnostic criteria for CRPS

1. Continuing pain that is disproportionate to any inciting event

2. Patient must report 1 symptom in 3 of the 4 following categories:

   a. Sensory: Reports of hyperesthesia and/or allodynia

   b. Vasomotor: Reports of temperature asymmetry and/or skin color changes and/or skin color asymmetry

   c. Sudomotor/edema: Reports of edema and/or sweating changes and/or sweating asymmetry

   d. Motor/trophic: Reports of decreased range of motion and/or motor dysfunction (weakness, tremor, dystonia) and/or trophic changes (hair, nail, and/or skin)

3. Patient must have 1 sign at the time of evaluation in 2 or more of the following categories:

   a. Sensory: Evidence of hyperalgesia to pin prick and/or allodynia to light touch and/or deep somatic pressure and/or joint movement

   b. Vasomotor: Evidence of temperature asymmetry and/or skin color changes and/or asymmetry

   c. Sudomotor/edema: Evidence of edema and/or sweating changes and/or sweating asymmetry

   d. Motor/trophic: Evidence of decreased range of motion and/or motor dysfunction (weakness, tremor, dystonia) and/or trophic changes (hair, nail and/or skin)

4. There is no other diagnosis that better explains the signs and symptoms

From Harden RN, Bruehl S, Perez RS, et al. Validation of proposed diagnostic criteria (the "Budapest Criteria") for complex regional pain syndrome. Pain 2010;150(2):274; with permission.

analog scales, and devices to quantify temperature and mechanical allodynia are available. Vasomotor findings are supported with a thermometer and Doppler measurement of vasomotor tone. Edema is quantitated with volumetry. Sudomotor function can be measured directly with quantitative sudomotor axon response testing, and indirectly with biopedance and skin potential fluctuations. Weakness and range of motion are measured by clinicians. Bone density testing is available. Small-fiber dropout via skin biopsy can be measured to validate a decrease in small nerve density.[10] Most of these technologies are not readily available in the office.

Diagnostic testing may include rheumatologic workup to assess for inflammatory arthritis. Electrodiagnostic testing serves to evaluate the peripheral nervous system, which can help in the diagnosis of CRPS II. Plain films may reveal advanced osteoporosis or fracture in the symptomatic limb with CRPS. Magnetic resonance imaging evaluates soft-tissue injuries and bone edema. A triple-phase bone scan is generally not diagnostic of CRPS.

Pain may or may not be mediated by the sympathetic nervous system. A fluoroscopic guided lumbar paravertebral block for the lower extremity and a stellate ganglion block for the upper extremity may be useful in determining how much sympathetic input contributes to a patient's symptoms. Because CRPS may or may not have a sympathetic component, a positive or negative response to a sympathetic block does not substantiate the diagnosis of CRPS.

PROGRESSION AND COURSE OF DISEASE

Schwartzman and colleagues[7] report that after 1 year most of the signs and symptoms are well developed. Most patients have abnormalities of pain processing such as allodynia, which is present in 90% of patients at 5 years and in 98% of patients by 15 years. Swelling is noted in 75% of patients at 5 years and 90% by 15 years. Loss of strength and difficult movement is seen in 90% of patients at 5 years. Spread of the pain occurs in 92% of patients.[7,11]

In a study of 27 patients with CRPS I, Maleki and colleagues[12] reported contiguous spread in all patients, 70% of whom had independent spread to another site, 15% mirror-image spread to the initial site, and 19% contiguous spread alone. Van Rijn and colleagues[13] reported that CRPS usually affects one limb but can spread to the contralateral or ipsilateral limb in 53% and 30% of cases, respectively. A diagonal spread was seen the least in 14% of cases. Aberrant regulation of neurogenic inflammation, maladaptive neuroplasticity, and genetic predisposition are theorized as the pathophysiology behind the spread of CRPS. Spontaneous spread is at the level of the spinal cord, as opposed to a systemic etiology.[13]

The CRPS Severity Score (CSS) was developed in an attempt to assess the severity of CRPS. The concept of staging CRPS has been abandoned owing to the lack of empirical statistical evidence to suggest the existence of the stages.[1,14] The CSS is based on the presence or absence of 17 clinically assessed signs and symptoms. Patients with higher CSS scores had greater reported pain intensity, distress, and functional impairments. Greater temperature asymmetry and abnormalities in thermal perception were seen more frequently.[14,15]

PSYCHIATRIC ISSUES

There is a debate as to whether patients who have CRPS are predisposed to develop the condition based on their psychiatric profile. Harden and colleagues[16] found that preoperative anxiety and severity of pain predicted the development of CRPS signs and symptoms following total knee arthroplasty. However, most studies do not find a unique relationship between CRPS and psychiatric factors. Shiri and colleagues[17] compared psychological profiles of patients with CRPS with those of patients suffering from conversion disorders. High somatization and depression and low anxiety scores were seen in both groups. Reedijk and colleagues[18] compared patients with CRPS I–related dystonia with those with conversion disorders and affective disorders. Although the CRPS patients did exhibit elevated scores for somatoform dissociation, traumatic experiences, general psychopathology, and lower quality of life compared with the general population, they also had lower total scores for personality traits, recent life events, and general psychopathology relative to the patients with conversion disorder and affective disorder. The investigators concluded that patients with CRPS I–related dystonia did not have a uniquely disturbed psychological profile as a group. Puchalski and Zyluk[19] reported that 62 patients who underwent distal radius fractures and developed CRPS did not exhibit significant differences in personality or depression scales relative to patients who did not develop CRPS. Monti and colleagues[20] compared 25 CRPS I patients with a control group with chronic back pain. Both groups exhibited similar findings of major depressive and personality disorders. It was concluded that the abnormal findings are a result of severe chronic pain and are not uniquely secondary to CRPS.

Beerthuizen and colleagues[21] conducted a systematic review of the literature since 1980, and concluded that there was no relationship between psychological factors and CRPS; they concluded that CRPS was associated only with patients who experienced more life events (divorce, death of spouse, vacation, and so forth). Geertzen and colleagues[22] also reported that a difficult time in life or a painful affective loss (stressful life event) is more common during the onset of CRPS when a group of patients with subacute CRPS were compared with a group of patients preparing for hand surgery over the next 24 hours.

TREATMENT

In 1997, consensus guidelines were generated for the functional restoration of CRPS. Medication, psychological counseling, and interventional options were reserved for patients who were failing to progress with physical and occupational therapy.[23] Current literature supports the use of medication, modalities, interventions, and psychological treatment more acutely.[24] Multiple articles support the use of physical therapy to treat CRPS.[25,26] Interdisciplinary treatment of CRPS is supported without high-level evidence by the aforementioned consensus-building conferences.[23,24] Interdisciplinary treatment of the more general category of chronic pain has been used for decades. The objectives of physical and occupational therapy in patients with CRPS are to minimize edema, desensitize a painful limb and normalize sensation, promote normal positioning, decrease muscle guarding, and increase functional use of the extremity. Edema management consists of specialized compressive garments along with manual edema mobilization techniques. Aquatic therapy has also been shown to aid in edema control and to facilitate early weight bearing.[27]

Desensitization can be achieved through a stress-loading program consisting of scrubbing and carrying techniques. Scrubbing involves using the affected limb to move a brush against a surface. Carrying involves a gradual weight-loading program whereby the patient carries objects and weights either in the hand or in a handled bag.[28] For the lower extremities, weight-shifting and balancing techniques are used to gradually stress the affected leg. Contrast baths can also be beneficial in mild cases of CRPS. Desensitization and improved circulation may be accomplished in the affected extremity by alternating vasodilation (heat) with vasoconstriction (cold).

Patient education involves explaining fear-avoidance models using the symptoms, beliefs, and behaviors of the individual patients. Patients are taught to view their various autonomic and vasomotor disturbances as a condition that can be self-managed, rather than a disease whereby the affected limb needs careful protection. Under therapist supervision, the patient identifies dangerous and threatening situations and gradually increases exposure to these activities as much as possible until anxiety levels have decreased.[29]

Mirror therapy, or mirror visual feedback, is conducted with the patient seated before a mirror that is oriented parallel to the midline. View of the affected limb is blocked behind the mirror. The patient first closes his or her eyes and describes both the affected and unaffected limb, followed by imagined movements of both extremities. When looking into the mirror, the patient sees the reflection of the unaffected limb positioned as the affected limb. The patient is then asked to look at the mirrored limb without movement. Finally, the patient moves the unaffected extremity through different planes of movement. Movement of or touch to the intact limb may be perceived as affecting the painful limb.[30]

Graded motor imagery (GMI) acts on the reorganization of cortical networks presumed to be involved in chronic pain and CRPS. GMI consists of a sequential set of brain exercises comprising laterality training, imagined hand movements, and mirror feedback therapy. The patient looks at a photograph of a hand or foot, then imagines moving the painful limb into the position in the photograph. This action is progressed to moving both limbs into the position while observing the unaffected limb in a mirror that obscures the affected limb.[30]

Alternative therapeutic techniques include acupuncture, Qigong therapy, and relaxation training. However, there is very low-quality evidence that any of these methods are effective in reducing CRPS I–related pain.[31] Hyperbaric oxygen therapy has been reported to reduce pain and edema in a placebo-controlled, randomized study of 71 CRPS patients.[32]

PHARMACOTHERAPY

There are many medication options for the treatment of CRPS. Unfortunately, there is a paucity of evidence to support their use in treating CRPS specifically. CRPS affects the vascular, neurologic, osseous, integumentary, and immunologic systems. In most cases, polypharmacy is required to manage the various symptoms of CRPS. The use of medications from complementary drug classes minimizes side effects from any one medication by lessening individual dosage requirements. As in any syndrome, it is important to analyze the efficacy and side effects of all drugs that are added to the treatment regimen.

Nonsteroidal anti-inflammatory drugs (NSAIDs) are used in a variety of pain conditions to manage inflammation. It is unclear whether the inflammatory component of CRPS follows the traditional cyclooxygenase (COX) pathway or is more neurogenic in nature (mediated by afferent nociceptors). NSAIDs inhibit COX, which is responsible for the production of prostaglandins that mediate inflammation and hyperalgesia. Their use may help block spinal nociceptive processing as well.[33] Small clinical trials looking at NSAID use in neuropathic pain have shown mixed results, and one study showed no benefit in the treatment of CRPS I.[33] The use of COX-2 selective inhibitors has not been formally studied in the treatment of CRPS, but there is some anecdotal mention in the literature.[34]

Clinical evidence supports the use of oral corticosteroids in cases of CRPS.[35] Improvements in symptoms of acute patients were seen in randomized controlled studies that used approximately 30 mg of corticosteroids per day for 2 to 12 weeks followed by a taper.[36,37] Their role in chronic CRPS in comparison with more acute cases is uncertain. Long-term use of steroids has not proved to be effective. Given the significant complications of steroids, it is not recommended that steroids be prescribed for long-term use.

Neuropathic pain is often related to increased excitability of neurons. Gabapentin and pregabalin work by blocking voltage-dependent calcium channels, and are effective in treating post-herpetic neuralgia and diabetic neuropathy. There are limited data addressing the effect of gabapentin on CRPS, and no studies are available to evaluate whether CRPS patients benefit from pregabalin.[1] Carbamazepine (Tegretol) is approved by the Food and Drug Administration (FDA) for the treatment of trigeminal neuralgia.[38] One randomized controlled trial showed pain reduction in CRPS symptoms after 8 days of carbamazepine when compared with placebo.[39] Oxcarbazepine (Trileptal), phenytoin (Dilantin), and lamotrigine (Lamictal) are alternative anticonvulsants.

Norepinephrine and, possibly, serotonin have been shown to mediate inhibition of the dorsal horn and block peripheral sodium channels. The tricyclic and heterocyclic drugs, such as amitriptyline, augment descending inhibition by blocking presynaptic reuptake.[40] These agents are considered a first-line option for neuropathic conditions but have not been formally studied in CRPS. Their antidepressant and sedative effects provide additional benefit to patients in chronic pain. Combined serotonin and norepinephrine reuptake inhibitors, such as venlafaxine, milnacipran, and duloxetine, are FDA-approved for several chronic pain conditions but have not been studied in CRPS.

Several studies document the safety and benefit of opioids in treating neuropathic pain.[41] However, neuropathic pain does not seem to respond as well to opioids as acute nociceptive pain. Opioids are considered second-line or third-line agents that should be used cautiously in conjunction with other medications. It is possible that tramadol and tapentadol may be more efficacious in treating neuropathic pain related to CRPS, owing to their ability to block the reuptake of serotonin and norepinephrine. Opioids for chronic benign pain syndromes remain controversial secondary to potential for abuse, misuse, diversion, and overdoses leading to death.

N-Methyl-D-aspartate receptor antagonists are a class of anesthetics that have been used in the treatment of neuropathic pain and CRPS. Ketamine, amantadine, and dextromethorphan have been studied, but toxicity at effective doses has generally been too high.[42,43] These agents are popular as recreational drugs because of their dissociative, hallucinogenic, and euphoric effects.

An outpatient subanesthetic course of intravenous ketamine over 5 days provided significant relief of pain for up to 3 months.[44] Quality of life did not change. Side effects included nausea, headache, tiredness, and dysphoria. Pain relief was obtained in 16 of 20 patients in an open-label phase II study of anesthetic-dose intravenous ketamine in patients with refractory CRPS,[45] with treatment lasting 5 days. Quality of life, associated movement disorder, and ability to work significantly improved in most patients at 6 months after the study. Anxiety, nightmares, and difficulties with sleep were observed in most patients. Epidural ketamine administration for CRPS[46] and topical ketamine gel for neuropathic pain[47] have also been evaluated.

Clonidine has been used orally, transdermally, and epidurally to treat sympathetically maintained pain in CRPS.[48] A systematic review found no convincing support for clonidine in the treatment of CRPS.[35] Two uncontrolled case series showed nifedipine, a calcium-channel blocker, to be effective in managing vasoconstriction in patients with CRPS.[49,50]

Phenoxybenzamine is an irreversible α-antagonist that has antiadrenergic effects and has been shown to be beneficial in treating CRPS. It is considered a third-line agent and works best in cases lasting less than 3 months.[49,51] At higher doses, side effects include orthostatic hypotension and inhibition of ejaculation.

CRPS is frequently associated with localized osteopenia/osteoporosis. Active bone resorption and remodeling may be seen on triple-phase bone scan, and results in nociceptive bone pain. In addition, disuse of the affected limb in CRPS can cause reduction in bone mineral density. Calcitonin reduces blood calcium levels and is usually administered nasally. Calcitonin can help to preserve bone mass and also has antinociceptive effects that have been found to be useful in treating both acute and chronic pain. A meta-analysis of a limited number of controlled studies supported the use of intranasal doses of 100 to 300 U per day for 3 to 4 weeks.[52] Other clinical trials have revealed equivocal evidence regarding the efficacy of calcitonin in treating CRPS.[53,54]

Bisphosphonates, such as alendronate, improve bone density by slowing the resorption of bone. Multiple high-quality studies support the benefits of some older short-acting bisphosphonates in treating CRPS-related pain.

Baclofen administration via intrathecal pump is effective for pain and dystonia while minimizing sedation. The long-term use of other muscle relaxants such as benzodiazepines and cyclobenzaprine are usually not effective or recommended.[1] Injection of botulinum toxin can be considered in focal areas of spasticity. Intradermal injections of botulinum toxin extended the duration of pain relief in a subset of patients with CRPS who received a sympathetic chain block with bupivacaine.[55]

Intravenous immunoglobulin (IVIG) is a potent anti-inflammatory and immune modulator. In CRPS, peripheral and central glial-mediated neuroimmune activation sustains chronic pain. A randomized, double-blind, placebo-controlled trial of 13 patients with chronic CRPS compared low-dose IVIG with treatment with intravenous normal saline. The 12 patients who completed the trial described some pain relief in the IVIG group at 6 to 19 days after treatment. Further research is needed to determine whether IVIG, which is relatively costly, has a role in treating CRPS.[56]

Topical medications for the treatment of local symptoms are an attractive option when treating limb pain. EMLA cream and Lidoderm patches are local anesthetics used to treat CRPS. Capsaicin is a compound found in chili peppers. Topical application overstimulates nociceptive nerve endings and causes a "dying-back" phenomenon that can decrease neuropathic pain locally. It is not well tolerated by patients secondary to burning pain. DMSO is a cream that acts as a scavenger of free radicals. A 2-month trial of 50% DMSO cream decreased pain in CRPS in comparison with placebo.[57]

INTERVENTIONAL AND SURGICAL TREATMENTS

Sympathetic blockade may be particularly beneficial if pain and swelling is limiting participation in therapy despite medication. These blocks involve the injection of local anesthetics along the lumbar sympathetic chain (for lower limbs) or stellate ganglion (for upper limbs) under fluoroscopic guidance. A good response includes an increase in temperature in the affected extremity, without a motor or sensory block, reduced pain, decreased allodynia, and improved range of motion.[58] Blocks may be repeated if there is short-term benefit. These blocks are most beneficial in patients who demonstrate sympathetically mediated symptoms. Response duration and efficacy is variable. Success would be expected to be greater in the patient who has a sympathetically maintained pain than in a patient who has sympathetic independent pain.

Cepeda and colleagues[59] conducted a systematic review on the role of sympathetic blockade in CRPS, and found 2 small randomized, double-blind, crossover studies that evaluated 23 subjects. The combined effect of the 2 trials produced a relative risk of 1.17 to achieve at least 50% of pain relief 30 minutes to 2 hours after the sympathetic blockade (95% confidence interval 0.80–1.72). It was not possible to determine the effect of sympathetic blockade on long-term pain relief because the investigators evaluated different outcomes in the 2 studies. No conclusion concerning the effectiveness of this procedure could be drawn.

Chemical or surgical sympathectomies may be performed for sympathetically maintained pain from CRPS in patients who have had good but transient relief from sympathetic blocks. Chemical sympathectomy is a procedure whereby alcohol or phenol injections serve as agents to destroy the sympathetic chain. Outcomes are variable, and the procedure has uncertain efficacy.[58] Surgical ablation can be performed by open removal or electrocoagulation of the sympathetic chain, or minimally invasive procedures using stereotactic thermal or laser interruption of the sympathetic chain. The effects may be longer lasting, up to 1 year, with radiofrequency ablation.[58] Nerve regeneration commonly occurs following both surgical and chemical ablation, but may take longer with surgical ablation.

Manjunath and colleagues[60] randomized 20 patients with lower limb CRPS I to either radiofrequency or phenol lumbar sympathectomy. There were statistically significant reductions from baseline in all the pain scores used in both treatment groups. A 2012 Cochrane review found that lower-quality evidence seems to suggest that sympathectomy for neuropathic pain can be effective. Complications of sympathectomy are common, including postsympathectomy neuralgia, hyperhidrosis, and Horner syndrome (in cases of upper limb CRPS). Because there is poor evidence for the long-term effectiveness of sympathectomy, it should be used with great caution and only after failure of other treatment options.[61]

Intravenous regional anesthesia (IVRA) involves injection of medication directly into the involved extremity. Numerous IVRA trials have been conducted using atropine, guanethidine, lidocaine, bretylium, clonidine, droperidol, ketanserin, and reserpine. Bretylium and ketanserin IVRA been proved to have some efficacy, although there is a high risk of false-positive results.[62] All other trials have proved to be ineffective.

Spinal cord stimulation (SCS) involves surgical placement of electrodes within the epidural space at the level of the cervical or lower thoracic spinal cord. Kemler and colleagues[63] performed a randomized study to compare SCS combined with physical therapy (SCT/PT) with physical therapy (PT) alone in 54 chronic CRPS I patients (pain of at least 6 months' duration) who had failed conventional treatment. Patients in the SCT/PT group underwent 1 week of test stimulation. The SCS system was implanted if they had a 50% reduction in their visual analog score or if they reported that they were "much improved" or "best ever" on the global perceived effect scale; 24 patients proceeded to permanent lead placement. Detection thresholds and pain thresholds for pressure, warmth and cold, and the extent of dynamic and static hyperalgesia were evaluated at baseline, and at 1, 3, 6, and 12 months after implantation. At 2 years, the SCS/PT group had statistically better results.[64] However, in the last follow-up at 5 years there were no statistical differences in any of the measured variables. Complications include pulse-generator failure, lead displacement, and pulse-generator pocket revision. Despite the diminishing effectiveness of SCS, 95% of patients responded that they would repeat the treatment for the same result.[65]

Successful results of SCS include significant reductions in pain perception, allodynia, and muscle dysfunction, and improvement in blood flow. When applied early in the course of the disease, SCS can greatly increase the functionality of the affected limb.[66]

CRPS as an indication for amputation remains controversial. The predominant reasons for amputation have been pain, dysfunctional limb, gangrene, infection, or ulcers. Recurrence of CRPS I in the residual limb following the amputation was reported in 48% of the patients in 14 studies. Phantom pain was reported in 41% of patients in 15 studies.[67] In a recent retrospective study, 21 patients with long-standing therapy-resistant CRPS I underwent amputation of the affected limb. Pain reduction and improvements in mobility and sleep were seen in most patients. Only 4 patients (14%) had recurrence of CRPS I in the residual limb.[68]

Amputation should be considered for therapy-resistant CRPS only when the patient has no major psychopathology and has a realistic point of view about the possible beneficial and adverse effects of an amputation. Further research is necessary.[67,68]

SUMMARY

CRPS is a formidable disease to diagnose and treat. It is important to apply the current diagnostic criteria in making the diagnosis. Treatment should be aggressive early in the disease, and a multidisciplinary approach is often required. Medication, sympathetic blocks, and SCS may also be beneficial.

REFERENCES

1. Harden RN, Oaklander AL, Burton AW, et al. Complex regional pain syndrome: practical diagnostic and treatment guidelines, 4th edition. Pain Med 2013;14(2): 180–229.
2. Dommerholt J. Complex regional pain syndrome—1: history, diagnostic criteria and etiology. J Bodyw Mov Ther 2004;8(3):167–77.
3. Mitchell SW, Morehouse GR, Keen WW. Gunshot wounds and other injuries of nerves. 1864. Clin Orthop Relat Res 2007;458:35–9.
4. Evans JA. Reflex sympathetic dystrophy. Surg Clin North Am 1946;8:260–3.
5. Harden RN, Bruehl SP. Diagnosis of complex regional pain syndrome: signs, symptoms, and new empirically derived diagnostic criteria. Clin J Pain 2006; 22(5):415–9.
6. Harden R, Bruehl S. Introduction and diagnostic considerations. Milford (CT): Reflex Sympathetic Dystrophy Syndrome Association; 2006.
7. Schwartzman RJ, Erwin KL, Alexander GM. The natural history of complex regional pain syndrome. Clin J Pain 2009;25(4):273–80.
8. Bruehl S. An update on the pathophysiology of complex regional pain syndrome. Anesthesiology 2010;113(3):713–25.
9. Harden RN, Bruehl S, Perez RS, et al. Validation of proposed diagnostic criteria (the "Budapest Criteria") for complex regional pain syndrome. Pain 2010;150(2): 268–74.
10. Harden RN. Objectification of the diagnostic criteria for CRPS. Pain Med 2010; 11(8):1212–5.
11. Sandroni P, Benrud-Larson LM, McClelland RL, et al. Complex regional pain syndrome type I: incidence and prevalence in Olmsted county, a population-based study. Pain 2003;103(1–2):199–207.
12. Maleki J, LeBel AA, Bennett GJ, et al. Patterns of spread in complex regional pain syndrome, type I (reflex sympathetic dystrophy). Pain 2000;88(3): 259–66.
13. van Rijn MA, Marinus J, Putter H, et al. Spreading of complex regional pain syndrome: not a random process. J Neural Transm 2011;118(9):1301–9.

14. Bruehl S, Harden RN, Galer BS, et al. Complex regional pain syndrome: are there distinct subtypes and sequential stages of the syndrome? Pain 2002; 95(1–2):119–24.
15. Harden RN, Bruehl S, Perez RS, et al. Development of a severity score for CRPS. Pain 2010;151(3):870–6.
16. Harden RN, Bruehl S, Stanos S, et al. Prospective examination of pain-related and psychological predictors of CRPS-like phenomena following total knee arthroplasty: a preliminary study. Pain 2003;106(3):393–400.
17. Shiri S, Tsenter J, Livai R, et al. Similarities between the psychological profiles of complex regional pain syndrome and conversion disorder patients. J Clin Psychol Med Settings 2003;10(3):193–9.
18. Reedijk WB, van Rijn MA, Roelofs K, et al. Psychological features of patients with complex regional pain syndrome type I related dystonia. Mov Disord 2008; 23(11):1551–9.
19. Puchalski P, Zyluk A. Complex regional pain syndrome type 1 after fractures of the distal radius: a prospective study of the role of psychological factors. J Hand Surg Br 2005;30(6):574–80.
20. Monti DA, Herring CL, Schwartzman RJ, et al. Personality assessment of patients with complex regional pain syndrome type I. Clin J Pain 1998;14(4):295–302.
21. Beerthuizen A, van 't Spijker A, Huygen FJ, et al. Is there an association between psychological factors and the complex regional pain syndrome type 1 (CRPS1) in adults? A systematic review. Pain 2009;145(1–2):52–9.
22. Geertzen JH, de Bruijn-Kofman AT, de Bruijn HP, et al. Stressful life events and psychological dysfunction in complex regional pain syndrome type I. Clin J Pain 1998;14(2):143–7.
23. Stanton-Hicks MM, Baron RD, Boas RM, et al. Complex regional pain syndromes: guidelines for therapy. Clin J Pain 1998;14(2):155–66.
24. Stanton-Hicks MD, Burton AW, Bruehl SP, et al. An updated interdisciplinary clinical pathway for CRPS: report of an expert panel. Pain Pract 2002;2(1):1–16.
25. Perez RS, Zollinger PE, Dijkstra PU, et al. Evidence based guidelines for complex regional pain syndrome type 1. BMC Neurol 2010;10:20.
26. Baron R, Wasner G. Complex regional pain syndromes. Curr Pain Headache Rep 2001;5(2):114–23.
27. Sherry DD, Wallace CA, Kelley C, et al. Short- and long-term outcomes of children with complex regional pain syndrome type I treated with exercise therapy. Clin J Pain 1999;15(3):218–23.
28. Carlson LK, Watson HK. Treatment of reflex sympathetic dystrophy using the stress-loading program. J Hand Ther 1988;1(4):149–54.
29. de Jong JR, Vlaeyen JW, Onghena P, et al. Reduction of pain-related fear in complex regional pain syndrome type I: the application of graded exposure in vivo. Pain 2005;116(3):264–75.
30. Moseley GL. Graded motor imagery for pathologic pain: a randomized controlled trial. Neurology 2006;67(12):2129–34.
31. O'Connell NE, Wand BM, McAuley J, et al. Interventions for treating pain and disability in adults with complex regional pain syndrome. Cochrane Database Syst Rev 2013;(4):CD009416.
32. Yildiz S, Uzun G, Kiralp MZ. Hyperbaric oxygen therapy in chronic pain management. Curr Pain Headache Rep 2006;10(2):95–100.
33. Geisslinger G, Muth-Selbach U, Coste O, et al. Inhibition of noxious stimulus-induced spinal prostaglandin E2 release by flurbiprofen enantiomers: a microdialysis study. J Neurochem 2000;74(5):2094–100.

34. Pappagallo M, Rosenberg AD. Epidemiology, pathophysiology, and management of complex regional pain syndrome. Pain Pract 2001;1(1):11–20.
35. Kingery WS. A critical review of controlled clinical trials for peripheral neuropathic pain and complex regional pain syndromes. Pain 1997;73(2):123–39.
36. Christensen K, Jensen EM, Noer I. The reflex dystrophy syndrome response to treatment with systemic corticosteroids. Acta Chir Scand 1982;148(8): 653–5.
37. Braus DF, Krauss JK, Strobel J. The shoulder-hand syndrome after stroke: a prospective clinical trial. Ann Neurol 1994;36(5):728–33.
38. Rull JA, Quibrera R, Gonzalez-Millan H, et al. Symptomatic treatment of peripheral diabetic neuropathy with carbamazepine (Tegretol): double blind crossover trial. Diabetologia 1969;5(4):215–8.
39. Harke H, Gretenkort P, Ladleif HU, et al. The response of neuropathic pain and pain in complex regional pain syndrome I to carbamazepine and sustained-release morphine in patients pretreated with spinal cord stimulation: a double-blinded randomized study. Anesth Analg 2001;92(2):488–95.
40. Sindrup SH, Jensen TS. Pharmacologic treatment of pain in polyneuropathy. Neurology 2000;55(7):915–20.
41. Dellemijn PL, van Duijn H, Vanneste JA. Prolonged treatment with transdermal fentanyl in neuropathic pain. J Pain Symptom Manage 1998;16(4):220–9.
42. Eide PK, Jorum E, Stubhaug A, et al. Relief of post-herpetic neuralgia with the N-methyl-D-aspartic acid receptor antagonist ketamine: a double-blind, crossover comparison with morphine and placebo. Pain 1994;58(3):347–54.
43. Nelson KA, Park KM, Robinovitz E, et al. High-dose oral dextromethorphan versus placebo in painful diabetic neuropathy and postherpetic neuralgia. Neurology 1997;48(5):1212–8.
44. Schwartzman RJ, Alexander GM, Grothusen JR, et al. Outpatient intravenous ketamine for the treatment of complex regional pain syndrome: a double-blind placebo controlled study. Pain 2009;147(1–3):107–15.
45. Kiefer RT, Rohr P, Ploppa A, et al. Efficacy of ketamine in anesthetic dosage for the treatment of refractory complex regional pain syndrome: an open-label phase II study. Pain Med 2008;9(8):1173–201.
46. Takahashi H, Miyazaki M, Nanbu T, et al. The NMDA-receptor antagonist ketamine abolishes neuropathic pain after epidural administration in a clinical case. Pain 1998;75(2–3):391–4.
47. Gammaitoni A, Gallagher RM, Welz-Bosna M. Topical ketamine gel: possible role in treating neuropathic pain. Pain Med 2000;1(1):97–100.
48. Rauck RL, Eisenach JC, Jackson K, et al. Epidural clonidine treatment for refractory reflex sympathetic dystrophy. Anesthesiology 1993;79(6):1163–9 [discussion: 27A].
49. Muizelaar JP, Kleyer M, Hertogs IA, et al. Complex regional pain syndrome (reflex sympathetic dystrophy and causalgia): management with the calcium channel blocker nifedipine and/or the alpha-sympathetic blocker phenoxybenzamine in 59 patients. Clin Neurol Neurosurg 1997;99(1):26–30.
50. Prough DS, McLeskey CH, Poehling GG, et al. Efficacy of oral nifedipine in the treatment of reflex sympathetic dystrophy. Anesthesiology 1985;62(6):796–9.
51. Ghostine SY, Comair YG, Turner DM, et al. Phenoxybenzamine in the treatment of causalgia. Report of 40 cases. J Neurosurg 1984;60(6):1263–8.
52. Perez RS, Kwakkel G, Zuurmond WW, et al. Treatment of reflex sympathetic dystrophy (CRPS type 1): a research synthesis of 21 randomized clinical trials. J Pain Symptom Manage 2001;21(6):511–26.

53. Bickerstaff DR, Kanis JA. The use of nasal calcitonin in the treatment of post-traumatic algodystrophy. Br J Rheumatol 1991;30(4):291–4.
54. Gobelet C, Waldburger M, Meier JL. The effect of adding calcitonin to physical treatment on reflex sympathetic dystrophy. Pain 1992;48(2):171–5.
55. Carroll I, Clark JD, Mackey S. Sympathetic block with botulinum toxin to treat complex regional pain syndrome. Ann Neurol 2009;65(3):348–51.
56. Goebel A, Baranowski A, Maurer K, et al. Intravenous immunoglobulin treatment of the complex regional pain syndrome: a randomized trial. Ann Intern Med 2010;152(3):152–8.
57. Zuurmond WW, Langendijk PN, Bezemer PD, et al. Treatment of acute reflex sympathetic dystrophy with DMSO 50% in a fatty cream. Acta Anaesthesiol Scand 1996;40(3):364–7.
58. Nelson DV, Stacey BR. Interventional therapies in the management of complex regional pain syndrome. Clin J Pain 2006;22(5):438–42.
59. Cepeda MS, Carr DB, Lau J. Local anesthetic sympathetic blockade for complex regional pain syndrome. Cochrane Database Syst Rev 2005;(4):CD004598.
60. Manjunath PS, Jayalakshimi TS, Dureja GP, et al. Management of lower limb complex regional pain syndrome type 1: an evaluation of percutaneous radiofrequency thermal lumbar sympathectomy versus phenol lumbar sympathetic neurolysis—a pilot study. Anesth Analg 2008;106(2):647–9.
61. Straube S, Derry S, Moore RA, et al. Cervico-thoracic or lumbar sympathectomy for neuropathic pain and complex regional pain syndrome. Cochrane Database Syst Rev 2010;(7):CD002918.
62. Jadad AR, Carroll D, Glynn CJ, et al. Intravenous regional sympathetic blockade for pain relief in reflex sympathetic dystrophy: a systematic review and a randomized, double-blind crossover study. J Pain Symptom Manage 1995;10(1):13–20.
63. Kemler MA, Barendse GA, van Kleef M, et al. Spinal cord stimulation in patients with chronic reflex sympathetic dystrophy. N Engl J Med 2000;343(9):618–24.
64. Kemler MA, De Vet HC, Barendse GA, et al. The effect of spinal cord stimulation in patients with chronic reflex sympathetic dystrophy: two years' follow-up of the randomized controlled trial. Ann Neurol 2004;55(1):13–8.
65. Kemler MA, de Vet HC, Barendse GA, et al. Effect of spinal cord stimulation for chronic complex regional pain syndrome Type I: five-year final follow-up of patients in a randomized controlled trial. J Neurosurg 2008;108(2):292–8.
66. Stanton-Hicks M. Complex regional pain syndrome: manifestations and the role of neurostimulation in its management. J Pain Symptom Manage 2006; 31(Suppl 4):S20–4.
67. Bodde MI, Dijkstra PU, den Dunnen WF, et al. Therapy-resistant complex regional pain syndrome type I: to amputate or not? J Bone Joint Surg Am 2011;93(19):1799–805.
68. Krans-Schreuder HK, Bodde MI, Schrier E, et al. Amputation for long-standing, therapy-resistant type-I complex regional pain syndrome. J Bone Joint Surg Am 2012;94(24):2263–8.

Discogenic Low Back Pain

Jeremy Simon, MD[a],*, Matthew McAuliffe, MD[b],
Fehreen Shamim, MD[b], Nancy Vuong, MD[b], Amir Tahaei, MD[b]

KEYWORDS

- Low back pain • Discogenic low back pain • Lumbar disk disease • Annular tear
- Lumbar disk herniation • Internal disk disruption

KEY POINTS

- The intervertebral disk can be a common source of acute or chronic low back pain.
- A thorough history and physical examination are needed to assess patients with discogenic low back pain.
- Lifestyle modifications including smoking cessation, proper lifting mechanics, ergonomics, and lower body mass index are helpful.
- Discogenic pain results from changes in the nucleus pulposus and tears in the annulus fibrosis.
- Psychological support, including treatment of underlying or coexistent depression, is highly recommended.
- Conservative treatment, including home exercise for chronic lower back pain, is recommended.
- Injection of corticosteroids for discogenic lower back pain shows mixed efficacy and should be performed judiciously.
- Surgery for this condition should be reserved for cases of significant refractory cases with profound disability and should be confirmed with diskography.

INTRODUCTION

Nature of the Problem

Chronic low back pain is a common and challenging problem presenting to a variety of practitioners. It is estimated that up to 90% of people experience significant lower back pain in their lifetime.[1] Although low back pain was traditionally believed to be self-limited in most cases, data have emerged showing that many low back pain sufferers have recurrences or go on to a more chronic course.[2]

Disclosures: None.
[a] Department of Physical Medicine and Rehabilitation, Rothman Institute, 925 Chestnut Street, Philadelphia, PA 19107, USA; [b] Department of Rehabilitation Medicine, Thomas Jefferson University Hospital, 25 South 9th Street, Philadelphia, PA 19107, USA
* Corresponding author.
E-mail address: jeremyisimon@gmail.com

Phys Med Rehabil Clin N Am 25 (2014) 305–317
http://dx.doi.org/10.1016/j.pmr.2014.01.006
1047-9651/14/$ – see front matter © 2014 Elsevier Inc. All rights reserved.

The economic burden of lower back pain is staggering. It is estimated that the annual cost in the United States for the treatment of lower back pain is between 20 and 50 billion dollars.[3] The pain can be debilitating in many cases and is a major reason for absence from work.[4]

In most cases of acute lower back pain, a definite pain generator cannot be defined.[5–7] For chronic low back pain sufferers, an estimated 39% of cases can be attributed to the intervertebral disk.[8,9] This situation is complicated because not all degenerated or herniated disks are painful.[10] Disk degeneration is a natural part of the aging process and normally begins about the third decade of life. In the right clinical setting, the disk can become a primary source of pain. The following sections address the challenging problem of pain emanating from the damaged and sensitized lumbar intervertebral disk.

Anatomy

The human intervertebral disk consists of a firm, collagenous exterior annulus fibrosis and a gelatinous interior nucleus pulposus. It is often compared with a jelly donut. This structure offers shock absorption and allows for the dispersion of axial and torsional forces at each level through the spine. The annulus is thicker anteriorly than superiorly, therefore herniations and tears are more common posteriorly.[11] The nerve supply to the human intervertebral disk consists of contributions from the sinuvertebral nerves and gray rami communicantes.[12–14] These nerves are segmental and from the dorsal ramus, but recent studies have shown some contributions from the sympathetic chain in a nonsegmental distribution.[15]

Pathophysiology

Pain from lumbar disks can occur from 3 main causes, as described extensively by Bogduk.[16] These causes include disk infection, torsion injury, and internal disk disruption (IDD). This review focuses on torsion injury and IDD.

Torsion injury is believed to result from forcible rotation of the intervertebral joint.[16] Rotational forces around an impacted zygapophysial joint produce a lateral shear force on the disk, which can lead to circumferential tears.[16–19] This cause of disk pain is difficult to prove with objective testing. It is a clinical diagnosis related to patient history, often related to a rotational strain injury.[16]

IDD results from lumbar disk degradation, its nuclear components, and development of radial fissures that extend from the nucleus into the annulus. IDD is believed to be the most common type of discogenic pain.[16] Disk disruption is not to be confused with degenerative changes, which are a normal part of aging.[16] Studies have suggested IDD to be independent of degenerative changes that are seen with aging.[20] Furthermore, it is well known that degenerative disk changes related to aging do not correlate with pain.[21]

The development of radial fissures is believed to be related to repetitive shear, axial loads, and compression of the disk. This process leads to vertebral endplate fractures, in which the fissures can develop followed by disk degradation over time as nuclear material leaks out of the disk or desiccates.[22]

Radial fissures may correlate with pain. A process of sensitization and neural ingrowth are proposed mechanisms of the development of IDD.[12,13] Pain-associated proinflammatory mediators including calcitonin gene-related peptide, tumor necrosis factor α, interleukin 1, interleukin 6, and substance P have been isolated from disks with this morphology.[12,13,23,24]

The modified Dallas diskogram scale is a descriptive way to categorize the severity of IDD after diskography (**Fig. 1**).[25] Using this scale, grade 1 and 2 fissures often produce no pain, whereas grade 3 and 4 fissures frequently produce pain.[26]

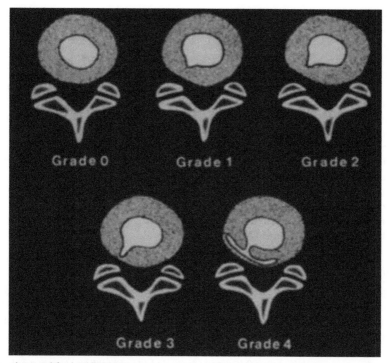

Fig. 1. The modified Dallas diskogram scale, in which grade 0 is described as a cotton-ball appearance with contrast staying in the disk, a grade 1 tear extends to inner third of disk, a grade 2 tear to middle third, a grade 3 tear to outer third, and a grade 4 tear with spread to outer third and circumferential spread greater than 30%. (*From* Aprill C, Bogduk N. High-intensity zone: a diagnostic sign of painful lumbar disc on magnetic resonance imaging. Br J Radiol 1992;65:365; with permission.)

Patient History

Patients may describe an injury such as a bending, lifting, twisting event and the sensation of a pop in the lower back. In some cases, no inciting event may occur.

The typical patient history is of pain in the center of the lower back with minimal radiation, usually to 1 or both buttocks. Radiation may occur to 1 or both sides of the lower back. The pain may have an absent or intermittent radicular component. The back pain is the most severe element of the syndrome. Pain may be reduced with extension and is better with standing and lying flat.

The pain is often described as a deep, dull ache. There is often tightness in the paraspinal and gluteal muscles. Pain is often worsened with sitting/driving, lumbar flexion, bending, twisting, Valsalva maneuver, and coughing. Increased intrathecal and intradiskal pressures are believed to play a role.[27–29] The pain in some cases can be constant or mechanical, often worse with activity and toward the end of the day. Bending and twisting may provoke symptoms.

Smokers, the obese, those with jobs requiring prolonged sitting, and those with physical jobs, especially with repetitive lifting and vibration exposure, are at increased risk of discogenic lower back pain and lumbar disk disease.[30–32]

Genetics may play a role in disk degeneration. One study of twins showed an increased relationship with disk degeneration.[33] A systematic review of 52 articles on degenerative disk disease looking at different genetic markers showed poor data and association.[34]

Physical Examination

- Observe the patient's posture, spinal curvature, and gait.
- Look for asymmetry or atrophy.
- Patients are often more comfortable standing than sitting in the examination room.
- Lumbar range of motion is often reduced in flexion, but may be reduced in all planes because of pain.
- Strength and sensation are usually normal. Reflexes are often normal, but may be blunted if there was a previous associated radiculopathy.
- Provocative maneuvers for neural tension such as straight leg raise, seated straight leg raise, and slump test may cause lower back or buttock pain that is concordant because of the flexion moment created in the lumbar region.
- Femoral nerve stretch test can be negative, because an extension moment is created with these maneuvers.
- Transmitting vibration via the spinous process may cause pain at the symptomatic level but is not sensitive or specific.[35]

Imaging and Additional Testing

Radiographs are often performed as an initial screening tool but are not sensitive or specific for discogenic low back pain. Radiographs are useful in determining if there is an associated spondylolithesis, compression fracture, sacroiliac sclerosis, some bony disease, or other potential mimickers. The only finding that may support discogenic lower back pain may be disk space narrowing.

Magnetic resonance imaging (MRI) can show disk degeneration. A commonly used grading system for disk degeneration was described by Pfirrman and colleagues.[36] This system assigns grades I to V to assess the degree of disk degeneration and looks at the structure, morphology of the annulus and nucleus, the signal intensity of the disk, and the disk height.[36] Degeneration, even a Pfirrman grade V, is not necessarily painful, and disk degeneration is considered a natural phenomenon of aging.[20]

Tears in the annulus may also be present and appear as a high signal in the posterior annulus on T2-weighted images, or high intensity zone.[25] These tears are shown to have a high incidence of concordant pain when stimulated during provocative diskography.[37] However, the presence of a high intensity zone on MRI does not necessarily mean the patient has pain.[38]

Provocative diskography remains the gold standard for the diagnosis of discogenic lower back pain.[39,40] This test was first performed in 1948 and remains a source of controversy.[41–44] It consists of accessing the intervertebral disk through the placement of needles into the nuclei with the use of fluoroscopy (**Fig. 2**). Contrast is administered under live or intermittent fluoroscopy, and pressures are measured with a manometer. Pain level on a visual analog scale, location of pain, similarity to typical pain, facial grimacing, and morphology of the disk after contrast administration are recorded. A positive disk reproduces the patient's typical pain (concordant pain) and is considered consistent with IDD. A negative disk causes no pain or production of dissimilar (discordant) pain. Control disks are also necessary for more accurate results. For example, if stimulation of the L5-S1 disk reproduces the patient's typical pain and has abnormalities on the fluoroscopy pictures, but the L4-5 and L3-4 disks do not, this would be considered a more reliable result.

The Derby criteria are a well-described method of interpreting diskography, in which concordant responses must produce pain greater than 6 out of 10 on a numeric pain scale at a pressure of less than 50 psi above the opening pressure of the disk and

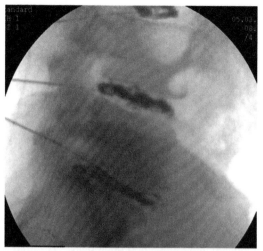

Fig. 2. A typical diskogram at L3-4, L4-5, and L5-S1. Needles and contrast are seen within the disks.

having a negative control disk.[45] The opening pressure is the manometry reading when dye is first observed to enter the disk. In addition, a nucleogram is performed after the disk stimulation, and this must be abnormal, showing a grade 3 tear or higher on the modified Dallas diskogram scale, to prove a diagnosis of IDD.

Patients with suspected IDD are identified and informed as to the risks and benefits of the procedure. The procedure need not be performed if the patient and physician are not seriously considering surgery or an intradiskal procedure as treatment (see later discussion). Because of the relatively avascular nature of the disk, infection is a serious potential risk. It is recommended that periprocedure intravenous antibiotics be administered and the procedure performed under sterile conditions. Many practitioners use a 2-needle technique, in which an introducer needle is placed through the skin and soft tissues and a spinal needle placed into the disk through the needle.

Diskography, when performed by skilled practitioners under sterile technique, has historically been viewed as a safe procedure.[46,47] In reviewing the usefulness in surgical planning, studies have supported its role.[48] However, Carragee and colleagues[49] recently followed patients who underwent lumbar diskography and found an increased risk of far lateral disk herniations and a more rapid rate of disk degeneration over a 10-year period compared with controls.

Management of Discogenic Low Back Pain

Goals of management of IDD are:

- Improvement in pain threshold, quantified on a pain rating scale
- Improvement in function, shown by a reduction in dependence on caregivers, return to work, and participation in recreational activities

Pharmaceutical management

Pharmacologic management is for analgesic purposes. The use of opioid medications is discouraged as a long-term treatment. Neuropathic pain agents may be used for concomitant radicular symptoms. For a complete discussion of medications, please refer to the separate medication section.

Acetaminophen Acetaminophen or paracetamol continues to be recommended by the American Pain Society (APS)/American College of Physicians (ACP) as a first-line pharmacologic option for back pain of any duration because of its comparable efficacy and safety considerations.[50] No clear difference has been established comparing acetaminophen with nonsteroidal antiinflammatory drugs (NSAIDs).[50]

NSAIDs NSAIDs have both antiinflammatory and analgesic properties via inhibition of the cyclooxygenase 2 enzyme, which confers efficacy in management of discogenic back pain.[50] A high-quality Cochrane review of 51 trials analyzing NSAIDs for acute low back pain found nonselective NSAIDs superior to placebo for global improvement and for not requiring additional analgesics.[51,52] This study did not show that any nonselective NSAID was superior to any other for pain relief. The review showed that there was no clear difference in efficacy between NSAIDs and opioid therapy, spinal manipulation, physical therapy, and bed rest when studying pain reduction.[51,52]

Skeletal muscle relaxants Skeletal muscle relaxants are medications grouped together because they are used for the treatment of spasticity and musculoskeletal conditions such as tension headaches and back pain.[50] A variety of skeletal muscle relaxants are available in the United States. Dantrolene, a peripheral calcium channel blocker, and baclofen, a γ aminobutyric acid modulator in the spinal cord, have not been shown to have any significant benefit in reducing back pain, which is logical given their mechanisms of action.[50] Some evidence supports the short-term use of muscle relaxants for acute lower back pain.[53] However, it remains unclear whether any of these medications truly relax muscles or if their effects on pain are related to sedation.

Tramadol Tramadol is a μ-opiate agonist and a norepinephrine and serotonin reuptake inhibitor. It has shown significant efficacy in the treatment of lower back pain.[54] It has the potential to have an effect on the radicular or neurogenic components, if present, with discogenic pain.

Tramadol has also shown significant potential in the combination setting, effectively addressing chronic lower back pain in a double-blind randomized controlled trial,[55] and allowing for dose-reduction with NSAIDs.[56]

Corticosteroids Many practitioners prescribe a short course of oral corticosteroids for an acute flare or episode of lower back pain. Typically, a tapering dose of methylprednisolone or prednisone is used. The appeal is the high potency of the antiinflammatory effects and the short duration (days) of treatment with few contraindications. However, data are lacking on the efficacy of this treatment.[57,58]

Opioids The role of opioids remains controversial, because they may lead to physical dependence and tolerance and have many undesirable effects when used chronically. There is some low-level evidence that for severe low back pain, opioids may have benefit.[59] Data on the effectiveness of long-term opioids for discogenic back pain are lacking, and studies indicate no significant reduction in pain or improvement in quality of life.[60] Extensive monitoring and close follow-up are crucial to safe use of opioids for analgesia.

Nonpharmacologic strategies

Physical therapy A variety of physical therapy approaches have been used to address discogenic back pain. Adams and colleagues[61] suggest that extension-biased therapy program may be superior. The McKenzie extension program[62] for lumbar disk herniations with associated radicular pain has been shown to be effective as well, but not so effective if the pain is purely axial.[63] There is also literature to suggest that combining physical therapy with education and manual therapy is superior to physical therapy alone.[64]

Cognitive behavioral therapy with pain education Although many consensus statements and a recent Cochrane review have recommended a cognitive behavioral approach to maximize physical and psychological well-being, the effect is often minimal and short-term.[65] Van Hooff and colleagues[66] sought to identify risk factors by multivariate analysis of a prospective study of the effect of combined physical and cognitive behavioral therapy (CBT) in patients with chronic low back pain. Patients' work status and lower pretreatment disability are important predictors of 1-year success after treatment.[66] This factor may help guide patient selection for this therapy.

Acupuncture Originating from traditional Chinese medicine, acupuncture is increasingly used as an adjunctive treatment in Western medical practice. Furlan and colleagues[67] examined the role of acupuncture in the treatment of acute and chronic lower back pain in a Cochrane review. This study showed no evidence for acupuncture in acute low back pain but some evidence suggesting that it may be better than no treatment or sham treatment of chronic low back pain. Per this meta-analysis, there was not sufficient evidence to conclude that acupuncture is more effective than other conventional treatments.

Similarly, multiple meta-analyses have concluded that true acupuncture is no more effective than sham acupuncture, but that both were significantly more effective than no treatment, thus highlighting the effect of the acupuncture experience as a whole, including the psychosocial context and the therapeutic milieu.[68,69] Benefits of acupuncture were also shown in the GERAC (German Acupuncture) trial compared with conventional treatments.[70]

Manual medicine: osteopathic and chiropractic manipulation Manual medicine is often used as adjunctive therapy with medical or interventional management and may have a role in improving back-specific functioning and patient satisfaction with therapy. It is difficult to study because of different techniques and the effects of clinician touch, and therefore, sham treatments as well as a study group and a nontreatment group are required. Studies are conflicting in terms of the efficacy of manual therapy for chronic back pain sufferers. A study showed comparative outcomes with osteopathic manipulation and standard medical treatments (analgesics, antiinflammatory medication, active physical therapy, or therapies such as ultrasonography, diathermy, hot or cold packs [or both], use of a corset, or transcutaneous electrical nerve stimulation) in treating subacute lower back pain.[71] A study by Zylbergold and Piper[72] showed no statistical difference comparing outcomes with manual therapy with flexion exercise or home care. However, an extension program rather than flexion program would have been more appropriate. A review of the literature found good evidence for moderate benefit in chronic low back pain sufferers, as well as CBT, exercise, and multidisciplinary rehabilitation.[73]

Self-management strategies
Yoga and tai chi
- Several randomized controlled studies have shown that yoga can help motivated individuals reduce back pain and improve back function.[74–76] Yoga shows more effectiveness in the short-term than in the long-term.[74] There are some data that it is superior to other self-help strategies, including books, but unclear if it is superior in the long-term over a therapeutic exercise program.[77,78]

- Tai chi incorporates exercise and meditation and attempts to create a mindfulness of the body.[79] Some data suggest that tai chi may be moderately effective in coping with lower back pain, but the studies are of low quality.[79]

Meditation
- There are inconclusive data that meditation is helpful for improving outcomes with chronic lower back pain.[80] Mind-body strategies have shown benefit compared with patient education.[81]

Interventional options
Because of the chronic and often debilitating nature of the condition, as well as the mixed data/patient responses as noted earlier, interventional options are considered in the treatment of IDD. These treatments include administration of corticosteroids either epidurally or into the disk itself, intradiskal procedures targeted at the annular tears, and surgery. There is little consensus and mixed data on these procedures. The risks and benefits must be weighed when considering any procedure, especially if the condition is not life threatening.

Lumbar Epidural Steroid Injections
- The logic behind the use of epidural steroid injection in the treatment of IDD is to deliver antiinflammatory corticosteroid to the outer annulus. As noted, studies have shown the presence of inflammatory mediators in the disrupted disk.[12,13,22,23] Studies have shown usefulness in the administration of epidural steroids via the caudal, interlaminar, or transforaminal route in the treatment of chronic lower back pain.[82–84] However, these studies are not specific to discogenic lower back pain.
- Intradiskal steroid injections have not shown convincing benefit and are not a routinely performed procedure for lower back pain.[85,86] One study showed a weak benefit of the administration of corticosteroids during diskography if degenerative endplate changes were also present.[87] Another study showed some short-term benefit of intradiskal steroid in patients with Modic endplate changes.[88]

Thermal Intradiskal Procedures
Various types of intradiskal procedures have been performed in the attempt to seal annular tears or coagulate the innervation to the disk. It is beyond the scope of this article to go into detail on each of these techniques, but some of the more common procedures are discussed.

- Intradiskal thermal annuloplasty (IDET) is a procedure in which a wire with contact points is placed through an introducer needle into the lumbar disk. This wire is then heated for 16 minutes to 90°C. The mechanism of action is unknown, but the theory is that heating denervates the nociceptors in the annulus and also increases collagen fiber stability in annulus fibers by modifying their shape. Complications include catheter breakage, nerve injury, post-IDET disk herniation, diskitis, and epidural abscess. Although the primary studies were promising, recent studies have not provided sufficient evidence for using IDET for discogenic back pain.[89,90] Further randomized clinical trials are needed to evaluate the efficacy of IDET in discogenic back pain treatment.
- Biacuplasty uses a radiofrequency current between 2 probes and creates heat in the posterior annulus.[91] The temperature increases gradually to 50°C while the patient is awake and alert for communication. Biacuplasty has some advantages

over IDET, including minimal damage to the tissue and easier targeting of the posterior annulus. Even although there were some promising results from pilot studies, further randomized clinical trials are required.[91]

SUMMARY

Discogenic lower back pain/IDD syndrome remains a common and challenging problem to treat. Several different pharmacologic and nonpharmacologic strategies are used, with varying degrees of success. The concept of *primum non nocere* and the weighing of potential risks and benefits should be considered in every patient presenting with chronic lower back pain of disk cause. Strong evidence is lacking in any of the treatments, but a healthy lifestyle, including exercise, lower body mass index, smoking cessation, exercise, and core strengthening, should be promoted as the first line. Physical and manual therapy may be considered. Yoga or tai chi may be used at home for maintenance, as well. Long-term medications should be questioned and used sparingly. Epidural steroid injections may be considered in refractory cases and used judiciously. The role of intradiskal steroids and procedures remains in question, and further studies are needed to determine efficacy.

REFERENCES

1. Frymoyer JW. Back pain and sciatica. N Engl J Med 1988;318:291–300.
2. Brennan G, Shafat A, Mac Donncha C, et al. Lower back pain in physically demanding college academic programs: a questionnaire based study. BMC Musculoskelet Disord 2007;8:67.
3. Pai S, Sundaram LJ. Low back pain: an economic assessment in the United States. Orthop Clin North Am 2004;35:1–5.
4. Nguyen TH, Randolph DC. Nonspecific low back pain and return to work. Am Fam Physician 2007;76:1497–502.
5. Comer C, Conaghan PG. Tackling persistent low back pain in primary care. Practitioner 2009;253:32–4, 3.
6. Rozenberg S, Foltz V, Fautrel B. Treatment strategy for chronic low back pain. Joint Bone Spine 2012;79:555–9.
7. Balague F, Mannion AF, Pellise F, et al. Non-specific low back pain. Lancet 2012; 379:482–91.
8. Anderson DG, Tannoury C. Molecular pathogenic factors in symptomatic disc degeneration. Spine J 2005;5:260S–6S.
9. Zhang YG, Guo TM, Guo X, et al. Clinical diagnosis for discogenic low back pain. Int J Biol Sci 2009;5:647–58.
10. Paajanen H, Erkintalo M, Kuusela T, et al. Magnetic resonance study of disc degeneration in young low-back pain patients. Spine 1989;14:982–5.
11. Parke WW, Schiff DC. The applied anatomy of the intervertebral disc. Orthop Clin North Am 1971;2:309–24.
12. Coppes MH, Marani E, Thomeer RT, et al. Innervation of annulus fibrosis in low back pain. Lancet 1990;336:189–90.
13. Coppes MH, Marani E, Thomeer RT, et al. Innervation of "painful" lumbar discs. Spine 1997;22:2342–9 [discussion: 2349–50].
14. Bogduk N, Tynan W, Wilson AS. The nerve supply to the human lumbar intervertebral discs. J Anat 1981;132:39–56.
15. Edgar MA. The nerve supply of the lumbar intervertebral disc. J Bone Joint Surg Br 2007;89:1135–9.

16. Bogduk N. Clinical and radiologic anatomy of the lumbar spine. 5th edition. New York: Churchill Livingstone; 2012.
17. Farfan HF, Cossette JW, Robertson GH, et al. The effects of torsion on the lumbar intervertebral joints: the role of torsion in the production of disc degeneration. J Bone Joint Surg Am 1970;52:468–97.
18. Farfan HF, Gracovetsky S. The nature of instability. Spine 1984;9:714–9.
19. Farfan HF, Huberdeau RM, Dubow HI. Lumbar intervertebral disc degeneration: the influence of geometrical features on the pattern of disc degeneration–a post mortem study. J Bone Joint Surg Am 1972;54:492–510.
20. Marinelli NL, Haughton VM, Anderson PA. T2 relaxation times correlated with stage of lumbar intervertebral disk degeneration and patient age. AJNR Am J Neuroradiol 2010;31:1278–82.
21. Bogduk N. Degenerative joint disease of the spine. Radiol Clin North Am 2012; 50:613–28.
22. Pezowicz CA, Schechtman H, Robertson PA, et al. Mechanisms of anular failure resulting from excessive intradiscal pressure: a microstructural-micromechanical investigation. Spine 2006;31:2891–903.
23. Kepler CK, Ponnappan RK, Tannoury CA, et al. The molecular basis of intervertebral disc degeneration. Spine J 2013;13:318–30.
24. Dongfeng R, Hou S, Wu W, et al. The expression of tumor necrosis factor-alpha and CD68 in high-intensity zone of lumbar intervertebral disc on magnetic resonance image in the patients with low back pain. Spine 2011;36:E429–33.
25. Aprill C, Bogduk N. High-intensity zone: a diagnostic sign of painful lumbar disc on magnetic resonance imaging. Br J Radiol 1992;65:361–9.
26. Vanharanta H, Sachs BL, Spivey MA, et al. The relationship of pain provocation to lumbar disc deterioration as seen by CT/discography. Spine 1987;12:295–8.
27. Park WM, Kim K, Kim YH. Effects of degenerated intervertebral discs on intersegmental rotations, intradiscal pressures, and facet joint forces of the whole lumbar spine. Comput Biol Med 2013;43:1234–40.
28. Wilke HJ, Neef P, Caimi M, et al. New in vivo measurements of pressures in the intervertebral disc in daily life. Spine 1999;24:755–62.
29. Nachemson AL. Disc pressure measurements. Spine 1981;6:93–7.
30. Jhawar BS, Fuchs CS, Colditz GA, et al. Cardiovascular risk factors for physician-diagnosed lumbar disc herniation. Spine J 2006;6:684–91.
31. Takatalo J, Karppinen J, Taimela S, et al. Body mass index is associated with lumbar disc degeneration in young Finnish males: subsample of Northern Finland birth cohort study 1986. BMC Musculoskelet Disord 2013;14:87.
32. Zawilla NH, Darweesh H, Mansour N, et al. Matrix metalloproteinase-3, vitamin D receptor gene polymorphisms, and occupational risk factors in lumbar disc degeneration. J Occup Rehabil 2013. [Epub ahead of print].
33. Battie MC, Videman T, Kaprio J, et al. The Twin Spine Study: contributions to a changing view of disc degeneration. Spine J 2009;9:47–59.
34. Eskola PJ, Lemmela S, Kjaer P, et al. Genetic association studies in lumbar disc degeneration: a systematic review. PLoS One 2012;7:e49995.
35. Vanharanta H, Ohnmeiss DD, Aprill CN. Vibration pain provocation can improve the specificity of MRI in the diagnosis of symptomatic lumbar disc rupture. Clin J Pain 1998;14:239–47.
36. Pfirrmann CW, Metzdorf A, Zanetti M, et al. Magnetic resonance classification of lumbar intervertebral disc degeneration. Spine 2001;26:1873–8.
37. Schellhas KP, Pollei SR, Gundry CR, et al. Lumbar disc high-intensity zone. Correlation of magnetic resonance imaging and discography. Spine 1996;21:79–86.

38. Park KW, Song KS, Chung JY, et al. High-intensity zone on L-spine MRI: clinical relevance and association with trauma history. Asian Spine J 2007;1:38–42.
39. Guyer RD, Ohnmeiss DD. Lumbar discography. Position statement from the North American Spine Society Diagnostic and Therapeutic Committee. Spine 1995;20:2048–59.
40. Maus TP, Aprill CN. Lumbar diskogenic pain, provocation diskography, and imaging correlates. Radiol Clin North Am 2012;50:681–704.
41. Simmons JW, Aprill CN, Dwyer AP, et al. A reassessment of Holt's data on: "The question of lumbar discography". Clin Orthop Relat Res 1988;(237):120–4.
42. Lindblom K. Diagnostic puncture of intervertebral disks in sciatica. Acta Orthop Scand 1948;17:231–9.
43. Carragee EJ, Lincoln T, Parmar VS, et al. A gold standard evaluation of the "discogenic pain" diagnosis as determined by provocative discography. Spine 2006;31:2115–23.
44. Holt EP Jr. The question of lumbar discography. J Bone Joint Surg Am 1968;50:720–6.
45. Derby R, Lee SH, Kim BJ, et al. Pressure-controlled lumbar discography in volunteers without low back symptoms. Pa Med 2005;6:213–21 [discussion: 222–4].
46. Wiley JJ, Macnab I, Wortzman G. Lumbar discography and its clinical applications. Can J Surg 1968;11:280–9.
47. Guyer RD, Ohnmeiss DD, NASS. Lumbar discography. Spine J 2003;3:11S–27S.
48. Colhoun E, McCall IW, Williams L, et al. Provocation discography as a guide to planning operations on the spine. J Bone Joint Surg Br 1988;70:267–71.
49. Carragee EJ, Don AS, Hurwitz EL, et al. 2009 ISSLS Prize Winner: does discography cause accelerated progression of degeneration changes in the lumbar disc: a ten-year matched cohort study. Spine 2009;34:2338–45.
50. Chou R. Pharmacological management of low back pain. Drugs 2010;70:387–402.
51. Roelofs PD, Deyo RA, Koes BW, et al. Nonsteroidal anti-inflammatory drugs for low back pain: an updated Cochrane review. Spine 2008;33:1766–74.
52. Roelofs PD, Deyo RA, Koes BW, et al. Non-steroidal anti-inflammatory drugs for low back pain. Cochrane Database Syst Rev 2008;(1):CD000396.
53. Toth PP, Urtis J. Commonly used muscle relaxant therapies for acute low back pain: a review of carisoprodol, cyclobenzaprine hydrochloride, and metaxalone. Clin Ther 2004;26:1355–67.
54. Schnitzer TJ, Gray WL, Paster RZ, et al. Efficacy of tramadol in treatment of chronic low back pain. J Rheumatol 2000;27:772–8.
55. Ruoff GE, Rosenthal N, Jordan D, et al, Protocol CAPSS-112 Study Group. Tramadol/acetaminophen combination tablets for the treatment of chronic lower back pain: a multicenter, randomized, double-blind, placebo-controlled outpatient study. Clin Ther 2003;25:1123–41.
56. Schnitzer TJ, Kamin M, Olson WH. Tramadol allows reduction of naproxen dose among patients with naproxen-responsive osteoarthritis pain: a randomized, double-blind, placebo-controlled study. Arthritis Rheum 1999;42:1370–7.
57. Friedman BW, Holden L, Esses D, et al. Parenteral corticosteroids for emergency department patients with non-radicular low back pain. J Emerg Med 2006;31:365–70.
58. Casazza BA. Diagnosis and treatment of acute low back pain. Am Fam Physician 2012;85:343–50.

59. Chaparro LE, Furlan AD, Deshpande A, et al. Opioids compared to placebo or other treatments for chronic low-back pain. Cochrane Database Syst Rev 2013;(8):CD004959.
60. Alford DP. Chronic back pain with possible prescription opioid misuse. JAMA 2013;309:919–25.
61. Adams MA, May S, Freeman BJ, et al. Effects of backward bending on lumbar intervertebral discs. Relevance to physical therapy treatments for low back pain. Spine 2000;25:431–7 [discussion: 438].
62. McKenzie RA. Manual correction of sciatic scoliosis. N Z Med J 1972;76:194–9.
63. Machado LA, de Souza M, Ferreira PH, et al. The McKenzie method for low back pain: a systematic review of the literature with a meta-analysis approach. Spine 2006;31:E254–62.
64. Mannion AF, Muntener M, Taimela S, et al. A randomized clinical trial of three active therapies for chronic low back pain. Spine 1999;24:2435–48.
65. Ostelo RW, van Tulder MW, Vlaeyen JW, et al. Behavioural treatment for chronic low-back pain. Cochrane Database Syst Rev 2005;(1):CD002014.
66. van Hooff ML, Spruit M, O'Dowd JK, et al. Predictive factors for successful clinical outcome 1 year after an intensive combined physical and psychological programme for chronic low back pain. Eur Spine J 2014;23(1):102–12.
67. Furlan AD, van Tulder M, Cherkin D, et al. Acupuncture and dry-needling for low back pain: an updated systematic review within the framework of the Cochrane collaboration. Spine 2005;30:944–63.
68. Yuan J, Purepong N, Kerr DP, et al. Effectiveness of acupuncture for low back pain: a systematic review. Spine 2008;33:E887–900.
69. Rubinstein SM, van Middelkoop M, Kuijpers T, et al. A systematic review on the effectiveness of complementary and alternative medicine for chronic non-specific low-back pain. Eur Spine J 2010;19:1213–28.
70. Haake M, Muller HH, Schade-Brittinger C, et al. German Acupuncture Trials (GERAC) for chronic low back pain: randomized, multicenter, blinded, parallel-group trial with 3 groups. Arch Intern Med 2007;167:1892–8.
71. Andersson GB, Lucente T, Davis AM, et al. A comparison of osteopathic spinal manipulation with standard care for patients with low back pain. N Engl J Med 1999;341:1426–31.
72. Zylbergold RS, Piper MC. Lumbar disc disease: comparative analysis of physical therapy treatments. Arch Phys Med Rehabil 1981;62:176–9.
73. Chou R, Huffman LH, American Pain Society, American College of Physicians. Nonpharmacologic therapies for acute and chronic low back pain: a review of the evidence for an American Pain Society/American College of Physicians clinical practice guideline. Ann Intern Med 2007;147:492–504.
74. Cramer H, Lauche R, Haller H, et al. A systematic review and meta-analysis of yoga for low back pain. Clin J Pain 2013;29:450–60.
75. Hill C. Is yoga an effective treatment in the management of patients with chronic low back pain compared with other care modalities - a systematic review. J Complement Integr Med 2013;10. http://dx.doi.org/10.1515/jcim-2012-0007.
76. Holtzman S, Beggs RT. Yoga for chronic low back pain: a meta-analysis of randomized controlled trials. Pain Res Manag 2013;18(5):267–72.
77. Sherman KJ, Cherkin DC, Erro J, et al. Comparing yoga, exercise, and a self-care book for chronic low back pain: a randomized, controlled trial. Ann Intern Med 2005;143:849–56.
78. Carneiro KA, Rittenberg JD. The role of exercise and alternative treatments for low back pain. Phys Med Rehabil Clin N Am 2010;21:777–92.

79. Peng PW. Tai chi and chronic pain. Reg Anesth Pain Med 2012;37:372–82.
80. Cramer H, Haller H, Lauche R, et al. Mindfulness-based stress reduction for low back pain. A systematic review. BMC Complement Altern Med 2012;12:162.
81. Morone NE, Rollman BL, Moore CG, et al. A mind-body program for older adults with chronic low back pain: results of a pilot study. Pa Med 2009;10:1395–407.
82. Peng BG. Pathophysiology, diagnosis, and treatment of discogenic low back pain. Worldview 2013;4:42–52.
83. Manchikanti L, Falco FJ, Pampati V, et al. Cost utility analysis of caudal epidural injections in the treatment of lumbar disc herniation, axial or discogenic low back pain, central spinal stenosis, and post lumbar surgery syndrome. Pain Physician 2013;16:E129–43.
84. Benyamin RM, Manchikanti L, Parr AT, et al. The effectiveness of lumbar inter-laminar epidural injections in managing chronic low back and lower extremity pain. Pain Physician 2012;15:E363–404.
85. Zhou Y, Abdi S. Diagnosis and minimally invasive treatment of lumbar disco-genic pain–a review of the literature. Clin J Pain 2006;22:468–81.
86. Kallewaard JW, Terheggen MA, Groen GJ, et al. 15. Discogenic low back pain. Pain Pract 2010;10:560–79.
87. Buttermann GR. The effect of spinal steroid injections for degenerative disc dis-ease. Spine J 2004;4:495–505.
88. Cao P, Jiang L, Zhuang C, et al. Intradiscal injection therapy for degenerative chronic discogenic low back pain with end plate Modic changes. Spine J 2011;11:100–6.
89. Pauza KJ, Howell S, Dreyfuss P, et al. A randomized, placebo-controlled trial of intradiscal electrothermal therapy for the treatment of discogenic low back pain. Spine J 2004;4:27–35.
90. Freeman BJ. IDET: a critical appraisal of the evidence. Eur Spine J 2006; 15(Suppl 3):S448–57.
91. Kapural L, Vrooman B, Sarwar S, et al. A randomized, placebo-controlled trial of transdiscal radiofrequency, biacuplasty for treatment of discogenic lower back pain. Pa Med 2013;14:362–73.

The Failed Back Surgery Syndrome
Pitfalls Surrounding Evaluation and Treatment

Carl M. Shapiro, DO

KEYWORDS

- Failed back surgery syndrome • Myofascial pain • Chronic neuropathic pain
- Interventional pain management techniques • Interdisciplinary pain management

KEY POINTS

- Failed back surgery syndrome (FBSS) is a multidimensional chronic pain syndrome that has significant myofascial and psychosocial components that are directly related to the high incidence of lumbar surgeries in the United States.
- The development of more sophisticated surgeries and interventional treatments has not made a measurable impact on outcomes relative to return to work or medication use.
- Physical examination and radiologic evaluation have to correlate and take into account the clinical overlap of various types of pain, including radicular pain, referred (myofascial) pain, and chronic neurogenic pain, when reviewing findings.
- Prevention is the most effective treatment and postoperative treatment requires realistic goals focusing on functional accomplishments, not complete pain relief.

INTRODUCTION

FBSS is persistent or recurring low back pain with or without lumbosacral radiculopathy after 1 or more spine surgeries.[1] The incidence of FBSS is reported as between 10% and 40% but ranges between 5% and 50% have been quoted for microlaminectomy alone.[1-4] The incidence is known to increase with more complex surgeries and has not improved with the development of less-invasive advanced surgical techniques.[1,5-7] The failure rate for lumbar fusion is reported between 30% and 46% based on previous reviews[1] whereas the failure rate for microdiskectomy is thought to range between 19% and 25%.[1] The financial costs are considerable.

Disclosures: Dr C.M. Shapiro serves as the medical director for The Pain Solutions Network, a CARF-accredited outpatient interdisciplinary pain center.
Tri-State Spine and Neuromuscular Associates, 10475 Montgomery Road, Suite 1J, Cincinnati, OH 45242, USA
E-mail address: cshapirodo@yahoo.com

Phys Med Rehabil Clin N Am 25 (2014) 319–340
http://dx.doi.org/10.1016/j.pmr.2014.01.014
1047-9651/14/$ – see front matter © 2014 Elsevier Inc. All rights reserved.

RISK FACTORS FOR FAILED BACK SURGERY SYNDROME

Chan and Peng[1] provide an excellent review of the risk factors for the development of FBSS. Specific psychosocial risk factors that have been found to result in poor outcome for spinal surgery are significant levels of depression, anxiety, poor coping, somatization, and hypochondriasis.[1,8] The presence of a worker's compensation claim is consistently cited in the literature as a risk factor associated with poor surgical outcomes and is often dismissed as due to secondary gain.[1] It is important to differentiate true secondary gain from symptom magnification imposed by inability to obtain timely diagnosis and treatment. In addition, FBSS patients often pursue disability claims after job loss to retain insurance coverage for ongoing treatment. FBSS is, therefore, a biopsychosocial problem where indirect and intangible costs play a significant role in defining morbidity.[4]

A major difficulty in preventing FBSS is that the ideal time to operate is not well defined in the literature.[1,3] Surgical decision making is clear when there is progressive motor loss or cauda equina syndrome. But the timing and indications for surgery when pain is the primary complaint are not well defined. A general dictum is that 6 to 12 weeks of conservative care is reasonable prior to surgery.

It has been stated that the 2-year outcome for patients treated with either laminectomy or microlaminectomy is the same as for those treated with conservative care.[1,9–11] The time to pain improvement is faster, however, with the surgical groups. If considerations for lost productivity and lifestyle compromise are openly discussed, surgery may be a reasonable option for refractory pain as an earlier option.

Earlier surgical intervention for low back pain may make sense in selected cases on a physiologic basis. Since the 1970's it has been accepted that untreated pain promotes persistent pain patterns in the central nervous system in as little as 3 months. This is often attributed to "wind-up phenomena" or central sensitization at the levels of the spinal cord and central nervous system. Once chronic pain patterns develop treatment because more complicated and the likelihood of a successful outcome diminishes.

Deciding on the ideal time to operate is further complicated by disuse atrophy and chronic inflammation promoting physical deconditioning,[3] making restoration of function and pain control more difficult after surgery. Prolonged pain and distress also may exacerbate preexisting psychosocial stressors, which is especially problematic with hypervigilant patients who have poor pain tolerance because they may simply refuse to normalize their activities, thereby creating a vicious cycle of pain and deconditioning. Thus, although an ounce of prevention may be worth a ton of cure, nihilism with respect to surgical decision making is not reasonable.

PREOPERATIVE RISKS

- Prior surgery
  - Spinal instability has been noted to occur in 12% of cases after a first surgery and increases to greater than 50% after 4 or more revisions.[12]
- Surgery based on imagining abnormalities without good clinical correlation[1]
- Nonsurgical causes of radiculopathy and neuropathy, including toxic-metabolic neuropathies (eg, diabetes), viral and inflammatory radiculitis, vascular disease, and plexopathies due to a pelvic mass or trauma

INTRAOPERATIVE RISKS

- Difficult radiographic localization intraoperatively during microsurgical cases or when there are segmentation defects[3] causing operation at the wrong level, thus leaving the true pain generator without intervention[1,3]

- Inadequate decompression may leave a pain generator intact.
- Aggressive decompression may lead to spinal instability and pain.[1]
- Loss of disk height after diskectomy may lead to vertical stenosis, compression, and pain.
- Unrecognized pathology, such as disk fragments in the neural foramen, kinking of the nerve root by the adjacent pedicle, root compression by the articular process, spinal stenosis, extraforaminal disk herniation, and conjoined nerve roots may frustrate a successful outcome.[1,3]
- Excessive retraction, bleeding, or use of cottonoid patties may lead to battered root syndrome.[1,3] Battered root syndrome is thought to occur in as many as 13% of cases with diskectomy and should be suspected if there is incomplete resolution of sciatic symptoms with or without progressive neurologic deficit that progresses over 3 to 6 months.[1,3] It may be more common if there are conjoined nerve roots.[1]
- Pars interarticularis fracture may occur during decompression.
- Use of methyl methacrylate as a primary means of stabilization or as a salvage technique for stripped screws may damage neural elements through compression or heat.[3]
- Roots may be damaged by graft extrusion after posterior lumbar interbody fusion (PLIF) or from excessive retraction.
- Finally, the aim of surgery may be difficult to achieve. Proper decompression for foraminal stenosis due to ligamentous hypertrophy or far lateral disk herniation may cause destabilization of the segment and postoperative pain.[1]

POSTOPERATIVE FACTORS

- Postsurgical complications
  - Hematoma or infection
  - Symptomatic pseudoarthrosis after fusion surgery
  - Epidural fibrosis may tether spinal nerve roots and interfere with cerebrospinal fluid–mediated nutrition of the nerve roots or interfere with the vascular supply of the nerve roots.
  - Pseudomeningocele, which can result from inadequate closure or inadvertent meningeal tear. This is a pseudocyst with no true meningeal lining that is secondary to postoperative dehiscence and can affect up to 2% of postlaminectomy patients. Patients with pseudomenigocele complain of wound swelling, headache, and focal neurologic symptoms, including radicular pain and cauda equina symptoms.[1,3,13]
  - Persistent irritation of the nerve roots may also result from postsurgical arachnoiditis and can result in both axial and lower limb pain.[1] MRI T2-weighted fast spin-echo sequences provide the best evaluation for arachnoiditis.[13] There are 3 patterns of presentation on MRI:
    - Type 1 is a conglomerate of nerve roots seen as nerve root clumping, and this pattern is associated with the mildest involvement.
    - Type 2 is due to peripheral adhesions of the nerve roots to the thecal sac producing the so-called empty sac appearance and is associated with moderate involvement.
    - Type 3 refers to an intermediate attenuation mass obliterating the subarachnoid space below the conus medullaris and is thought to produce the most severe presentation.[13]
- Anatomic or biomechanical alterations

- Spinal instability has been noted to occur in 12% of cases after a first surgery and increases to greater that 50% after 4 or more revisions.[14]
- Loss of disk height after diskectomy may lead to vertical stenosis, compression, and pain.
- Transition syndrome,[1,15–17] or adjacent level disease, is due to altered biomechanics that imposes increased load across adjacent spinal segments after diskectomy, thereby accelerating preexisting disk degeneration. Similar mechanisms are thought to predispose to sacroiliac (SI) dysfunction, especially after fusion,[16,17] and this is thought to occur in up to 36% of patients after lumbar fusion.[1,16]
- Recurrent disk herniations are known to occur in approximately 15% of patients at the site of operation or in adjacent segments because of altered load distributions.[1,18] Altered load distributions may exacerbate adjacent level spondylolisthesis or further stenosis as part of a transition syndrome.[1,13]
- Myofascial pain

Myofascial pain may result from dissection or prolonged retraction of the paraspinals during surgery, causing denervation and atrophy. Altered postural changes postoperatively may also create permanent chronic strain.[1] There are no large studies to demonstrate that development of minimally invasive fusion surgeries, such as PLIF, axial lumbar interbody fusion, and transforaminal lumbar interbody fusion, have an impact on the incidence of FBSS or this component of FBSS, despite that these surgeries do not disrupt the dorsal musculature extensively. The author's anecdotal experience over 10 years in a university-affiliated spine center is that there is little if any difference.

Fusion disease is a form of myofascial pain that has been attributed to compensatory hyperextension of the lumbar spine exacerbating poor posture. It has been attributed to paraspinal and hamstring muscle spasm or atrophy.[1] In the author's experience, however, flexed posture and difficulty arising from sitting is even more common after low lumbar fusion. Short-term relief can be afforded with manipulation and focused physical therapy but recurrent and persistent pain, spasm, and limited of range of motion is common. In the author's view, the recurrence of these symptoms is most likely due to a combination of permanently altered postural biomechanics from fusion hardware constructs and self-perpetuating muscle imbalances with the hip flexors overpowering the multifidi, short lumbar rotators, paraspinals, and transversus abdominis.

The difficulty demonstrated by long-term treatment of this problem emphasizes that myofascial pain is a complex problem demanding an individualized approach that targets specific deficits. Complicating factors include

- Differentiating referred versus true radicular pain
- Differentiating the role of osteoligamentous structures versus the role of neuromuscular coordination (motor control) for pain-free motion[19]
- Understanding how predominantly tonic muscles and phasic muscles respond to injury[20]

Myofascial referred pain can be easily confused with radicular pain. The description of chronic ligamentous strain or musculotendinous pain as deep burning ache is similar to dysesthesia and the patterns of pain can also confound diagnosis. Travell and Simons[21] provide several examples of pain patterns responsive to trigger point therapy that seem indistinguishable from dermatomal radicular pain, for example, trigger points in the gluteus minimus and gluteus medius that mimic L5 radiculopathy.

The clinical presentation of myofascial pain is important for 2 reasons: (1) it is not responsive to many of the treatments commonly offered to chronic FBSS patients, such as opioids and interventional spine techniques; and (2) if left untreated, it becomes worse, making it more difficult to resolve. This is important because it feeds patient perceptions of incapacity and hopelessness and contributes to the vicious cycle of pain and deconditioning commonly seen with FBSS patients. There are 2 dominant theories of myofascial pain propagation. One focuses on peripheral mechanisms where damaged motor endplates locally propagate more trigger points, and the other posits that central sensitization in the dorsal horn causes expanded receptive fields in the spinal cord[22] and amplifies perception. The issues of posture and balance most likely also play a significant role.

Another major consideration, relative to lumbar myofascial pain, is the issue of motor control if overloading of muscles, tendons, ligaments, disks, and joints are to be minimized. Motor control is the regulation of coordinated muscular activity allowing efficient transfer of loads to joint services. Motor control requires (1) accurate instantaneous feedback from mechanoreceptors at the joint/soft tissue interface, (2) appropriate interpretation of this input, and most importantly, (3) modulation and timing of the responses to accomplish specific tasks.[19,20] The loss or perturbation of these neuromuscular adaptations can result in refractory pain, inefficient movement, and inappropriate force closure of joints during motion.[23] These, in turn, can lead to articular microtrauma and inflammation, ligamentous laxity, and disuse atrophy, which can mimic neurogenic weakness.

The role of the inner ring muscles, consisting of the multifidus, thoracolumbar fascia, and transverses abdominis, and, their interaction with the diaphragm and pelvic floor muscles to create a cylindrical supporting system for the lumbar spine through the regulation of intra-abdominal pressure is especially important.[19] This is not an issue of strength but rather of timing and coordination, which are fundamentally important because the posterior portion of this ring, the multifidus, receives its innervation from the posterior rami and medial branches of the lumbar roots. Consequently, if there is injury to the lumbar roots, coordination of the multifidus can be compromised. Richardson and colleagues[19] presented persuasive data that these timing issues play an important role and are common denominators in many cases of chronic low back pain. Motor control is generally regulated by reflex mechanisms at the level of the spinal cord but it can be affected by supraspinal influences, such as mood and arousal,[19] and this too is consistent with chronic pain variability.

The propagation of myofascial pain is also affected by how tonic and phasic muscles respond to injury. Physicians learn that muscle fibers can be categorized histologically and by their speed of contraction:

- Type I, or slow oxidative muscle fiber, has high mitochondrial content.
- Type IIa, or fast glycolytic muscle fiber, has low mitochondrial content.
- Type IIb, or fast oxidative muscle fiber, has a high mitochondrial content like type I fiber, but, it has a lower glycogen content than type IIa fiber and an intermediate range of fatigue between type I and type IIa fiber.[24]

Most human skeletal muscle is not truly represented by any of these types, however. A more functional classification characterizes muscles as either predominantly tonic or phasic. Tonic muscles are postural and not susceptible to early fatigue. Phasic muscles provide ballistic function (movement) and are less suited to endurance activities. Some muscles serve both functions depending on situational context, such as the vastus medialis, which stabilizes the knee during loading and standing (tonic function) but also extends the leg ballistically during activities, such as drop kicking a football (phasic activity). The point of this classification is how these muscle types respond to overloading and injury.[20] Tonic muscles tend to shorten with injury and overloading. Phasic muscles tend to weaken with injury and overloading. Examples of tonic muscles include the erector muscles of the lumbar spine, piriformis, and hip flexors. Examples of phasic muscles include the abdominal muscles, knee extensors, and gluteus muscles. The important point is that shortened tonic muscles can inhibit phasic antagonists and synergists, thereby preventing maximal activation and optimal trainability.[20] Consequently, a vicious cycle is created and compounded by faulty substitution patterns that develop after injury and surgery. This situation is especially problematic after denervation or if fusion constructs prevent range of motion, because normal muscle balance may not be recoverable. Consequently, any successful rehabilitation strategy has to account not only for strength and flexibility but also for posture and motor control issues. Treatment of myofascial pain is also thought dependent on improving a patient's aerobic capacity.[25]

EVALUATION OF THE POSTOPERATIVE SPINE: HISTORY AND PHYSICAL

History and physical examination are the most important parts of evaluating FBSS. There is considerable overlap, however, of the types of pain associated with this syndrome. The potential anatomic and pathologic processes responsible for postoperative pain complaints are difficult to differentiate. The types of pain include myofascial pain, arthropathic joint pain, and radicular pain that follows true dermatomal patterns associated with dysesthesia, loss of sensation, or loss of power. Chronic neural pain of any kind, whether visceral, sympathetically mediated, or phantom pain, is diffuse, poorly localized, and not well described anatomically. It is sometimes described with combinations of cramping, aching, and tight or burning sensations and is, therefore, similar to myofascal pain; it is ill described. It may also be associated with hyperalgesia or allodynia, which is important because, like myofascial pain, chronic neural pain is less responsive to opioids and better treated with adjuvant medications and therapies.

Physical examination typically focuses on neurologic findings, such as deep tendon reflexes and motor and sensory examination.[1,3] Musculoskeletal examination, however, should include flexibility and tests of hip mobility, seated and standing trunk rotation, lumbar flexion and extension, lumbar side-bending, and palpation of the SI joints and trochanters. The entire spine should be examined and concomitant disease causing myelopathy with increased tone, clonus, and Babinski and Hoffmann signs should be ruled out. Spondylosis is a generalized condition and does not affect the lumbar spine in isolation.

Side-to-side asymmetry of motion is more important than measured range of motion. Straight leg raise and femoral nerve stretch test are also important with respect to the postoperative spine. True radicular pain with numbness or dysesthesia in dermatomal patterns is important to differentiate from decreased flexibility and discomfort due to lost range of motion from chronic injury or postsurgical guarding. A good representative neurologic examination is available from the American Spinal Injury Association, and the American College of Rheumatology has excellent materials on trigger/tender point examination. Patients should be assessed for leg length discrepancies and focal weakness, especially footdrop, because orthotics and bracing may be necessary to minimize repetitive strain over the kinetic chain. Finally, screening tests for motor control and stabilization are also recommended. Two easy tests include

- Assessing balance from the hands and knee position with opposite arm and leg extension (the pointer dog test)
- Maintaining a stable prone plank position from a modified push-up position where the patient starts prone and elevates to the elbows and balls of the feet[19]

The entire physical examination should not take more than 8 to 10 minutes of office time. Evaluation of functional potential is more important than immediate relief of pain. The initial cause of surgery, prior symptoms and neurologic deficits, type of surgery, current symptoms, and time since surgery are critical to know to evaluate the advantages and limitations of particular imaging studies, further work-up, and treatment modalities.[1,13] It is also imperative to assess compliance with previous treatments and rehabilitation efforts to appreciate any psychosocial overlay that has an impact on care.

EVALUATION OF THE POSTOPERATIVE SPINE: WORK-UP

Radiographic evaluation is an important tool because it may reveal anatomic aberrations, allowing for definitive treatment and better prognostication, such as residual lateral recess stenosis. Diagnostic studies may also provide reassurance that serious pathology is not present and that neurologic deterioration is not likely to occur with increased activity.

Radiologic findings specific to FBSS should not be confused with postoperative normal variants. Small seromas and edema of the subcutaneous tissue after surgery should be expected and herniation of the thecal sac through a new laminectomy defect may produce a mass effect that is normal if it is seen to decrease on serial films over the first 30 to 60 days.[1,3,13]

MRI demonstrating epidural fibrosis has to be interpreted with caution because most patients with epidural fibrosis are asymptomatic. Nerve root enhancement is often seen in asymptomatic patients for 6 months after surgery, but if nerve root thickening and displacement are seen, the positive predictive value of imaging improves.[1,26,27] The main differential in this setting is recurrent disk herniation, and recurrent disk herniation needs to be ruled out in symptomatic patients.[13]

Similarly, postoperative inflammation and fibrosis due to disruption of the annulus fibrosis and epidural edema may simulate recurrent disk herniation with noncontrast MRI studies.[13] Vertebral endplates can demonstrate edema and enhancement in 19% of patients between 6 and 18 months after surgery and nerve root enhancement may linger for 6 weeks or longer in 20% to 62% of patients after surgery.[13] Consequently, careful correlation with progressive clinical signs and symptoms is mandatory during any investigation for postoperative or persistent pain.

MRI is generally the modality of choice in the postoperative setting because it allows for evaluation of soft tissues, bone marrow, and intraspinal content.[13] Metallic hardware may lead to magnetic artifact but this can be minimized with fast spin-echo sequences, short echo time, and longer repetition time. Titanium and vitallium hardware produce less artifact than stainless steel on MRI. T2-weighted sequences should also afford better visualization with less artifact and short time inversion recovery sequences and should be used for fat suppression to improve homogeneity of the image.[13]

Contrast administration with T1 imaging is useful to distinguish inflammatory tissue from recurrent disk herniation.[1,13] Contrast is also useful when infection is suspected because bacterial diskitis is associated with particularly intense contrast enhancement compared with normal inflammatory change that can be seen postoperatively.[13] A heightened index of suspicion for infection should arise if fluid collections are seen in paraspinal areas or the anterior epidural space; if they are located adjacent to the disk involved; or if there is psoas enhancement.[13] Contrast-enhanced MRI with fat saturation is the modality of choice when infection is suspected because it allows for evaluation of bone edema and diskitis earlier than other modalities.[13] Contrast-enhanced CT allows for assessment of associated bone involvement, phlegmons, and abscesses and both CT and ultrasound are useful for guiding biopsies.[13]

CT is the modality of choice for bone and abnormal calcification assessment. Intravenous iodine contrast is required to investigate suspected infection. Metal artifact can be reduced with attenuation techniques, and software manipulation and orthopedic hardware with lower attenuation coefficients are known to produce less distortion. Titanium produces less distortion than stainless steel, which, in turn, produces less distortion than cobalt-chrome.[13]

CT is particularly useful for investigating suspected misplaced or loosened hardware. Root irritation can be seen with misplaced pedicle screws encroaching on the lateral recess or foramen. In general, root irritation is associated with low or medial screw placement. Loosening of hardware can be seen with infection or stress fatigue and is associated with a halo or hypoattenuation greater than 2 mm around the hardware.[13]

Conventional radiographs are particularly useful when there is hardware because there is no metallic artifact.[13] Anteroposterior, lateral, oblique views and flexion/extension views are all useful when planning diagnostic or therapeutic interventional procedures and to diagnose structural problems, such as postoperative loss of disk height or spondylolisthesis with instability.[27]

Electrodiagnostic evaluation of the postoperative spine can be useful for both localization and prognosis, especially if there is a preoperative study to compare with. A change in compound motor action potential and increase in peripheral membrane irritability may reflect worsening postoperative axonopathy. Similarly, membrane irritability may localize to the involved nerve root when there is multilevel disease. The presence of membrane irritability that correlates with at least one grade of motor loss on physical examination may assist treatment considerations if differentiating motor loss from involuntary guarding is difficult. For example, assistive devices and lifestyle management may be more appropriate in the presence of extensive neurogenic atrophy whereas aggressive strengthening exacerbates joint pain and instability.

Interpreting electrodiagnostic evaluations requires some caution. Sampling size always has an impact on recognition of membrane irritability and both positive and negative findings have to be measured against the clinical picture and radiology. As a rule, MRI is more sensitive than electromyogram (EMG) for diagnosing the cause of radiculopathy but EMG is more specific for the presence of radiculopathy. If both sensory and motor nerve conduction abnormalities are seen, a peripheral nerve problem is more likely than a preganglionic root problem. It is, however, possible for vertical stenosis or a large lateral disk herniation to affect the dorsal root ganglion and cause sensory nerve conduction abnormalities too, most commonly at L5.[28]

Paraspinal denervation does not always equal lumbar disease. It can be seen in diabetics[29] and, if associated with extensive denervation in more than the expected peripheral myotomes, the differentials for myopathic, neuropathic, or motor neuron diseases should come to mind. Finally, irritability in the paraspinals may persist because of incisional muscle damage and therefore, muscle sampling should be further than 2 cm from an incision line and interpretation must still be made with caution.[28]

TREATMENT

The goals of treatment are to maximize neuromuscular and musculoskeletal efficiency with activity, control pain, and interrupt and reverse the progression of debility.

Medical therapy should be advanced with the goal of increasing physical activity and community involvement. Pharmacologic management includes

1. Nonsteroidal antiinflammatory drugs or acetaminophen
2. Muscle relaxants, such as cyclobenzaprine, methacarbamol, and metaxalone
3. True antispastic medications, such as baclofen or tizanidine
4. Antidepressants, such as tricyclics, selective serotonin reuptake inhibitors, and combined serotonin and norepinepherine reuptake inhibitors
5. Gabapentinoids
6. Tramadol
7. Opioids[1]

Medication prescription should take into account mechanisms of action, presumed modification of specific symptom complexes, and side-effect profiles. In actuality, off-label indications, trial and error, and empiric decision making are common in community medicine settings; for example, low-dose amitriptyline or tizanidine may prescribed at hour of sleep to promote better sleep hygiene and improve myofascial pain.

The American Pain Society has published clinical practice guidelines for chronic low back pain but not specifically for FBSS.[1,30] Cochrane reviews are also available for symptomatic relief of low back pain but again these do not specifically address FBSS.[1,31] There is at least 1 case report of decreased pain and improved function with gabapentin as monotherapy for FBSS, but there are no formal studies of gabapentinoids and the effect on FBSS.[1,32] Side effects and drug interactions often limit these therapies, and polypharmacy increases the risk of serious complications, such as serotonin syndrome. Consequently, opioids are commonly prescribed.

All of these medications have been well reviewed in Braddom's textbook, Physical Medicine and Rehabilitation, 4th ed, with respect to mechanisms of action and dosage ranges. Another focused review is available from the American Pain Society/American College of Physicians Clinical Practice Guideline.[30]

Nonopioid medications are considered adjunctive pain medications and are usually insufficient in the setting of FBSS. Opioids are generally considered safe and effective for moderate to severe pain[1] but the use of opioids for chronic noncancer pain is becoming more controversial. This is especially true in the setting of FBSS, especially in the setting of instrumented lumbar fusion. Chan and Peng comment on a recent publication investigating mortality after lumbar fusion:

> In this study, the leading cause of mortality (accounting for 31% of all deaths) was analgesic related. The overwhelming majority of deaths were related to opioids (20/22 patients with analgesic related death). While the majority were accidental, three deaths were the result of suicide. Of those patients who suffered from analgesic related mortality, all had undergone either instrumented fusion or intervertebral cage procedure. No patient with receiving lumbar fusion from autograft or allograft suffered from analgesic related death. While more investigation is required to determine why patients with instrumentation may be more prone to serious complications of opioid analgesia, this finding should caution the physician to be careful when prescribing analgesics for FBSS and to undertake close monitoring of patients on chronic opioids for pain.[1]

FBSS patients are often pushed aside and told that their surgeons have little to offer them after their surgeries were unsuccessful. These patients are generally managed by community-based physicians, including primary care physicians, anesthesiologists, physiatrists, and neurologists. Scope of practice and the limits of a patient's third party coverage influence the pharmacologic management, interventional therapies, and physical therapy treatments that are offered. Once treatment options are expended, FBSS patients are often told to seek out a physician who will prescribe pain medications chronically.

Treatment of FBSS demands recognition that it is a chronic pain syndrome. One reason that FBSS is a difficult-to-treat syndrome and a public health problem is that the antecedent back pain did not respond to intervention and was often augmented with additional pain complaints caused by the surgery. The psychosocial burden for individuals is huge, especially if there is job loss or loss of function physically. Many of the immediate postoperative pharmacologic strategies complicate the situation further by altering the patient sensorium, mood, affect, and even libido. Opioid-induced hyperalgesia is probably under-recognized and under-reported.

Prescription opioid abuse is now considered a major public health problem in itself. Ten years after pain was recognized as the fifth vital sign, primary care physicians and specialists alike are being placed under scrutiny for excessive opioid prescribing. As of the time of this writing, states, including Washington, Utah, Ohio, Indiana, Kentucky, and New York, all regulate and monitor opioid prescribing carefully and this trend can be expected to continue.

Patients often become chronically habituated to opioids and underinsured after job loss, leading to further marginalization by institutions and practitioners, who of necessity are becoming more focused on competitive cost containment and the potential for clinical censure. These patients are often viewed as doctor shopping when they are unable to obtain adequate relief and most do not have good insight into the nature of their problem. Despite high doses of opioids, many patients still report 10/10 pain during clinical interviews. This clinical observation has been corroborated by a study from 2007 where opioids did not give patients a significant reduction in pain from baseline.[1,33]

Therapeutic encounters need to emphasize that complete pain relief may not be reasonable, but pain control allowing increased activity and enjoyment may be attainable. In general, long-acting opioids should be preferred to short-acting opioids to decrease peaks and troughs that stimulate craving, and patients need to be monitored for aberrant drug behavior, including secondary financial gains from diversion. Patient education addressing the deleterious effects of prolonged immobility and deconditioning is essential if the vicious cycle of pain and deactivation is to be interrupted.

INTERVENTIONAL PAIN TREATMENTS AND SURGERY FOR TREATMENT OF FBSS

Interventional pain management techniques are frequently used to treat FBSS because pharmacologic interventions have significant morbidities of their own. More importantly, a ceiling effect is often reached before a patient has satisfactory relief. Some of these modalities, such as medial branch blocks, selective foraminal epidurals, and SI joint injections, offer further diagnostic insight. Others are clearly salvage techniques to minimize the deleterious effects of oral pain medicines, improve quality of life, or substitute for revision surgery. The justification for these procedures is derived from the extensive morbidity associated with FBSS and these patients experiencing permanent loss with respect to their earning capability, activity level, and life enjoyment. Treatment algorithms are designed to address either predominantly axial or radicular pain[1] and are aimed at arthroidal or neural structures.

Facet Interventions

Zygapophysial joint injection, medial branch block, and radiofrequency neurotomy/ablation (RFA) are used to address axial back pain. When strict criteria are followed, these procedures can provide important diagnostic information even if they are not therapeutically successful. Repeated successful diagnostic medial branch block followed by radiofrequency ablation of the facet joint(s) is generally preferred to intra-articular facet injection because of difficulty entering the joints,[34] potential epidural spread, or venous uptake, which has been documented as occurring in as many as 6.1% of cases.[34] Similarly, chemical medial branch neurotomy with alcohol or phenol is now discouraged because of potential epidural spread. A positive diagnostic response for medial branch block is 80% pain reduction after 2 blinded blocks with concordant responses. RFA should then be expected to provide sustained analgesia. Efficacy has been reported to offer 60% of patients 90% relief at 12-month follow-up, and 87% of patients have greater than 60% relief over a similar time span.[35] Other investigators cite similar statistics, and previous surgery has not been found to have an effect on the efficacy of radiofrequency neurotomy.[8,35]

Facet-mediated pain has been attributed to 16% of FBSS[36] cases and RFA is now used widely throughout the United States. It does not offer a permanent fix to facet-mediated pain, which should raise concern with regard to overutilization. More importantly, there are other potential confounding variables that raise questions as to whether it is counterproductive. One of these is the physiologic effect of RFA on the multifidus muscle. This is important because the multifidus forms the posterior portion of the inner muscular ring responsible for spine stabilization. RFA lesioning is targeted proximal to the branch point for facet and multifidus innervations and, therefore, the muscle is denervated along with the facet. One method to determine whether RFA lesioning is effectively accomplished is to obtain a baseline EMG of the multifidus and then perform a repeat study 4 weeks after RFA lesioning. Denervation can be considered successful if there is a decrease of more than 90% muscle activity registered with the second study.[37]

Retraining this muscle with motor control techniques is at the core of most presurgical or postsurgical spine rehabilitation strategies[19,38–40] and therefore, premature RFA may be more damaging than helpful. RFA usually offers only temporary relief for approximately 10.5 to 12 months before the effect diminishes.[1,8,36,37] Consequently, RFA should be reserved for the most refractory cases as a quality of life salvage procedure. This author has never seen a patient successfully perform either of the stabilization tests (described previously) after RFA. However, 100% of these patients were seen for refractory or recurrent pain that was predominantly axial.

Epidural Steroid Injection

Epidural steroid injection (ESI) is indicated for radicular pain. It is considered effective for epidural fibrosis, disk disruption, and spinal stenosis and, therefore, addresses several of the causes attributed to FBSS.[1,8,41] Proposed mechanisms of action include an antiinflammatory effect by addressing phospoholipase A2 elicited from disk material, sodium channel blockage, and an effect on vascular permeability.[1,41] In a study comparing caudal ESI with just local anesthetic versus local anesthetic plus steroid, however, both groups had greater than 50% pain relief in 60% of the patients from either arm of the study.[8] Functional improvement was noted in 55% to 70% of the patients, with no significant differences at 1-year follow-up. Understanding regarding the mechanisms responsible for the therapeutic effect of epidural injections is further questioned in recent literature.[41]

Bicket and colleagues[41] evaluated randomized, double-blind studies comparing high doses of steroid with lower doses in which the steroid was replaced by saline or local anesthetic. This review is remarkable for a consistent failure to demonstrate any significant differences between treatment groups. They noted another systematic review by Rabinovitch and colleagues[42] where larger injectate volumes provided a statistically significant benefit over smaller injectate volumes irrespective of the injectate contents, suggesting several other mechanisms of action for the therapeutic effect of ESI, including suppression of ectopic discharges from inflamed nerves, enhanced blood flow to ischemic nerve roots, lysis of iatrogenic and inflammatory adhesions, washout of proinflammmatory cytokines, and reversing peripheral and central sensitization.[42]

Steroid delivery to the lumbar epidural space can be accomplished with reasonable certainty when the target pain generator is L4/5 or below with one of several approaches. These include translaminar, transforaminal, and caudal approaches. Fluoroscopic guidance is recommended to assist placement. The presence of epidural fibrosis, instrumentation, and other anatomic alteration after surgery makes needle placement more difficult and increases the risk of dural puncture, which has been reported as high as 20%.[1] Even if the needle is placed properly, medication may not reach the pain generator due to scarring, fibrosis, and altered anatomy.[1] Because the posterior longitudinal ligament is taken during laminectomy, loss of resistance technique is compromised with translaminar approaches at the operative level. In general, if this approach must be used, the next level caudal is used.

Transforaminal approaches are often cited as more effective than translaminar approaches because they access the anterior epidural space and are thought more selective relative to the disk and root exit zone in the foramen. They have also been assessed as more efficacious with respect to pain relief based on the Numeric Rating Scale.[8] Dye flow to adjacent levels, however, is often seen with this approach and, therefore, specificity is questionable.

Caudal ESI offers a more global medication delivery and the roots forming the entire lumbosacral plexus up to the L4/5 level can be bathed at once. Large-volume caudal ESI has also been compared with epiduroscopy to treat epidural fibrosis.[43] Epiduroscopy is a technique where a specialized RK needle is inserted percutaneously, allowing a Racz catheter to be threaded into the epidural space. The Racz catheter is then advanced to the area of fibrosis and injectate is then delivered focally to lyse adhesions. Other wire-bound catheters can also be used to mechanically lyse adhesions and there are several protocols and injectates that have been reviewed in the literature.[44,45] These are specialized techniques not commonly performed in community settings. In contrast, caudal ESI is a commonly used technique throughout the United States.

Manchikanti and colleagues[46,47] proposed a protocol in 2010 to evaluate the comparative effectiveness of large-volume caudal ESI versus percutaneous epiduroscopy and reported results in 2012 with a cohort of 120 randomized subjects who received multiple procedures over a 2-year period. There was a significant and dramatic difference between the 2 groups with respect to duration of relief after each procedure and a statistically significant change in pain and functional status was noted between the 2 groups. The caudal ESI cohort fared worse but benefit between 3 and 6 months was noted in both groups. Opioid decreases, measured in morphine equivalents, dropped from baseline in both groups but never extinguished, and no significant differences were noted between the 2 groups.

Evaluation of epiduroscopy by Takeshima in 2009[48] noted similar trends. Twelve weeks of improvement in the Roland-Morris questionnaire were noted whether the nerve roots were mechanically separated or not by the procedure, but better long-term improvement was noted if the nerve roots were mechanically separated by the procedure.

The evidence supporting the use of ESIs and epiduroscopy is controversial. There have been several summaries of the literature since 2005 with evaluations of the strength of the evidence,[8,49–51] and the consistent trends are that short-term relief is better than long-term relief for all modalities; acute pain and subacute pain are better relieved than chronic pain (ie, lasting greater than 3 months); and, overall, 60% to 70% have a good response of some duration and 30% have little or no benefit at all. These procedures are, therefore, at best, an adjunct in the treatment of FBSS and should not be expected to return patients to employment, decrease oral medication usage significantly over the long term, or affect disability in the setting of FBSS. The use of ESI is, therefore, at best limited as an adjunct to control exacerbations of radiculopathy in FBSS patients, allowing them to return to baseline functionality and medication levels.

Like medial branch blocks, ESI may also provide diagnostic insight. Consider a patient with postoperative persistent pain and radiographic evidence of foraminal compromise that correlates well with the clinical presentation. A foraminal block with alleviation of symptoms of any duration argues for a potentially reversible process, such as reherniation or incomplete decompression of the lateral recess. Therefore, reoperation with decompression may be a reasonable and definitive alternative as opposed to placement of a spinal cord stimulator for refractory postsurgical neuropathic pain.

Sacroiliac Injections

SI injections are the gold standard for diagnosing SI pain.[1] SI pain is thought to occur between 16% and 43% postoperatively in the setting of lumbosacral fusion.[52] It has been estimated that approximately 14.5% of patients presenting to spine surgeons before operation have SI joint pain.[52] SI joint pain is important in the preoperative and postoperative differential because it is often associated with referred pain down the leg and can mimic radiculopathy. The general dictum that SI referred pain does not go below the knee is disputed. Schwarzer and colleagues[53] contend that pain below the knee and into the foot are as common in SI joint pain as other sources.[53] A potential confounding variable in this study is that when diagnostic SI joint blocks are performed, up to 24% of the time dye can be seen in sacral foramina.[54] Physical examination testing and imaging are not considered reliable for diagnosing SI joint pain.[53,55,56] In asymptomatic patients greater than 50 years old, 24.5% of were found to have abnormal SI joints on plain radiographs. Abnormal CT findings, such as sclerosis, erosions, and narrowing have a sensitivity of 58% and a specificity of 69% compared with pain relief from diagnostic local anesthetic injection.[52]

SI joint pain has been attributed to ligamentous or capsular tension, shear forces, extraneous compression, hypomobility or hypermobility, aberrant joint mechanics, and myofascial or kinetic chain imbalances, resulting in inflammation and pain. Ivanov and colleagues[17] postulated a model where fusion increased angular motion and stress across the SI joint and maintains that because the ligaments around the SI joint articulation are richly innervated, even small increases in motion trigger pain.[17,52]

Innervation of the SI joint is derived from the lumbar plexus and sacral nerve roots. Radiofrequency lesioning can be performed at the L4/5 and L5/S1 dorsal rami along with the sacral foramina, at the joint itself, or with a combination of neural and ligamentous approaches. A 50% reduction in pain is considered therapeutic.[57–59] Pain relief of 50% or greater has been reported to last from 6 weeks to as long as 12 months.[60]

SI joint injections with local anesthetic and steroid can be therapeutic but the duration of efficacy has been noted shorter in patients with a history of lumbar fusion.[52] Like epidurals, SI joint injections show an approximately 60% success rate at decreasing preprocedure pain by 50% and, therefore, can be a useful adjunct in the setting of exacerbated pain associated with FBSS. Diagnostic SI joint injections should be concordant and replicate or increase a patient's typical pain with pressure loading of the joint, and at least 50% pain relief should be noted to correlate with the expected duration of the local anesthetic. Other strategies to manage SI joint pain include the use of pelvic belts and physical therapy and manipulation.[52] The goal of physical therapy for SI joint pain, and all lumbosacral spine problems, is to restore motor control and postural and dynamic muscle balance, stabilize the pelvis, equalize flexibility, centralize referred and/or radicular pain, and correct gait abnormalities.[52]

Intrathecal Pumps and Spinal Cord Stimulators

With the exception of caudal ESI and epiduroscopy, most interventional procedures are aimed at specific structures. After these have failed, systemic pain control for quality of life can be augmented with implantable pain pumps or spinal cord stimulation (SCS). Revision surgery is usually not recommended unless a surgically correctable lesion can be identified because success rates are unusually low and continue to decline with each additional surgery. Successful outcomes have been reported in only 22% to 40% of patients who undergo revision surgery,[1] leading to an expanded use of intrathecal pumps and spinal cord stimulators, which are less invasive and less costly and have an added advantage of being potentially reversible procedures.

Until recently, intrathecal delivery systems were reserved for cancer pain. The popularity of these systems, however, has increased for chronic nonmalignant pain.[1] Analgesia has been found effective in FBSS and 88% to 92% of patients have reported satisfaction with these devices globally in several observational studies.[1] Winkelmuller and Winkelmuller[61] evaluated the therapeutic response relative to nociceptive somatic pain versus neuropathic pain. Short-term follow-up revealed better pain reduction in the nociceptive group at 77%. Some decrease in efficacy at long-term follow-up was noted, with only 68% achieving long-term results, whereas only 62% of the cohort with deafferentation pain achieved significant pain relief.[1,61] In another study, a long-term reduction in total morphine dose of 23% was noted when comparing intrathecal opioid plus local anesthetic administration to intrathecal opioid alone.[1,62] Two other reviews concluded that intrathecal delivery systems resulted in improvements for 30% to 56% of patients with better than 50% pain relief and function.[1,63]

None of these studies is a randomized controlled trial (RCT) and side effects can be formidable, including urinary retention, constipation, equipment malfunction, and catheter tip granulomas.[1] Therefore, intrathecal infusion can be recommended only when all other viable options have failed and side effects from oral medications have become intolerable.[1] Psychological evaluation and a trial with a temporary catheter are recommended before permanent implantation to assure effectiveness. Some patients may be unresponsive to intrathecal opioids if they have had to escalate their oral opioids because of tachyphylaxis.[1]

SCS has become a regularly used treatment of refractory FBSS. The proposed mechanism of action is via the gate control theory and modulation of neurotransmitter release in the dorsal horn.[63] A subcutaneously buried pulse generator is connected to electrodes placed in the epidural space over the dorsal columns and the location, frequency, and intensity of the electrical stimulation is adjusted to provide coverage to the painful area(s).[1,8,63] Results are considered better for radicular/neuropathic pain than axial/somatic/nociceptive pain.[1]

Several randomized controlled studies have influenced the upsurge in popularity for this modality. North and colleagues[64] have published data based on self-reported pain relief along with patient satisfaction comparing SCS with reoperation for FBSS.[2,65] The overall conclusion is that SCS is more successful than reoperation.[64] The total number of patients was 60 with cohorts of 30 in each arm of this RCT. What makes these data compelling is that the follow-up data extend to approximately 3 years and there was significant crossover to the SCS group from the revision surgery group.

Prospective Randomized Controlled Multicenter Trial of the Effectiveness of Spinal Cord Stimulation (PROCESS) compared SCS in conjunction with conventional medical management (CMM) to CMM alone. The population size was 100 patients and an outcome measure of greater than 50% pain relief was followed at 6, 12, and 24 months. Both groups showed improvement but the difference is noteworthy: 48% for the SCS group versus 18% for the CMM group. A 32% complication rate was also noted, however, in the SCS group at 6 months.[66] Relatively low morbidity complications can occur after implantation. These may necessitate explantation and reimplantation and include local wound infection, pain at the generator site or subcutaneously burrowed lead tract, and paddle or lead migration.[67]

Higher morbidity complications that may be associated with the initial implantation itself include wet tap with spinal headache, total spinal block due subarachnoid injection, local anesthetic toxicity, epidural hematoma, midline or generator pocket seromas, and subsequent epidural abscess.[63,67] Relative contraindications to SCS trial and placement include inability to pass the leads past scar tissue or scoliosis; untreated infection; presence of a cardioverter, defibrillator, or cardiac pacemaker; anticoagulation; and antiplatelet therapy. Absolute contraindications to implantation include pregnancy, previous dorsal root entry zone lesions, critical central stenosis along the lead pathway, serious neurologic deficit with surgically correctable pathology, anatomic spine instability at risk for progression, coagulopathy or immunosuppression, requirement for therapeutic diathermy, substance abuse, and severe cognitive impairment or failed psychological screening.[63] The need for future MRI is also listed as an absolute contraindication[63] and should be considered carefully in the decision-making process leading up to SCS implantation, especially in younger patients, given the likelihood of developing adjacent level disease over the course of a normal lifetime.

One of the factors leading to the increase in popularity of SCS in community settings is that it is considered cost effective, based on prospective modeling and assuming that the benefit is maintained over the lifetime.[68,69] Kumar and colleagues[69] noted in 2002 that 9 patients (15%) from the treatment group who received SCS plus CMM returned to some form of gainful employment compared with none of the patients in the control group, who received CMM alone. The average cost of drug therapy for pain (in Canadian dollars) was also noted to decrease from $78.00/month to $25.00/month after SCS implantation, whereas the average cost remained higher at $72.00/month over 5 years for the control group. Projected long-term modeling assigning economic quality-of-life cost values has also been performed in both Canada[65] and the United Kingdom,[2] with cost savings purported as an alternative to CMM or repeat surgery.

Two studies from the University of Washington, however, with a cohort of 51 workers' compensation patients,[70,71] question both the effectiveness and cost savings of SCS versus usual care (UC) or pain clinic care (PC). The investigators concluded that few patients in any group achieved success at follow-up with respect to less daily opioid use or improvement in leg pain and function. At 6 months, the SCS group showed modest improvement in leg pain and function but higher rates of opioid use, and by 12 months, these differences disappeared. In addition, 19% of the SCS group had their stimulators removed by 18 months and complications were noted with both trial and permanent implantations. The follow-up cost-effectiveness study maintained that the high cost of SCS was not counterbalanced by lower costs of subsequent care.[70,71] The median cost for the SCS group in US dollars was $52,091, which was $17,291 higher than the PC group and $28,128 higher than the UC group.[70,71]

Reconciling these disparities is not easy. The Kumar and North studies are randomized controlled studies with mixed population bases and were managed in university clinics. The University of Washington studies are population-based cohort studies and consisted of only workers' compensation patients from community referrals with community-based management and telephone questionnaire follow-up. Ostensibly, these were higher-risk patients without as tight monitoring. Finally, all the patients in the Kumar and North studies underwent preimplantation psychological screening and only 25% of the University of Washington patients did so. Consequently, Kumar and North conceivably screened out patients who would have failed prior to implantation, thereby contributing to better outcomes. All these studies evidenced significant complication rates and the cohort groups are remarkably small, suggesting that the issues surrounding cost benefit are far from settled and that the increasing use of this modality for FBSS needs to be reassessed over time.

Currently, approximately 20,000 spinal cord stimulators per year are placed in the United States.[72] Since introduced in the 1967 as a salvage procedure for refractory debilitating pain,[8] its use is becoming widespread in community settings. At present, it is not clear whether best practice guidelines for implantation are adhered to and what the ultimate impact of this procedure on FBSS outcomes will be. Reliance on preimplantation psychological testing prior to stimulator implantation has not changed the significant rate of stimulator removal or failure rates seen in these studies.

A final disconcerting issue regarding the literature for SCS, and probably all interventional procedures for FBSS, is that many of the data are dependent on patient self-reporting of pain scales. The modest incremental changes in opioid use, the minimal return to work rate, and the statistically significant but not dramatic changes in disability scales and depression scales pose the question of whether the right questions are asked clinically both before and after initial spine surgeries.

THE RATIONALE FOR A GLOBAL APPROACH

Kelly and colleagues[73] noted that "while subjective self-report assessment is vital in providing patientcentered opinion on treatment success, objective outcome measures are necessary to supplement these findings and quantify change." Their publication reviewed multiple studies with respect to patient self-reports and measurable functional scales and concluded that most were level C evidence studies and, consequently, generalizations to large diagnostic groups must be interpreted with reservation. The lack of consistency between clinical observation and patient self-reporting has to be reconciled if the pain literature is meaningful. Supporting addenda to this article offer a summary of validated instruments for self-reporting as well as objective outcome measures of physical function that are available today.[73]

The problem with these instruments is that time constraints preclude their use in a nonresearch setting. Another problem is that there is less control of patient follow-through, and, in general, communication between clinicians is not well integrated in community settings. In addition, each clinician has a different vantage point: surgeons see a structural problem to be corrected; physical therapists see motor function and flexibility issues to address; manual medicine practitioners see motion barriers to remove; interventionalists see inflammatory cycles or pain patterns that need to be interrupted; and psychotherapists see anxiety and perceptual issues that undermine care. All have legitimate concerns.

Interventional and pharmacologic treatments are based on narrow disease/impairment models where patients are recipients of passive care.[74] FBSS, like most presurgical low back pain, is a biopsychosocial phenomenon. Cost mitigation and clinical success have to be predicated on functional outcomes and specific goal setting, not just reported pain alleviation. Complete pain relief is not often possible either before or after surgery. Rehabilitation strategies must be individualized to improve physical function and reduce disability in the context of daily activities because improved physical function is linked to improved psychosocial function and mood.[74] The overall goal is to interrupt the cycle of pain, guarding, anxiety, disuse atrophy, and deactivation commonly seen with these patients.[74]

FBSS is a challenge to treat because there are multiple physical and psychosocial problems that have to be addressed. It is the prototypical chronic pain syndrome. It is poorly defined anatomically and there is significant overlap of the types of pain presentations. There is a disproportionate emphasis in the medical literature regarding drug, interventional, and surgical treatments and these options clearly have the most corporate support for research.

Interdisciplinary approaches have been shown to achieve clinical and cost-effective improvements in patient function,[24,38,40,75] but they are perceived as costly. The Commission on Accreditation of Rehabilitation Facilities (CARF) recognizes and accredits outpatient interdisciplinary programs where different disciplines collaborate. Evaluation, goal setting, and treatment are all monitored as part of these programs and are much less costly than the traditional inpatient/outpatient centers of the 1980s. But they are few and far between.

The author has an affiliation with the only CARF-accredited interdisciplinary pain center within an approximately 100-mile radius of Cincinnati. The cost for this individually tailored 20-day outpatient program, including physical therapy, occupational therapy, and psychological support, is approximately $15,000 (Pain Solutions Network, personal communication, 2013). This is similar to the cost for a single-level laminectomy not requiring a hospital stay and is substantially less costly than the direct costs for lumbar fusion when hospital, hardware, surgeon, and anesthesia costs are added up.

As a chronic pain syndrome, FBSS demands a global set of clinical skills that is different from that needed for the evaluation and management of acute pain. Most therapies and interventions described in the medical literature are discussed with respect to back pain treatment and do not distinguish between presurgical or postoperative care. It is important that the evaluating physician evaluate the physiology and physical limitations of the back problem and not just the imaging. Treatment becomes dangerous when it is overly influenced by symptoms that are magnified by the prospect of job loss, the expectation of a perfect cure, or other psychosocial issues. A global evaluation of a patient's life situation and a discussion of the morbidities associated with potential interventions are required, along with specific goal setting during every stage of treatment. A more appropriate question for patients is not, How is your pain on a 1 to 10 scale? but rather, What is your pain preventing you from doing?

Many clinicians and patients have a perception that if there is an abnormal imaging study associated with persistent back pain and radiculopathy, it requires a surgical evaluation. The rate of spine surgery in the United States is double that of Australia, Canada, and Finland and 5 times the rate of spine surgery performed in the United Kingdom.[1,76] Population-based outcomes are not very different. One study found that in the state of Maine, the best results from spine surgery (pain and function) occurred in the areas with the lowest surgical rates and the worst outcomes occurred in areas with high surgical rates.[1,77] Most back pain patients do not require surgery. Similarly, cost constraints should not preclude an interdisciplinary pain program trial, if elective fusion surgery is being planned without clear-cut indications—especially for predominantly axial low back pain, given that the occurrence of FBSS in this population is between 30% and 46%.[1]

Prevention of FBSS requires setting clear expectations of what a proposed surgery offers:

- The kind of pain relief to expect—whether axial or radicular
- The expected healing time and reconditioning needs
- Activity limitations or work restrictions, along with their expected duration

In addition, some form of psychological assessment and treatment or vocational counseling should be offered both prior to and after surgery, if the expected outcome is not full return of function.

Multiple reviews of the literature have demonstrated that FBSS is ill defined and difficult to manage. In 1997, 317,000 lumbar surgeries were performed in the United States with a cost of $4.8 billion for the surgeries alone.[1] In 2002, there were more than 1 million spine procedures performed in the United States and 400,000 were instrumented.[1] Between 1990 and 2010, there was a 220% increase in the number of spinal fusions performed with no demonstrated increase in efficacy.[4] The increasingly large influence of the cost of fusion surgery on total cost of care is reflected by the $16 billion for hospital charges alone that occurred with spinal fusions in the United States by 2004.[1]

Similarly, between 1994 and 2001, Medicare data revealed a 271% increase in the number of epidural injections and a 231% increase in the number of facet interventions performed in the United States without a concordant increase in the health status for Medicare low back patients demonstrated.[50] Virtually every review of the literature regarding spine surgery and interventional procedures demonstrates significant treatment failures of approximately 30%. It should be clear that thinking about back pain and FBSS, in particular, is too parsimonious and that a more global approach is necessary.

In summary, there are several generalizations that can be made regarding pitfalls to avoid in the treatment of FBSS:

- First, interventional procedures should only be used to control flares of pain, returning patients to preinjection baselines; to allow them to partake in restorative physical therapy; or as diagnostic measures that may guide other treatments.
- Second, the role of pharmacotherapy can be expected to change because of increased recognition of opioid-induced hyperalgesia and the regulatory climate surrounding opioids.
- Third, although no specific physical therapy recommendations can be universal, it is clear that the complications of immobility and deactivation make restoration of function imperative.
- Finally, medical education is going to have to be broadened so that physicians learn to focus on functional performance and avoid assigning importance to terms that are diagnostically ambiguous, such as degenerative disk disease, or assigning significance to MRI findings without confirming correlation to pain complaints, loss of motor function, or bowel and bladder instability.

REFERENCES

1. Chan C, Peng P. Failed back surgery syndrome. Pain Med 2011;12:577–606.
2. Taylor R, Ryan J, ODonnell R, et al. The cost effectiveness of spinal cord stimulation in the treatment of failed back surgery syndrome. Clin J Pain 2010;26: 463–9.

3. Grossman RG, Loftus CM, editors. Priniciples of neurosurgery. 2nd edition. Philadelphia: Lippincott- Raven; 1999. p. 422–30.
4. Taylor RS, Taylor RJ. The economic impact of failed back surgery syndrome. British Journal of Pain 2012;6:174–81.
5. Asch HL, Lewis PJ, Moreland DB, et al. Prospective multiple outcomes of outpatient microdiscectomy: should 75-85% success rate be the norm? J Neurosurg 2002;96:34–44.
6. Peul WC, van Houwelingen HC, van den Hout WB, et al, The Hague Spine Intervention Prognostic Study Group. Surgery versus prolonged conservative treatment for sciatica. N Engl J Med 2007;356:2245–56.
7. Peul WC, van den Hout WB, Brand R, et al. Prolonged conservative care versus surgery in patients with sciatica caused by lumbar disc herniation: Two year results of a randomized control trial. BMJ 2008;336:1355–8.
8. Hussain A, Erdek M. Interventional pain management for failed back surgery syndrome. Pain Pract 2013;14(1):1–12.
9. Amundsen T, Weber H, Nordal H, et al. Lumbar spinal stenosis: conservative or surgical management? A prospective 10-year study. Spine 2000;25:1424–36.
10. Weinstein JN, Lurie JD, Tosteson TD, et al. Surgical versus non-surgical treatment for lumbar degenerative spondylolisthesis. N Engl J Med 2007;356:2257–70.
11. Weinstein JN, Tosteson TD, Lurie JD, et al, SPORT Investigators. Surgical versus non-surgical lumbar spinal stenosis. N Engl J Med 2008;358:794–810.
12. Fokter SK, Yerby SA. Patient based outcomes for the operative treatment of degenerative lumbar spinal stenosis. Eur Spine J 2006;15:1661–9.
13. Herrara HI, Moreno de la Presa R, Gutierrez RG, et al. Evaluacion de la columna lumbar posquirurgica. [Evaluation of the postoperative lumbar spine]. Radiologia 2013;55:12–23.
14. Fritch EW, Heisel J, Rupp S. The failed back surgery syndrome-reasons, intraoperative findings and longterm results: a report of 182 operative treatments. Spine 1996;21:626–33.
15. Kumar MN, Baklanov A, Chopin D. Correlation between sagittal plane changes and adjacent level degneneration following lumbar spine fusion. Eur Spine J 2001;10:314–9.
16. Onesti ST. Failed back syndrome. Neurologist 2004;10:259–64.
17. Ivanov AA, Kiapour MS, Ebraheim NA, et al. Lumbar fusion leads to increases in angular motion and stress across sacroiliac joint. Spine 2009;34(5):E162–9.
18. Ross JS, Robertson JT, Frederickson RC, et al. Association between peridural scar and recurrent radicular pain after lumbar discectomy: magnetic resonance evaluation. Neurosurgery 1996;38:855–63.
19. Richardson C, Jull G, Hodges P, et al. Therapeutic exercise for spinal segmental stabilization in low back pain. London: Harcourt Publishers Limited; 1999. p. 11.
20. Spring H, Illi U, Kunz H, et al. Stretching and strengthening exercises. New York: Thieme Medical Publishers; 1991. p. 112–7.
21. Travell JG, Simons DG. Myofascial pain and dysfunction. The trigger point manual, vol. 2. Baltimore (MD): Williams and Wilkins; 1992.
22. Hong CZ, Simons DG. Mechanism of myofascial trigger point. Arch Phys Med Rehabil 1998;79:863–72.
23. Jones LH. Strain and counterstrain. (CO): The American Academy of Osteopathy. Colorado Springs; 1981.
24. Braddom RL. Physical medicine and rehabiltiation. 4th edition. Philadelphia: Elsevier Saunders; 2011. p. 412, 414: 935–69.

25. Delisa JA. Rehabilitation medicine priniciples and practice. 3rd edition. Philadelphia: Lippincott-Raven; 1998. p. 1442.
26. Bosscher HA, Heavner JE. The incidence o epidural fibrosis after back surgery: an endoscopic study. Pain Pract 2010;10:18–24.
27. Rabb CR. Failed back surgery and epidural fibrosis. Spine J 2010;10:454–5.
28. Kimura J. Electrodiagnosis in diseases of nerve and muscle: principles and practice. 3rd edition. New York: Oxford University Press; 2001. p. 640–1.
29. Zochodne DW. Diabetes mellitus and the peripheral nervous system: manifestations and mechanisms. Muscle Nerve 2007;36:144–56.
30. Chou R, Huffman LH. Medications for acute and chronic low back pain: a review of the evidence for an American Pain Society/American College of Physicians Clinical Practice Guideline. Ann Intern Med 2007;147:505–14.
31. Noble M, Treadwell JR, Tregear SJ, et al. Long-term opioid management for chronic noncancer pain. Cochrane Database Syst Rev 2010;(20):CD006605.
32. Schnitzer TJ, Gray WL, Paster RZ, et al. Efficacy of tramadol in treatment of chronic low back pain. J Rheumatol 2000;27:772–8.
33. Martell BA, O'Connor PG, Kerns RD, et al. Systematic review: opioid treatment for chronic back pain: prevalence, efficacy, and association with addiction. Ann Intern Med 2007;146:116–27.
34. Lennard TA. Pain procedures in clinical practice. 2nd edition. Philadelphia: Hanley and Belfus; 2000. p. 277–8.
35. Cohen SP, Hurley RW, Christo PJ, et al. Clinical predictors of success and failure for lumbar facet radiofrequency denervation. Clin J Pain 2007;23:45–52.
36. Klessinger S. Zygoapopysial joint pain in post lumbar surgery syndrome. The efficacy of medial branch blocks and radiofrequency neurotomy. Pain Med 2013;14:374–7.
37. Masala S, Nano G, Mammucari M, et al. Medial branch neurotomy in low back pain. Neuroradiology 2012;54:737–44.
38. Moseley L. Combined physiotherapy and education is efficacious for chronic low back pain. Aust J Physiother 2002;48:297–302.
39. Bystrom MG, Rassmussen-Barr E, Grooten WJ. Motor control exercises reduces pain and disability in chronic and recurrent low back pain: a meta-analysis. Spine 2013;38:E350–8.
40. Sanders H, Harden N, Vicente PJ. Evidence-based clinical practice guidelines for interdisciplinary rehabilitation of chronic nonmalignant pain syndrome patients. Pain Pract 2005;5:303–15.
41. Bicket MC, Gupta A, Brown CH, et al. Epidural injections for spinal pain: a systematic review and meta-analysis evaluating the "control" injections in randomized controlled trials. Anesthesiology 2013;119:907–31.
42. Rabinovitch DL, Peliowski A, Furlan AD. Influencw of lumbar epidural injection volume on pain relief for radicular leg pain and/or low back pain. Spine J 2009;9:509–17.
43. Manchikanti L, Singh V, Cash RT, et al. A comparative effectiveness evaluation of percutaneous adhesiolysis and epidural steroid injections in managing lumbar post surgery syndrome: a randomized controlled trial. Pain Physician 2009;12:E355–8.
44. Helm S, Benyamin RM, Chopra P, et al. Percutaneous adhesiolysis in the management of chronic low back pain in post lumbar surgery syndrome and spinal stenosis: a systematic review. Pain Physician 2012;15:E435–62.
45. Hayek S, Helm S, Benyamin RM, et al. Effectiveness of spinal endoscopic adhesiolyisis in post lumbar surgery syndrome: a systematic review. Pain Physician 2009;12:419–35.

46. Manchikanti L, Singh V, Cash KA, et al. Management of pain of post lumbar surgery syndrome: one- year results in a randomized, double-blind, active controlled trial of fluoroscopic caudal epidural injections. Pain Physician 2010;13:509–21.
47. Manchikanti L, Singh V, Cash KA, et al. Assessment of effectiveness of percutaneous adhesiolysis and caudal epidural injections in managing post lumbar surgery syndrome: 2-year follow-up of a randomized, controlled trial. J Pain Res 2012;5:597–608.
48. Takeshima N, Miyakawa H, Okuda K, et al. Evaluation of the therapeutic result of epiduroscopic adhesiolysis for failed back surgery syndrome. Br J Anaesth 2009;102:400–7.
49. Manchikanti L, Salahadin A, Atluri S, et al. An update of comprehensive evidenced-based guidelines for interventional techniques in chronic spinal pain. Part II: Guidance and recommendations. Pain Physician 2013;16:S49–283.
50. Chou R, Atlas S, Stanos S, et al. Nonsurgical interventional therapies for low back pain: a review of the American Pain Society clinical practice guideline. Spine 2009;34:1078–93.
51. Abdi S, Datta S, Lucas LF. Role of epidural steroids in the management of chronic spinal pain: A systematic review of effectiveness and complications. Pain Physician 2005;8:127–43.
52. Yoshihara H. Sacroiliac joint pain after lumbar/lumvosacral fusion:current knowledge. Eur Spine J 2012;21:1788–96.
53. Schwarzer AC, April CN, Bogduk N. The sacroiliac joint in chronic low back pain. Spine 1995;20:31–7.
54. Fenton DS, Cervionke LF. Image guided spine intervention. Philadelphia: Saunders; 2003. p. 127.
55. Dreyfuss P, Michaelson M, Pauza K, et al. The value of medical history and physical examination in diagnosing sacroiliac pain. Spine 1996;21:2594–602.
56. Potter NA, Rothstein JM. Intertester reliability for selected clinical tests of the SIJ. Phys Ther 1999;651:1671–5.
57. Cohen SP, Hurley RW, Buchenmeier CC 3rd, et al. Randomized placebo controlled study evaluating lateral branch radiofrequency denervation for sacroiliac joint pain. Anesthesiology 2008;109:279–88.
58. Ferrante FM, King LF, Roche EA, et al. Radiofrequency sacroiliac joint denervation for sacroiliac syndrome. Reg Anesth Pain Med 2001;26:137–42.
59. Gevargez A, Groenemeyer D, Schirp S, et al. CT guided percutaneous radiofrequency denervation of the sacroiliac joint. Eur Radiol 2002;12:1360–5.
60. Burnham RS, Yasui Y. An alternative method of radiofrequency neurotomy of the sacroiliac joint: a pilot study of the effect on pain, function, and satisfaction. Reg Anesth Pain Med 2007;32:12–9.
61. Winkelmuller M, Winkelmuller W. Long term effects of continuous intrathecal opioid treatment on chronic pain of non-malignant etiology. J Neurosurg 1996; 85:458–67.
62. Deer TR, Caraway DL, Kim CK, et al. Clinical experience with intrathecal bupivicaine with opioid treatment for the chronic pain related to failed back surgery syndrome and metastatic cancer pain of the spine. Spine J 2002;2:274–8.
63. Kreis PG, Fishman SM. Spinal cord stimulation percutaneous implantation techniques. New York: Oxford University Press; 1999. p. 3–5 preface. 13–8, 71–92, 115–9,131–45.
64. North RB, Farrokhi F, Piantadosi SA. Spinal cord stimulation versus repeated lumbosacral spone surgery for chronic pain: a randomized controlled trial. Neurosurgery 2005;56(1):98–106.

65. Kumar K, Rizvi S. Cost-effectiveness of spinal cord stimulation therapy in the management of chronic pain. Pain Med 2013;14:1–19.

66. Kumar K, Taylor RS, Jacques L, et al. Spinal cord stimulation versus conventional medical management for neuropathic pain: a multicentre randomized controlled trial in patients with failed back surgery syndrome. Pain 2007;132: 179–88.

67. Mekhail NA, Mathews M, Nageeb F, et al. Retrospective review of 707 cases of spinal cord stimulation: indications and complications. Pain Pract 2011;11: 148–53.

68. North RB, Kidd D, Shipley J, et al. Spinal cord stimulation versus reoperation for failed back surgery syndrome: a cost effectiveness and cost utility analysis based on a randomizred, controlled trial. Neurosurgery 2007;61:361–8.

69. Kumar K, Malik S, Demeria D. Treatment of chronic pain with spinal cord stimulation versus alternative therapies: cost-effectiveness analysis. Neurosurgery 2002;51:106–16.

70. Turner JA, Hollingsworth W, Comstock BA, et al. Spinal cord stimulation for failed back surgery syndrome: outcomes in a worker's compensation setting. Pain 2010;148:14–25.

71. Hollingsworth W, Turner JA, Welton NJ, et al. Costs and cost effectiveness of spinal cord stimulation (SCS) for failed back surgery syndrome. Spine 2011; 36:2076–83.

72. Celestin J, Edwards RR, Jamison RN. Pretreatment psychosocial variables as predictors of outcomes following lumbar surgery and spinal cord stimulation: a systematic review and literature synthesis. Pain Med 2009;10:639–53.

73. Kelly GA, Blake C, O'Keefe D, et al. The impact of spinal cord stimulation on physical function and sleep quality in individuals with failed back surgery syndrome: a systematic review. Eur J Pain 2012;16:793–802.

74. Harding VR, Simmonds MJ, Watson PJ. Physical therapy for chronic pain. Pain 1998;6(3):1–4.

75. Guzman J, Esmail R, Karjalainen K, et al. Multidisciplinary rehabilitation for chronic low back pain: systematic review. BMJ 2001;322:1511–6.

76. Cherkin DC, Deyo RA, Loeser JD, et al. An international comparison of back surgery rates. Spine 1994;19:1201–6.

77. Keller RB, Atlas SJ, Soule DN, et al. Relationship between rates and outcomes of operative treatment of lumbar disc herniation and spinal stenosis. J Bone Joint Surg Am 1999;81:752–62.

Diagnosis of Myofascial Pain Syndrome

Robert D. Gerwin, MD[a,b,*]

KEYWORDS

- Myofascial pain • Trigger points • Active trigger points • Latent trigger points
- Muscle • Referred pain • Diagnosis

KEY POINTS

- Myofascial pain is a common condition that occurs as a primary source of pain as well as a comorbid pain with other conditions.
- The source of pain in myofascial pain is the myofascial trigger point that is a small region of hardness and tenderness in a taut band of muscle.
- Many of the pain syndromes are caused by pain referred from the trigger point region.
- The diagnosis of myofascial pain in the clinical setting is best made by palpation of the trigger point, moving in a cross-fiber direction perpendicular to the direction of the fibers.
- Evaluation of the patient must include an assessment of those factors that either predispose the patient to the development of myofascial pain or that are comorbid with it.

INTRODUCTION

Myofascial pain (MP) is a widespread and universal cause of soft tissue pain. Physicians commonly overlook this condition because of lack of awareness and training but it is a relatively simple diagnosis. The central feature of MP syndrome (MPS) is the myofascial trigger point (MTrP), a very small, localized area of muscle contraction that is hard to the touch, and that is very tender. The trigger point is always located on a discrete band of hardness located within a muscle. The diagnosis of MPS is made by palpation of the MTrP.

FEATURES OF THE MTRP

The MTrP is always located on a tight or taut band of muscle. An MTrP that causes pain is always tender to palpation. When stimulated mechanically by palpation or by

---

Disclosure: The author reports no conflict of interest and nothing to disclose.
[a] Department of Neurology, Johns Hopkins University School of Medicine, Baltimore, MD, USA;
[b] Pain and Rehabilitation Medicine, 4405 East-West Highway, Suite 502, Bethesda, MD 20814, USA
* 7424 Hampden Lane, Bethesda, MD 20814.
E-mail address: gerwin@painpoints.com

Phys Med Rehabil Clin N Am 25 (2014) 341–355
http://dx.doi.org/10.1016/j.pmr.2014.01.011
1047-9651/14/$ – see front matter © 2014 Elsevier Inc. All rights reserved.

needling, it contracts sharply, referred to as local twitch response (LTR). The taut band limits stretch of a muscle and produces weakness that is rapidly reversed as the trigger point is inactivated. It can activate autonomic activity, such as vasodilation or constriction, goose bumps, or piloerection (**Box 1**).

The MTrP, like other physical sources of chronic pain, refers pain to distant sites and leads to central nervous system sensitization. Central sensitization results in a lower pain threshold and in tenderness, and in an expansion of painful areas, including an increase in MTrPs. MTrPs can be spontaneously painful (so-called "active" MTrPs) or they can be nascent or quiescent (so-called "latent" MTrPs), inactive until physical activity converts them to active MTrPs.

Diagnosis

The diagnosis of MPS is based on a pertinent history and physical examination. Objective means of identifying the MTrP exist, but are generally not used in clinical practice because they are costly, time-consuming, and are not available to most practitioners. Now that high-definition ultrasound (HDUS) is more widely available, there is interest in using it to guide the practitioner in performing injection or deep dry needling of difficult muscles using HDUS guidance.[1] The experienced hand is faster and quite adequate at identifying the site to be needled.

History

MP can be acute pain or chronic muscle pain. The nature of the pain in both cases is dull, deep, aching, and poorly localized. It is rarely sharp and stabbing, although acute episodes of stabbing pain can occur, even on a background of chronic pain. It mimics radicular or visceral pain. Somatic pain from trigger points in the abdomen, for example, can feel like irritable bowel, bladder pain, or endometrial pain. Trigger points in the gluteus minimus muscle refer pain down the side and back of the leg, like L5 or S1 radicular pain. It can be accompanied by a sensory component of paresthesias or dyesthesias but does not present in this manner. Paresthesias, such as tingling, when present, are generally distributed in the dermatome of the nerve root(s) innervating the muscle harboring the relevant trigger point. Pain is often experienced as referred to other regions, such as the head, the neck, or the hip, as referred pain (RP). MP can also be the presenting symptom for radiculopathy, or major joint pain (shoulder or hip). MPS persists long after the initiating cause of pain has resolved. Hence, the story of a remote injury can be relevant.

Box 1
Features of the myofascial trigger point: the first 3 are essential for diagnosis; the last 5 are not required to make a diagnosis

1. Taut band within the muscle

2. Exquisite tenderness at a point on the taut band

3. Reproduction of the patient's pain

4. Local twitch response

5. Referred pain

6. Weakness

7. Restricted range of motion

8. Autonomic signs (skin warmth or erythema, tearing, piloerection [goose-bumps])

Thus, the onset of the pain, the regions involved, the timing and pace of progression, and the quality of the pain, are important elements of the history. In addition, there are certain predisposing factors that make MP more likely to occur. These include iron deficiency (most commonly caused by menstrual blood loss in women, but also from dietary insufficiency), hypothyroidism, and deficiency of vitamin D or B12. Lyme disease, hypermobility, and spondylosis also predispose to the development of MP. Parasitic infections can manifest as widespread trigger point pain. Questions about travel and backpacking are therefore relevant as well.

Physical Examination

The diagnosis of MPS is made by the identification of an MTrP and relating it to the patient's pain complaint (**Box 2**). A MTrP is identified by palpation. The MTrP is characterized by the presence of a taut band palpable within muscle. The taut band can be palpated in almost every muscle, with some initial guidance and practice. It is also tender when it is the immediate cause of the patient's pain. Thus, MTrP-containing muscle has a heterogeneous feel of hard and soft areas, rather than a homogeneous uniform consistency. The intense contraction of the trigger point results in a sensory phenomenon of localized, exquisite pain that is always associated with the taut band. Moreover, some taut bands are not painful to palpation, but have functional consequences, such as altering the normal sequence of muscle activation.[2] The taut band must be palpated cross-fiber, that is, perpendicular to the direction of the muscle fiber. The direction of muscle fiber may not be obvious, especially in pectoral muscles, the infraspinatus muscle, and the gluteal muscles.

Palpating the Taut Band

An MTrP is always palpated perpendicular to the direction of the muscle fiber so as to detect the taut band. Palpation overlying a firm or bony structure is palpated by compressing the muscle against it (**Fig. 1**). When the muscle can be grasped between the fingers, the muscle is palpated by a pincer grip with the thumb and the index and long fingers (**Fig. 2**). When a taut band is identified, the examining fingers move along the band to identify the small region of greatest hardness, the area of least compliance to compression. It is this area that is most tender. This is the center or heart of the trigger point. Stimulation of this area induces RP. It is in this area that mechanical stimulation elicits the LTR. The farther away stimulation is from this center, the more difficult it is to elicit RP and the LTR, until they cannot be elicited at all.[3] The LTR cannot be elicited at all when the taut band is stimulated 3 cm or more from the trigger point zone. The

---

Box 2
Procedure for identifying trigger points

1. History and pain diagram: the history identifies the areas affected by pain

2. Examination of muscles whose trigger points can refer pain to the affected areas

3. Palpate the muscle for taut bands, using either flat palpation or pincer palpation

4. Move the fingers along the taut band to find the hardest and most tender spot (the trigger point)

5. Compress the trigger point manually and ask (1) if the spot is tender or painful, and if so, (2) does the pain resemble the patient's usual pain

6. Compress the trigger point for 5–10 seconds and then ask if there is pain or some sensation away from the trigger point (referred pain)

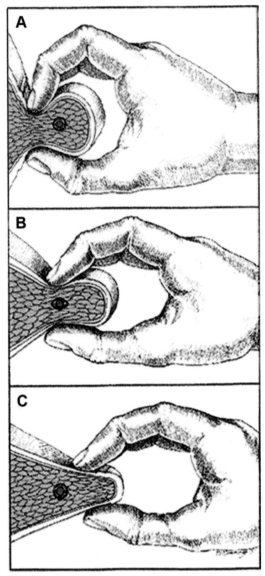

Fig. 1. (A–C) The palpating finger rolls over a trigger point taut band. Flat palpation compresses the trigger point between the skin and an underlying hard, bony structure. Palpation is always perpendicular to the direction of the fiber. (*From* Simons DG, Travell JG, Simons LS. Travell & Simons' Myofascial Pain and Dysfunction: The Trigger Point Manual, 2nd ed. Philadelphia: Lippincott Williams & Wilkins, 1996; with permission.)

importance of locating the area of greatest hardness in the taut band, which is the area of greatest tenderness, is that this is the area that is to be treated. Compression of the trigger zone for 5 to 10 seconds can induce referred pain, or pain that is at a distance from the point of stimulation because RP represents central activation or central sensitization. It requires activation of interneurons and spreads rostrally and caudally in the spinal cord, which does not occur instantaneously. Hence, 5 to 10 seconds of

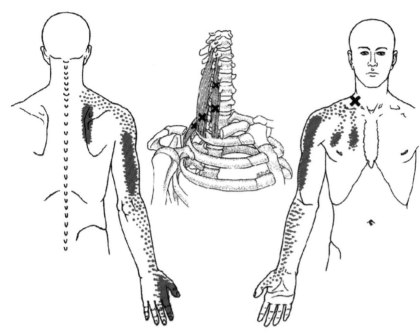

Fig. 2. An example of referred pain, in this case from trigger points in the anterior scalene muscle. (*From* Simons DG, Travell JG, Simons LS. Travell & Simons' Myofascial Pain and Dysfunction: The Trigger Point Manual, 2nd ed. Philadelphia: Lippincott Williams & Wilkins, 1996; with permission.)

compression is needed to be certain that the palpated MTrP induces RP. Once the MTrP is identified, determined to be tender, and RP is confirmed, the patient is asked if the pain or tenderness, local or referred, reproduces or is like all or part of his or her usual pain. That relates a particular MTrP to a patient's complaint. Identifying an MTrP that is related to the presenting or another complaint aids in determining which trigger points need to be treated and in what order.

A tender trigger point is an indication that there is hyperalgesia or allodynia. Pain at the MTrP is due to the release of neuropeptides, cytokines, and inflammatory substances, such as substance P, calcitonin gene–related peptide, interleukin-1α, and bradykinin,[4] and protons that create local acidity. Models for *acute* muscle pain have been developed and have yielded information about the generation of local and referred pain.[5] However, most clinically relevant muscular pain syndromes last far longer than the conditions studied in animals or humans under laboratory conditions. Therefore, there is great interest in studying longer-lasting and chronic pain in humans.

Taut Bands

A taut band does not need to be tender because MTrPs are dynamic, being quiescent (when they do not cause pain) or resolve with rest, massage, or stretch. They are activated with movement or action, including psychological stress. When they are quiescent, the MTrP does not reproduce pain (ie, spontaneously cause pain), but that was nonetheless tender to palpation. A taut band that is not tender to palpation will not, of course, reproduce pain unless it does so by causing RP. Such taut bands restrict movement because taut bands are not innocuous with deleterious functional effects.

Lucas and colleagues[2] have shown a latent MTrP disrupts the normal sequence of muscle activation. They can activate central effects, such as decreasing the threshold for pain activation distally.[6,7] They limit muscle lengthening and have a role in activating other MTrPs. Hence, determination of treatment is to be made to treating taut bands, whether latent or not. The decision requires a judgment about whether a taut band is clinically relevant or not. This is not always clear and, therefore, the taut band may be treated more often than not.

Additional Trigger Point Characteristics

LTR is elicited by mechanical stimulation of the taut band causing local contraction. This is differentiated from a Golgi tendon reflex, which involves contraction of an entire muscle in response to stretch. The LTR is a brief (25–250 ms), high-amplitude, polyphasic electrical discharge. The discharge is attenuated when the stimulation is remote from the trigger zone. The twitch response is dependent on an intact spinal cord reflex arc. Severing the peripheral nerve completely abolishes the local twitch response, whereas transecting the spinal cord does not abolish the twitch response.[8] Thus, the local twitch response is mediated through the spinal cord, and is not affected by supraspinal influences. The twitch response is unique to the MTrP and is not seen in healthy muscle.

Referred Pain

RP represents spread through a central nervous system that has been activated (ie, spread that is facilitated by central sensitization).[5] It is most common in the distribution of the nerve innervating the muscle with the trigger point being activated. Thus, a trigger point arising in the infraspinatus muscle, primarily innervated by the C5 nerve root, tends to refer pain to other C5-innervated muscles, with a spillover to C4 and C6 innervated muscles. The primary referral patterns reflect the arborization and spread of incoming first-order neuronal axons within the spinal cord. The nociceptive spread or arborization of incoming axons is far greater than that of touch and position sense. Hence, there is the potential for greater spread of pain than for perception of touch. Moreover, as incoming nociceptive impulses become more intense and the duration of central nociceptive neurons becomes longer, central sensitization results in a greater extent of increased synaptic efficacy through more distant spinal segments, a result of the neuroplastic changes that accompany central sensitization and RP encompasses ever far-reaching parts of the body. RP can be felt over many spinal cord segments, and in extreme cases can appear to be bizarre and body wide. MTrP points in the ventral (anterior) trunk muscles can even refer to the dorsal (posterior or back) muscles.

Limited Range of Motion

Limited range of motion (ROM) is due to pain on lengthening a muscle harboring an MTrP and to the limitations imposed by the shortened taut band. ROM testing can be misleading because of the potential multiple pathologies that can limit motion about a joint, and, additionally, normal ROM is variable depending on the individual, such as hypermobile individuals.

Examination of ROM can be a useful clue in determining which muscles harbor trigger points. Limited rotation of the head and neck to the left can implicate the left sternocleidomastoid and/or trapezius muscles, or the right splenius cervicis and oblique capitis inferior muscles, all muscles that have to lengthen to accomplish this movement. An additional limitation of head and neck side bending right would focus attention on the left sternocleidomastoid and trapezius muscles.

WEAKNESS

Weakness is often but not always evident in a muscle harboring a trigger point. Weakness in affected muscles is rapidly reversed as the trigger point is inactivated. Hence, weakness does not represent a neuropathic or myopathic process, but appears to be a form of muscle inhibition that may be central. This phenomenon has not been well studied.

AUTONOMIC CHANGES

Vascular dilation and constriction occur as a result of autonomic nervous system activation, resulting in erythema or blanching, and warm or cool areas usually in the distribution of the nerve innervating an affected muscle.

Diagnostic Criteria

There is some debate in the literature as to what is needed to diagnose an MTrP (and hence, diagnose MPS). Articles often state that the diagnosis of MP is made using the criteria of Simons and colleagues.[9] Simons and colleagues[9] described at least 7 features of the trigger point: (1) taut band, (2) exquisite tenderness on the taut band, (3) reproduction of pain, (4) local twitch response, (5) restricted ROM, (6) autonomic symptoms, and (7) RP. To this is often added a nodular hardness at the trigger point. Not all features described are present at any one time, and not all are necessary to identify a trigger point and make a diagnosis. This question has not been answered definitively at this time, but the presence of a taut band that is tender and that reproduces the patient's pain complaint in full or in part is sufficient to base a treatment program. These criteria, a tender, taut band that reproduces the patient's pain, allow the clinician to select a trigger point for treatment. The proof of efficacy is that treatment based on these criteria alone is sufficient to reduce or eliminate pain, which is our experience, although there has not been a study confirming this.

One can ask if identification of a taut band is enough to make a diagnosis. However, to diagnose a pain syndrome, one must have pain, so that it makes sense that tenderness or pain must be elicited by examination so as to diagnosis MPS. However, a nontender taut band should be treated in a patient with trigger point pain syndrome when it is likely to have significant clinical effects, like restricting motion or producing weakness.

There are a number of studies that have shown inter-rater reliability of the physical examination of an MTrP, starting with the study by Gerwin and colleagues.[10] Subsequent studies were more sophisticated and showed that clinicians could agree on the identification of the same trigger point, not just the muscle(s) that harbored MTrPs. Sciotti and colleagues[11] showed that examiners could independently identify the same taut band region. Interrater reliability of MTrP palpation in shoulder muscles was demonstrated by Bron and colleagues.[12]

A number of reviews have been published questioning the data and purporting to show that physical examination is not reliable, but these reviews show a fundamental lack of understanding of the anatomy and physiology of the MTrP, which biases the author's conclusions. For example, one such review discounted a number of positive studies because the investigators did not specify that they looked for a "nodule" in the taut band, a feature they said was mentioned as essential by MP "experts."[13] In fact, "all" the experts they were referring to turned out to be Dr David Simons. Simons[9] was referring to the area of tender hardness on the taut band. One has to identify the taut band and to elicit tenderness, but there is no need to identify the region as nodular rather than linear to make a diagnosis. Simons never made a point that identifying a nodularity in the taut band was necessary for identifying a trigger point. The MTrP may simply be described as a sense of swelling, but often all that the palpating finger feels is hardness on the taut band.

Diagnostic Inactivation of the Trigger Point

An active MTrP is symptomatic and can be assessed for a particular complaint of pain, like headache pain or shoulder or low-back pain. Reproduction of the patient's pain complaint is important in determining if a particular trigger point is clinically significant. When there is doubt about the clinical significance of a particular trigger point, it can be inactivated either manually, by using a laser, by deep dry needling, or by a trigger point injection. An immediate (with 2–3 minutes) unequivocal decrease in pain is good evidence that the MTrP in question is clinically relevant. Sometimes the relief of pain can be dramatic, as in piriformis syndrome, and readily leads to an effective treatment plan (**Box 3**).

OBJECTIVE IDENTIFICATION OF TRIGGER POINTS

Identification of the taut band is now possible with a number of objective techniques. The taut band and the twitch response can be visualized by ultrasound.[14–16] Newer ultrasound devices produce high-resolution images of the taut band, and may be

---

Box 3
Case history: myofascial syndrome or pinched nerve?

History: A 56-year-old woman complained of pain in the right leg 6 months after lumbar spine surgery to remove a herniated disc and decompress an S1 nerve root. She had continued pain after surgery with no period of decreased pain. Pain was down the outside of the leg to the dorsum of the foot. Her pain was the same after surgery as it was before surgery. Her preoperative imaging studies showed a right-sided L5–S1disc herniation. The postoperative study showed the same herniated disc findings.

Examination: She could not bear weight on the right leg. She came down the hall on a walker, not stepping on the right leg. She had moderately full low-back flexion, limited extension. She had to use her hands to lift the right leg onto the examination table. She had full straight leg raising with pain on the right side, but only to the buttock, not felt in the back; normal 2+ knee and ankle reflexes; there was no sensory loss. Right leg strength could not be assessed because of pain. Examination of the right buttock musculature showed linear hardness and tenderness (increased resistance to palpation) over the right piriformis muscle.

Diagnostic test: A diagnostic inactivation of the piriformis muscle with a trigger point injection using lidocaine 0.25% resulted in a marked decrease in pain within 1–2 minutes. She was able to get off the examination table on her own and walked out of the office without assistance. Pain relief lasted 30 minutes.

Outcome: She was treated with deep dry needling of the piriformis trigger point twice weekly for 6 weeks, by which time she was free of pain, ambulating normally. There was no recurrence for the remaining 10 years of her life.

Comment: The diagnosis of piriformis muscle trigger point was suspected by the history. That she did not have any improvement after surgery suggests that the trigger point was symptomatic at that time. The referral of pain down the leg in a sciatic nerve distribution is consistent with entrapment of the sciatic nerve, peroneal branch, otherwise known as a piriformis muscle syndrome. The dramatic reversal of pain with release of the trigger point by lidocaine injection was highly suggested of a piriformis syndrome. The outcome after treatment confirmed the diagnosis. It is not possible to tell if a component of her pain came from an S1 nerve root compression that was relieved by surgery.

useful in future research studies of the MTrP. MTrPs can also be identified by magnetic resonance imaging.

Magnetic Resonance Elastography

Magnetic resonance elastography is a new technique that can differentiate tissues of varying densities. The technique involves using phase contrast to identify tissue distortion when cyclic energy waves like vibration are introduced into the muscle. Shear waves travel more rapidly in stiffer tissues. The harder taut band can be distinguished from the surrounding normal muscle by this technique.[17,18] MR elastography will likely emerge as an effective tool for the identification of the MTrP's taut band.

Ultrasound

The combination of vibration sonoelastography with ultrasound imaging localizes hypoechoic, elliptical, focal areas that corresponded to a palpable trigger point nodule in the trapezius muscle.[15] The trigger point taut band can be imaged in latent and active trigger points. A nonsymptomatic trigger point has not been systematically sought, although changes in "normal muscle" that may represent such taut bands may be seen. A reversal of capillary flow that most likely represents shunting of blood away from an area of trigger point–induced vascular compression has also been shown by ultrasound sonoelastography.[19]

Thus, there are a number of ways in which trigger points can be imaged objectively. The practical application of these approaches is just beginning to be explored, like ultrasound guidance of the needle when treating a deep muscle like the psoas muscle. Computerized tomography and electromyographic localization of the trigger point are presently available for guidance in trigger point needling, but rarely used. Ultrasound localization of the trigger point for needling guidance is presently being evaluated, and may be useful for muscles that are difficult to palpate. These techniques have already confirmed beyond a doubt the existence of the MTrP that previously was identifiable only by palpation.

ELECTROMYOGRAPHY

Hubbard and Berkoff[20] described a signature electromyographic signal associated with the trigger point as a persistent, low-amplitude, high-frequency discharge found at the MTrP region in active MTrP. This activity, which initially came to be known as spontaneous electrical activity (SEA), is associated with the MTrP region.[21,22] As the recording electrode is moved away from the trigger zone, the SEA diminishes. Likewise, the SEA diminishes as the needle is placed outside the taut band.[3] A needle placed 1 cm away from the trigger zone and outside the taut band does not display SEA.[20]

The electrical activity associated with the trigger point most likely arises from the motor endplate,[9] and has been named endplate noise by Simons.[23] There has been controversy about the nature of this electrical activity, but the low-amplitude, constant discharges are consistent with the small, monophasic negative waveform of less than 50 μV called miniature endplate potentials (MEPPs). The higher-amplitude waveforms seen only in active trigger point zones are consistent with endplate spikes.[24] MEPPs are thought to be the result of spontaneous release of acetylcholine from motor nerve potentials. Botulinum toxin reduces the endplate noise in rabbit myofascial trigger points, supporting the postulated role of acetylcholine release from the motor nerve terminal in the generation of endplate noise.[25] The low-amplitude activity is thought to be the result of the release of acetylcholine sufficient only to generate subthreshold endplate depolarization in close proximity to the electrode. The endplate spike of several hundred microvolts' amplitude represents temporal summation of MEPP sufficient to reach or exceed the membrane threshold value.[24] The studies by Hubbard and Berkoff,[20] and subsequently others, compared the spontaneous electrical activity at the trigger zone with a control point a centimeter or so away from the index electrode. The absence of electrical activity at the control electrode confirms the lack of anterior horn cell motor action potentials and therefore establishes the resting state of the muscle. Endplate noise is 5 times more frequent in endplate zones in the trigger point than in endplate regions outside the trigger point zone and the taut band.[21]

Endplate noise intensity is directly correlated with the degree of trigger point irritability as measured by pressure pain threshold.[26] Thus, motor endplate activity is greater in active, spontaneously painful trigger points, than in latent trigger points. Greater endplate activity and consequently greater focal muscle sarcomere compression can be thought of as being associated with greater local muscle injury and local release of nociceptive substances.

Hence, endplate noise is now well described as an electrical phenomenon unique to the trigger point. Nevertheless, electromyography is not used for the clinical identification of trigger points because it is not readily available to many clinicians treating trigger points, it is costly, and it is a far less efficient way to identify MTrPs than palpation. One can examine the entire body for trigger points in minutes, something that is not feasible by any laboratory means of detecting MTrPs.

LABORATORY

Laboratory studies are not used to make a diagnosis of MPS or of the MTrP because there is no laboratory or imaging study that has clinical utility in diagnosis. Rather, laboratory studies are used to identify conditions that seem to be associated with MPS. The most common conditions that are thought to predispose to, and perpetuate, MTrPs, are iron deficiency, hypothyroidism, vitamin D deficiency, vitamin B12 deficiency, parasitic infestation, and recurrent vaginal yeast infections. A list of symptoms that should make one think of underlying disease and the tests that are commonly used are found in **Table 1**.

MULTIPLE DEFICIENCY STATES

If 2 or more nutritional (iron, vitamin D, vitamin B12) deficiency states are present or if one is present, but does not respond to supplementation, malabsorption syndromes must be considered. Antitissue transglutaminase (anti-TTG) immunoglobulin (Ig)A antibodies are present and increased in 90% of cases of malabsorption syndrome. Serum IgA is also measured, as 3% of the population has little to no IgA. In that case, one must specify that the anti-TTG antibodies should be IgG antibodies. In a few cases, patients have had normal anti-TTG antibodies, but responded to a gluten-free diet by eliminating their pain symptoms (Gerwin RD, unpublished data, 2013).

If iron deficiency is found, the cause must be identified. Iron supplementation alone is not an adequate approach. Iron deficiency is generally seen in only women, as a result of menstrual blood loss with insufficient dietary iron intake. Male iron insufficiency is uncommon. There must be a specific reason found, like excessive use of nonsteroidal anti-inflammatory drugs causing gastritis, or cancer.

DIFFERENTIAL DIAGNOSIS

The diagnosis of MPS with trigger point tenderness and referred pain is enough to initiate treatment at a symptomatic level. However, the diagnosis of MPS is only the

Table 1
Commonly used laboratory tests in the evaluation of myofascial pain syndromes

Condition	Symptoms	Test	Threshold
Hypothyroidism	1. Diffuse muscle pain 2. Widespread MTrPs 3. Deep coldness 4. Fatigue 5. Constipation	1. TSH 2. Serum cholesterol	TSH >2.25 μIU/mL
Iron insufficiency	1. Diffuse muscle pain 2. Widespread MTrPs 3. Fatigue 4. Deep coldness	1. Serum ferritin 2. Serum iron, IBC, percent saturation 3. Hemoglobin, hct, differential count	1. Ferritin <25 ng/mL 2. Low serum iron, high IBC, saturation <18% 3. hct <28, MCH and MCHC low
Vitamin D insufficiency	1. Diffuse pain 2. Widespread MTrPs 3. Fatigue 4. Weakness	1. 25-OH vitamin D 2. PTH if vitamin D is very low	1. 25-OH vitamin D <30 ng/mL 2. PTH if 25-OH vitamin D <18 ng/mL
Vitamin B12	1. Diffuse pain 2. Weakness 3. Impaired vibration and position sense in the great toes	1. Vitamin B12 level 2. CBC	1. Serum vitamin B12 level <350 pg/mL 2. Macrocytic anemia
Parasitic infestation	1. Diffuse myalgia 2. Widespread MTrPs 3. Gastrointestinal symptoms	1. 3 stools on different days for ova and parasites	Stool positive for ova and/or parasites
Candida	1. Recurrent vaginal itching and discharge 2. Widespread pain 3. Diffuse muscle tenderness	1. History of recurrent episodes of vaginal candida 2. History of repeated use of antibiotics	Vaginal examination may or may not be positive for candida

Abbreviations: CBC, complete blood count; hct, hematocrit; IBC, iron-binding capacity; MTrP, myofascial trigger point; PTH, parathyroid hormone; TSH, thyroid-stimulating hormone.

beginning of the diagnostic and treatment process. Additional steps are necessary to fully address a patient's pain. The cause of the MP must be explored by history, physical examination, and by laboratory testing. Thus, the evaluation of a patient with apparent MPS must consider those conditions that have a similar presentation and that constitute the differential diagnosis of MPS (**Table 2**).

LOOK-ALIKES

One problem associated with the diagnosis of MP is that referred pain from MTrPs can be similar to referred pain from other conditions and from pain generated directly by other conditions. For example, one of the first signs of radiculopathy can be the development of MTrPs that precede the appearance of signs of neurologic impairment. Trigger point pain can mimic radicular pain. The clinician must be aware of these 2 possibilities. Referred pain that radiates into upper and lower limbs from muscle trigger points also typically affects the neck or back, the shoulder, or hip region. Thus, the pain pattern from the MTrP is no different from radicular pain from nerve

Table 2
Differential diagnosis of regional pain syndromes

Pain Region	Examine for Signs and Symptoms of Regional Disorders	Muscles with Trigger Point Referred Pain Patterns that Reproduce the Regional Pains in Column 2
Head and neck	Headache features (laterality, character of headache [sharp, stabbing, dull, throbbing, etc.] and clinical feature as dizziness, photophobia, and phonophobia); the presence of neurologic signs (weakness, absent tendon reflexes, sensory loss). Range of motion of neck, loading tests for facet joints, imaging for spondylosis and instability	Upper trapezius, levator scapulae, posterior cervical (splenius capitis and cervicis, semispinalis, and oblique capitis inferior), sternocleidomastoid, facial muscles (masseter, temporalis)
Shoulder	Shoulder and acromioclavicular joint dysfunction signs, shoulder impingement, and rotator cuff syndrome signs	Trapezius, supraspinatus, levator scapulae, supraspinatus, infraspinatus, posterior serratus superior, rhomboids, subscapularis, teres major and minor, latissimus dorsi, deltoid, pectoralis major and minor
(Noncardiac) Chest	History and signs of tracheobronchial and esophageal disease, including carcinoma, cardiac disease, especially angina	Pectoralis major, abdominal obliques rectus femoris, back muscles
Low back	Spondylo-arthropathies, spondylolisthesis, disc disease, spinal stenosis, myelopathies (cord compression, tethered cord), hypermobility syndromes	Psoas, quadratus lumborum paraspinal muscles (iliocostalis, longimus thoracis, multifidi), abdominal oblique, rectus femoris
Pelvic/hip	Internal organ disease: painful bladder, irritable bowel, endometriosis, menstrual cramps, prostatitis, vulvovaginitis, carcinoma, radicular pain from the lumbo-sacral spine	Abdominal muscles, psoas, quadratus lumborum, gluteal muscles, including the piriformis muscle, thigh adductors, including the pectineus muscle, hamstrings, especially the upper semitendinosis muscle, the short extensor muscles of the thigh (obturators, gemellae)
Knee	Intrinsic knee joint disease, radicular pain from the low back	Quadriceps muscle (especially the vastus medialis) for medial knee pain, vastus lateralis for lateral knee pain, hamstrings and gastrocnemius muscles for back of knee pain
Ankle/foot	Intrinsic joint pain, radicular pain from the low back	Anterior and posterior leg muscles, (gastrocnemius, soleus, fibularis, anterior tibialis, long flexor and extensor muscles of the leg), intrinsic foot muscles

root compression and is similar to the pain referral from facet joint arthropathy in that it often has an axial component and referral down a limb. In fact, the problem is more complicated because either or both conditions can occur as comorbidities with MTrP pain (see the following section, Comorbidities).

COMORBIDITIES

MTrPs can occur in association with a large number of other clinical conditions, both conditions then occurring as comorbidities (**Box 4**). This applies even if it is thought that the MTrP is a result of another condition. Increasing awareness of mild hypothyroidism with thyroid-stimulating hormone levels as low as 2.25 μIU/mL has led to the identification of individuals with widespread trigger point pain that resolves with the administration of thyroid hormone. Awareness of the coexistence of MTrPs with internal organ disease can uncover such diverse etiologies as cancer, infection (parasitic and Lyme disease are 2 outstanding examples), acute and chronic radiculopathy, nerve entrapment, endometriosis, painful bladder syndrome, and Ehlers-Danlos syndrome, to name some comorbid conditions. Common comorbid conditions are listed in **Box 4**. In some cases, trigger points may persist along with the conditions that may have led to their creation. This is particularly true of spinal disorders, such as radicular syndromes and facet arthropathies (see the preceding section, Differential diagnosis). The astute clinician will pursue the underlying cause or predisposing conditions that need to be addressed for a successful outcome. Patients who experience relief from their pain when treated by such an astute clinician are eternally grateful.

Box 4
Common conditions that are comorbid with myofascial pain syndrome

1. Migraine headache
2. Tension-type headache
3. Temporomandibular joint disorder
4. Fibromyalgia
5. Hypermobility syndromes
6. Painful bladder syndrome
7. Irritable bowel syndrome
8. Pelvic pain syndrome
9. Vulvovaginitis
10. Prostatitis
11. Endometriosis
12. Dysmenorrhea
13. Hypothyroidism
14. Vitamin D deficiency
15. Vitamin B12 deficiency
16. Iron deficiency
17. Parasitic infection
18. Celiac disease of malabsorption

In some cases, MTrPs can produce a well-described clinical condition, such as migraine or chronic tension-type headache, and then coexist with it as a comorbid condition.[27,28] In this case, elimination of the trigger point may be essential to resolving the headache if it is the primary trigger for the headache.

Rounded shoulders and forward head posture asymmetrically shorten the trapezius and sternocleidomastoid muscles, creating a mechanical dysfunction that promotes the development of trigger points in these muscles.

SUMMARY

MTrP is common and readily identified by a trained examiner. The diagnosis is made by suspecting the possibility of MPS from the history then confirmed by identifying the MTrP by physical examination. Provocative factors and factors that may perpetuate the condition are investigated. Comorbid conditions are identified and treated. Thus, the evaluation of the patient is comprehensive and is not limited simply to identification of a specific MTrP causing a specific pain. A comprehensive evaluation is necessary to reach a diagnosis and develop a successful comprehensive treatment plan.

REFERENCES

1. Turo D, Otto P, Shah JP, et al. Ultrasonic characterizations of the upper trapezius muscle in patients with chronic neck pain. Ultrason Imaging 2013;35:173–87.
2. Lucas KR, Rich PA, Polus B. Muscle activation patterns in the scapular positioning muscles during loaded scapular plane elevation: the effects of latent myofascial trigger points. Clin Biomech 2010;25:765–70.
3. Hong CZ, Torigoe Y. Electrophysiologic characteristics of localized twitch responses in responsive taut bands of rabbit skeletal muscle. J Muscoskel Pain 1994;2:17–43.
4. Shah JP, Phillips TM, Danoff JV, et al. An in vitro microanalytical technique for measuring the local biochemical milieu of human skeletal muscle. J Appl Phys 2005;99:1977–84.
5. Mense S. Central nervous system mechanisms of muscle pain: ascending pathways, central sensitization, and pain-modulating systems. In: Mense S, Gerwin RD, editors. Muscle pain: understanding the mechanisms. Heidelberg (Germany): Springer; 2010. p. 105–76.
6. Ge HY, Madeleine P, Cairns B, et al. Hypoalgesia in the referred pain areas after bilateral injections of hypertonic saline in the trapezius muscles of men and women: a potential experimental model of gender-specific differences. Clin J Pain 2006;22:37–44.
7. Xu YM, Ge HY, Arendt-Nielsen L. Sustained nociceptive mechanical stimulation of latent myofascial trigger point induces central sensitization in healthy subjects. J Pain 2010;12:1348–65.
8. Hong CZ, Torigoe Y, Yu J. The localized twitch responses in responsive taut bands of rabbit skeletal muscle fibers are related to the reflexes at spinal cord level. J Muscoskel Pain 1995;3(1):15–33.
9. Simons DG, Travel JG, Simons LS. Myofascial pain and dysfunction: the trigger point manual. Baltimore (MD): Williams & Wilkins; 1999.
10. Gerwin RD, Shannon S, Hong CZ, et al. Interrater reliability in myofascial trigger point examination. Pain 1997;69:65–73.
11. Sciotti VM, Mittak V, DiMarco L, et al. Clinical precision of myofascial trigger point location in the trapezius muscle. Pain 2001;95:259–66.

12. Bron C, Frenssen JL, Wensing M, et al. Interobserver reliability of palpation of my-ofascial trigger points in shoulder muscles. J Man Manip Ther 2007;15:203–15.
13. Lucas N, Macaskill P, Irwig L, et al. Reliability of physical examination for diag-nosis of myofascial trigger points. Clin J Pain 2009;25:80–9.
14. Gerwin RD, Duranleau D. Ultrasound identification of the myofascial trigger point. Muscle Nerve 1997;20:767–76.
15. Sikdar S, Shah JP, Gilliams E, et al. Assessment of myofascial trigger points (MTrPs): a new application of ultrasound imaging and vibration sonoelastogra-phy. Proceedings of the 30th Annual International IEEE EMBS Conference. Van-couver (Canada): 2008. p. 5585–8.
16. Turo D, Otto P, Shah JP, et al. Ultrasonic tissue characterization of the upper trapezius muscle in patients with myofascial pain syndrome. Conf Proc IEEE Eng Med Biol Soc 2012;2012:4386–9.
17. Chen Q, Bensamoun S, Basford J, et al. Identification and quantification of myo-fascial taut bands with magnetic resonance elastography. Arch Phys Med Reha-bil 2007;88:1658–61.
18. Chen Q, Basford J, An KN. Ability of magnetic resonance elastography to assess taut bands. Clin Biomech 2008;23:623–9.
19. Sikdar S, Shah JP, Bebreah T, et al. Novel applications of ultrasound technology to visualize and characterize myofascial trigger points and surrounding soft tis-sue. Arch Phys Med Rehabil 2009;90:1829–38.
20. Hubbard DR, Berkoff M. Myofascial trigger points show spontaneous needle EMG activity. Spine 1993;18:1803–7.
21. Simons DG, Hong CZ, Simons LS. Prevalence of spontaneous electrical activity at trigger points and at control sites in rabbit skeletal muscle. J Muscoskel Pain 1995;3(1):35–48.
22. Hong CZ, Simons DG. Pathophysiologic and electrophysiologic mechanisms of myofascial trigger points. Arch Phys Med Rehabil 1998;79:863–72.
23. Simons DG. Do endplate noise and spikes arise from normal motor endplates? Am J Phys Med Rehabil 2001;80:134–40.
24. Dumitru D, King JC, Stegeman DF. Endplate spike morphology: a clinical and simulation study. Arch Phys Med Rehabil 1998;79:634–40.
25. Kuan TS, Chen JT, Chen SM, et al. Effect of botulinum toxin on endplate noise in myofascial trigger spots of rabbit skeletal muscle. Am J Phys Med Rehabil 2002; 81:512–20.
26. Kuan TS, Hsieh YL, Chen SM, et al. The myofascial trigger point region: correla-tion between the degree of irritability and the prevalence of endplate noise. Am J Phys Med Rehabil 2007;86:183–9.
27. Fernandez-de-las-Peñas C, Simons D, Gerwin RD, et al. Muscle trigger points in tension-type headache. In: Fernandez-de-las-Peñas C, Arendt-Nielsen L, Gerwin RD, editors. Tension-type and cervicogenic headache. Boston: Jones and Bartlett; 2010. Chapter 6.
28. Graven-Nielsen T, Ge HY, Arendt-Nielsen L. Neurophysiologic basis of muscle-referred pain to the head. In: Fernandez-de-la-Peñas C, Chaitow L, Schoenen J, editors. Multidisciplinary management of migraine headache. Bos-ton: Jones and Bartlett; 2013. Chapter 7.

Myofascial Pain Syndrome Treatments

Joanne Borg-Stein, MD*, Mary Alexis Iaccarino, MD

KEYWORDS

- Myofascial pain syndrome • Regional muscle pain • Treatment
- Myofascial trigger points • Pharmacotherapy

KEY POINTS

- Myofascial pain syndrome is a painful condition arising from myofascial trigger points.
- Treatment of myofascial pain syndrome consists of pharmacologic and nonpharmacologic interventions.
- Exercise and education are the mainstay treatments for all patients.
- Medications, physical modalities, dry needling, and trigger point injection are adjunct therapies that are appropriate in some patient subsets to treat myofascial pain and associated symptoms.

INTRODUCTION

Myofascial pain syndrome (MPS) is a painful condition of myofascial trigger points (MTrPs) in the skeletal muscle.[1] It can occur alone or in combination with other pain generators. MTrPs are focal areas of taut bands found in skeletal muscle that are hypersensitive to palpation. When manual pressure is applied over an MTrP, it produces a distinct local and referred pain that is consistent with the patient's presenting pain symptoms.[2] MPS is often grouped with other pain syndromes; however, it is distinct from diagnoses such as fibromyalgia in that it is focal, does not require multiple pain generators, and involves a taut band in skeletal muscle.[3]

EPIDEMIOLOGY

The prevalence of myofascial pain varies in the general population. In internal medicine and orthopedics clinics, the estimated prevalence is 21% to 30%. In a nationwide German study of more than 300 physicians experienced in treating patients with pain, 46% of patients had active MTrPs.[4] In other specialty pain clinics, estimates as high as 85% to 90% have been reported.[5] Unlike other chronic pain

Department of Physical Medicine and Rehabilitation, Harvard Medical School, 300 First Avenue, Boston, MA 02129, USA
* Corresponding author.
E-mail address: jborgstein@partners.org

Phys Med Rehabil Clin N Am 25 (2014) 357–374
http://dx.doi.org/10.1016/j.pmr.2014.01.012
1047-9651/14/$ – see front matter © 2014 Elsevier Inc. All rights reserved.

disorders, which are more prevalent in women, men and women are equally affected by MPS. However, studies in nationalized health care systems have found women to be more limited by musculoskeletal pain, with higher pain scores and more frequent absence from work.[6]

CLINICAL PRESENTATION

For a detailed review of clinical presentation, the reader is referred to the article on MPS diagnosis elsewhere in this issue by Dr Gerwin. Topics relevant to determining appropriate treatment of myofascial pain are discussed here.

MPS can be of insidious onset or occur as a result of trauma or injury. Patients complain of varying degrees of pain from mild to severe, characterized as deep and aching. Pain is focal and can have discrete referral patterns, which can help identify the muscle that contains the causative MTrP.[1] Patients may report associated autonomic dysfunction. Diaphoresis, lacrimation, flushing, dermatographia, pilomotor activity, and temperature change are common in MPS.[7] Cervical myofascial pain has been associated with vestibular symptoms, such as dizziness, blurred vision, and tinnitus.[8] Hyperesthesia, numbness, tingling, and twitching may occur if nearby nerves are irritated by the MTrPs. Decreased work tolerance, muscle fatigue, weakness, and other functional complaints may be present, and over time, mood and sleep disturbance can develop.[9–11] Eliciting associated symptoms and assessing their degree of impact on the patient is helpful in guiding treatment strategies.

Physical examination aids diagnosis and may guide treatment, particularly if local trigger point therapy is being considered. A thorough medical, neurologic, and musculoskeletal examination should be performed. Myofascial pain can be caused by postural stress, muscle imbalance, and repetitive overuse. Therefore biomechanics, joint function, and posture should be evaluated to assess their contribution.[12] Myofascial pain is associated with restricted range of motion. Muscles around the restricted area should be palpated for active MTrPs. To identify MTrPs, the examiner applies gentle pressure perpendicular to the muscle fibers. A taut band should be palpable, and direct pressure should produce significant pain, which reproduces the patient's local and referred symptoms.[12]

Laboratory studies may be useful to exclude systemic diagnoses, particularly when the clinical presentation is not definitive. In MPS, blood counts, chemistry and liver panel, erythrocyte sedimentation rate, and C-reactive protein levels are normal. A thyroid panel may be used to exclude thyroid disease as a cause of muscle pain. Radiography and advanced imaging may show concurrent osteoarthritis, diskogenic disease, neural irritation, and other mechanical changes. The relevance of these findings must be determined in individual cases based on the clinical scenario.

DIFFERENTIAL DIAGNOSIS

MPS and other muscle pain diagnoses can have overlapping and related symptoms. MTrPs occur insidiously or secondary to mechanical dysfunction and other disease states. Determining both primary and secondary causes of myofascial pain helps formulate a treatment plan. The following are questions that may aid clinicians in identifying contributing factors.

- Is there regional myofascial pain with trigger points present?
- Is myofascial pain the primary pain generator or are there other coexisting or underlying structural diagnoses?

- Is there a nutritional, metabolic, psychological, visceral, or inflammatory disorder contributing to the myofascial pain?
- Is there widespread pain that does not resemble the pattern associated with regional myofascial pain?

Table 1 provides a list of common differential diagnoses for myofascial pain. This list is not exhaustive. For a list of differential diagnoses by region of pain, please refer to the article on diagnosis of MPS elsewhere in this issue.

In difficult-to-treat cases with refractory pain symptoms, consider MPS when other diagnoses have been exhausted. In the literature, MPS has had uncommon presentations. It has been implicated in patients with chronic unilateral shoulder pain, lateral epicondylalgia, and chronic tension-type headache.[13–15] It has been found concurrently in the affected limb in patients with complex regional pain syndrome.[16] In a review of pelvic pain, symptoms of dysuria, dyspareunia, dyschezia, constipation, and

Table 1 Differential diagnosis for MPS	
Joint disorders	Zygapophyseal joint disorders Osteoarthritis Loss of normal joint motion
Inflammatory disorders	Polymyositis Polymyalgia rheumatica Rheumatoid arthritis
Neurologic disorders	Radiculopathy Entrapment neuropathy Metabolic myopathy
Regional soft tissue disorders	Bursitis Epicondylitis Tendonitis Cumulative trauma
Diskogenic disorders	Degenerative disk disease Annular tears Disk protrusion or herniation
Visceral referred pain	Gastrointestinal Cardiac Pulmonary Renal
Mechanical stress	Postural dysfunction Scoliosis Leg length discrepancy
Nutritional, metabolic, and endocrine disorders	Vitamin deficiency (B_1, B_{12}, D, calcium, folic acid, iron, magnesium) Alcoholic and toxic myopathy Hypothyroidism
Psychological disorders	Depression Anxiety Disordered sleep
Infectious disease	Viral illness Chronic hepatitis Bacterial or viral myositis
Widespread chronic pain	Fibromyalgia

From Borg-Stein J. Treatment of fibromyalgia, myofascial pain, and related disorders. Phys Med Rehabil Clin N Am 2006;17(2):491–510, viii; with permission.

testicular pain can be presenting symptoms of pelvic floor myofascial pain.[17] In a study of patients with suspected carpal tunnel syndrome, approximately one-third were found to have infraspinatus trigger points and normal nerve conduction studies, suggesting that MPS may mimic or be concurrent with carpal tunnel syndrome.[18] Postoperative myofascial pain after thoracotomy and mastectomy has also been described.[19–22]

TREATMENT OF MPS

Treatment of MPS targets MTrPs and aims to correct the structural and mechanical imbalance that prompted MTrP formation. Treatment should also address sympathetic dysfunction, identify emotional stressors, and treat late complications. The following is a discussion of therapeutic interventions for MPS. Education, pharmacotherapy, local needle therapy, and exercise serve to reduce pain and associated symptoms. Most often a combination of therapies is used simultaneously or in sequence and appropriate initial therapy is patient and provider dependent.

EDUCATION

- Based on the patient's symptoms and pain characteristics, a firm diagnosis of MPS should be made.
- Build rapport with the patient by approaching them with an attitude of empathy and understanding. Validate their concerns and reassure them that their symptoms are real and not psychogenic.
- In difficult-to-treat or refractory cases of pain, the patient may have had other diagnoses. The patient should be educated on the symptoms of MPS, and explanation should be provided as to why other diagnoses are less likely.
- Unnecessary tests should be avoided.
- Probable mechanisms of pain should be discussed in simple terms, emphasizing that the muscle pain associated with MPS is not dangerous and does not cause tissue damage.
- Inquire about associated symptoms.
- Determine what is most aggravating to the patient: intolerance to pain, loss of function, lack of sleep, or fear of underlying structural or catastrophic disease. Associated symptoms vary from patient to patient but help guide individual management.
- Educate the patient on each proposed modality of treatment: pharmacotherapy, manual modalities such as osteopathy or manual release, and injection.
- Recognize and address underlying psychosocial factors, such as depression, anxiety, stress at home or work, and poor coping skills.
- Educate the patient that psychological factors exacerbate pain. A few patients may require referral to mental health providers.
- Educate patients on the importance of restful sleep, cardiovascular fitness, and body mechanics to overall lifestyle.
- Promote behavioral modification through education, including cognitive behavioral techniques.

PHARMACOLOGIC MANAGEMENT

The pathophysiology of MPS is not completely understood. However, it is believed that there are local muscle, peripheral nerve, and central nervous system components. Therefore, medications that target each of these areas may be effective in treating

MPS. For each medication, it is important to consider mechanism of action and side effect profile, which is discussed in the addendum, in the context of individual patients. The adage of starting at a low dose and slowly increasing is important to patient tolerance and compliance. The side effect profile of medications is outlined in the article on side effects of commonly prescribed analgesic medications elsewhere in this issue.

Nonsteroidal Antiinflammatory Drugs

There is a paucity of literature on the use of oral nonsteroidal antiinflammatory drugs (NSAIDs) for MPS. Several studies show effectiveness for chronic pain and fibromyalgia in combination with other medications such as diazepam, alprazolam, cyclobenzaprine, and amitriptyline, but little is known on the efficacy of oral NSAIDs in MPS.[23–26] Topical NSAIDs have been shown to be useful in MPS. In general, they have fewer systemic side effects than oral NSAIDs but are often more expensive.[27] A study of diclofenac patch use in patients with upper trapezius myofascial pain found a significant reduction in pain based on visual analog scale, neck range of motion, and cervical disability index.[28] Despite limited evidence, NSAIDs are often part of MPS treatment because they are readily available and many patients are comfortable using them without physician input. Until further evidence is offered, providers should inquire about frequency of patient use, advise on the common side effects, monitor use in patients who find it helpful, and encourage discontinued use for those who find it ineffective.

Muscle Relaxants

Muscle relaxants are a group of drugs with varying pharmacology that act on the central nervous system to disrupt nociceptive pain.[29]

Cyclobenzaprine targets muscle relaxation without affecting muscle function. Its mechanism of action is not known, but its structure is similar to that of a tricyclic antidepressant. It is often used for both pain relief and sleep, because it has a sedating effect. In 41 patients with myofascial jaw pain, cyclobenzaprine was slightly better than clonazepam or placebo in pain relief but not more effective at improving sleep.[30] A Cochrane review in 2009[31] found that because of insufficient studies, there is not enough evidence to support its use in MPS. However, cyclobenzaprine is commonly prescribed for musculoskeletal pain and is well tolerated. In MPS, prescribing this medication at night can provide analgesia and promote sleep.

Tizanidine, an α_2-adrenergic agonist, acts centrally at the level of the spinal cord to inhibit spinal polysynaptic pathways and reduce the release of substance P.[32] Studies in animal models show that, in the thalamus, it reduces the release of neurotransmitters in ascending pathways involved in central sensitization.[33,34] In a prospective study of 29 women with MPS treated with tizanidine for 5 weeks,[35] pain, sleep, and disability all significantly improved. Tizanidine has a sedating effect and can cause hypotension, therefore dosing at night may limit noticeable side effects and aid sleep. This medication is also used for spasticity, with doses titrated up to 36 mg daily. In MPS, available studies have used lower doses of tizanidine with success.[36,37]

Benzodiazepines

Clonazepam and diazepam are benzodiazepine derivatives with multiple applications as anxiolytics, anticonvulsants, and muscle relaxants and are used in the treatment of MPS.[38] Most studies of MPS treatment with benzodiazepines were performed in a subset of patients with orofacial and temporomandibular pain.[26] In 2000, an open trial of clonazepam in patients with MPS from a multidisciplinary pain facility found a significant reduction in visual analog scale pain scores. However, of 46 participants, about 20% dropped out of the study because of intolerable side effects before reaching an effective dose.[39] The success of benzodiazepines on MPS may be targeting not only pain but also commonly associated symptoms, including muscle tension, anxiety, restless leg syndrome, and sleep disturbance. However, disadvantages to their use include a potent side effect profile, including ataxia, weakness, cognitive impairment, memory dysfunction, fatigue, depression, and adverse withdrawal symptoms.[29,40]

Serotonin and Norepinephrine Selective Reuptake Inhibitors and Tricyclic Antidepressants

There is an increasing role for antidepressants in the treatment of chronic pain, including tricyclic antidepressants, selective serotonin reuptake inhibitors (SSRIs), and serotonin norepinephrine reuptake inhibitors (SNRIs). Trials examining chronic tension headache and myofascial pain found amitriptyline to be effective for many patients.[41,42] A systematic review by Annaswamy and colleagues[43] supported the use of amitriptyline in some MPS conditions. Fewer studies have assessed the efficacy of nortriptyline.

An increasing body of evidence exists for the use of SSRIs and SNRIs in the treatment of fibromyalgia and other pain disorders.[44–46] There is little research on their use in regional muscle pain, such as MPS. However, these agents, particularly SNRIs, are used to treat regional myofascial pain. The rationale for their use stems from the fact that regional and widespread muscle pain have some overlap in signs and symptoms and approach to treatment. Thus, extrapolating from the chronic pain literature, SSRIs and SNRIs may be beneficial adjuvant pharmacotherapy. Should patients show signs and symptoms of mood disturbance in combination with MPS, antidepressant therapy may be warranted along with referral to a mental health professional.[47]

Tramadol

Tramadol is a weak opioid agonist and inhibits reuptake of serotonin and norepinephrine in the dorsal horns of the spinal cord. There are no published studies to support the use of tramadol in myofascial pain. However, several studies support its use in chronic widespread pain, chronic low back pain, and osteoarthritis, which are commonly associated with regional MPS.[48–51]

Lidocaine Patch

The lidocaine patch is a transdermal application of a local anesthetic with effective local penetration and limited systemic absorption. It has been proposed as an alternative treatment to needle injection of local anesthetics in patients with hypersensitivity associated with MPS. In a randomized control study, the lidocaine patch was effective in treatment of MPS. It did not generate as great a pain reduction score as needle infiltration, but patients were satisfied with its analgesic effect, and its use was associated with less discomfort than needle infiltration.[52]

Over-the-Counter Agents

There are a surplus of over-the-counter or nonprescription topical agents that are recommended for joint and muscle pain. Many of these products, such as Biofreeze, Salonpas, Icyhot, Tiger Balm, and others, use the active ingredient methyl salicylate or menthol to create a cool or warm sensation that dulls pain. Although published evidence for their use in myofascial pain is limited, some patients find that these medications have an analgesic effect. They can be used in combination with oral medications, although they should not be mixed or coadministered with other topical agents. In general, they are well tolerated and have minimal side effects.

NONPHARMACOLOGIC MANAGEMENT
Exercise for Myofascial Pain

Exercise is one of the most important aspects of rehabilitation and management of musculoskeletal pain. It helps to improve flexibility, increase functional status, optimize mood, and reduce pain.

Initiating a stretching exercise program is fundamental in MPS treatment. Stretching lengthens the tight bands of skeletal muscle that have become shortened and are causing pain. Stretching improves joint range of motion, leading to decreased pain, increased mobility, and restoration of normal activity. After optimal muscle length is restored and pain is reduced, adding strengthening to the exercise program can help establish new movement patterns and increase muscle endurance.[1] This goal can be achieved with the assistance of physical therapy to strengthen weak muscle groups, correct posture, and provide feedback so as not to overuse dominant muscle groups. For example, overuse of the upper trapezius and levator scapulae for shoulder motion can be corrected by stretching of the overactive muscles, and strengthening of scapular stabilizers, such as latissimus dorsi, rhomboids, and the lower trapezius. Patients should be encouraged to maintain an active lifestyle and incorporate a cardiovascular and aerobic fitness program into their routine. Educating patients on manual techniques, exercises, and stretches that relieve pain empowers patients to self-manage symptoms and effectively move from formal physical therapy to a home exercise program.[53] As pain relief improves, patients can resume normal activity, which improves function and prevents recurrence of MTrPs.

For some patients, the pain associated with MPS may preclude an effective exercise program, and other treatments, such as trigger point injection (TPI), may be required first. However, exercise should be incorporated into the treatment plan for all patients with MPS. Clinical experience suggests that leaving a muscle in a shortened position aggravates MTrPs and prevents resolution of symptoms.[2]

Postural, Mechanical, and Ergonomic Modifications

In occupational health and ergonomics research, there is evidence that repetitive loads in undesirable positions cause muscle pain and predispose workers to injury.[54–57] Theoretically, the overused or poorly conditioned muscle develops microtrauma and myofascial shortening, placing the muscle at risk of MTrP formation. Based on this theory, it is standard clinical practice to recommend correction of postural and ergonomic abnormalities.[58] Incorporating postural training for workers[59] and patients with temporomandibular joint pain has led to improvement in pain symptoms.[60] However, there are limited long-term efficacy data to support postural change as an effective treatment of myofascial pain. Nevertheless, in occupation-related injury or a situation in which a specific repetitive or strenuous task cannot be avoided, ergonomic modifications to correct abnormal postures are encouraged.

Stress Reduction

There are many types of interventions to reduce stress in MPS, including cognitive behavioral therapy (CBT), mediation and relaxation training, and biofeedback (**Table 2**). It is theorized that autonomic innervation to muscles may provide a link between stress and muscle pain. Thus, strategies to reduce emotional and physical stress may aid in treatment of MPS. McNulty and colleagues[61] found a higher increase

Table 2	
Stress reduction interventions	
CBT	A psychotherapy technique that facilitates behavior change by altering patients' beliefs or thought patterns
Meditation	Encompasses a variety of practice all with the similar goal of facilitating a sense of personal well-being or relaxation
Biofeedback	Any technique or device that increases awareness of physiologic changes in the body to improve emotions or change behavior

in needle electromyographic activity in trapezius MTrPs than in other areas of the muscle during psychological stress. A small study of patients with myofascial jaw pain found stress reduction intervention to be as effective as transcutaneous electrical nerve stimulation (TENS).[62] A randomized control trial of 3 months of CBT in chronic temporomandibular joint pain found improvements in pain, function, and activity after 1 year.[63] Stress reduction methods have also been shown to treat chronic pain, such as fibromyalgia.[64–66] Extrapolating from the fibromyalgia literature and incorporating the few studies on regional myofascial pain, stress reduction techniques and behavioral medicine may be useful adjunct therapies. However, further research would help to validate this intervention in the treatment of MPS.

Acupuncture

Acupuncture has been shown to be effective in treating myofascial pain.[67–72] In 2 Cochrane systematic reviews, acupuncture showed short-term benefit in mechanical neck pain and chronic low back pain when compared with sham acupuncture or no treatment.[67,68] Birch and Jamison[69] found that acupuncture alone over painful areas in the neck had better outcomes than NSAID treatment combined with acupuncture over nonpainful areas.

There are still several clinical questions about acupuncture that are unanswered, including number of needles used, duration of effect, and the mechanism by which it produces an antinociceptive effect. There is a close relationship between acupuncture points and trigger points, making the distinction between treatment with dry needling of MTrPs and local acupuncture more difficult to differentiate.[73] Overall, there is some evidence for the use of acupuncture as an adjunctive therapy for MPS, but further research is needed to determine treatment course and specific needling procedure.

Massage, Electrotherapy, and Ultrasonography

Massage is often sought as an alternative therapy for MPS. Anecdotal evidence and small clinic studies report it as an effective treatment; however, large vigorous trials are lacking. Two studies have found that combined with stretching, massage is helpful in reducing pain intensity and number of MTrPs.[74,75]

Several electrotherapies have been investigated for pain reduction of MTrPs, including TENS, electrical muscle stimulation (EMS), frequency-modulated neural stimulation (FREMS), and electrical twitch-obtaining intramuscular stimulation (ETOIMS). Compared with EMS or placebo, TENS has been found to be superior in pain reduction.[76–78] However, its effects seem limited to immediately after treatment, with 1 study finding no reduction in symptoms at 1 and 3 months after treatment.[78] In comparison, FREMS is shown to be as effective as TENS for myofascial pain, and its effect persisted at 3 months, whereas the TENS group did not.[79] ETOIMS, an emerging electrotherapy technique, acts on deep motor end plates to produce a muscle twitch. It has been used in MPS, but there are few studies and limited evidence on pain reduction.[80–82]

Ultrasound applies mechanical and thermal energy to tissue, and is believed to increase circulation, improve metabolism, and increase tissue pliability. Several studies have found that ultrasound alone, or in combination with exercise, improves pain in MPS.[75,83–85] Ay and colleagues[85] conducted a blinded randomized controlled trial, in which ultrasound was found to improve pain and number of MTrPs better than sham ultrasound. This study also found ultrasound alone to be as effective as ultrasound with diclofenac. Other studies of heat and antiinflammatory use with ultrasound have reported positive effect on pain in MPS.[86,87] In conclusion, ultrasound can be an effective adjunct therapy for MPS, and some patients may benefit from the addition of heat or antiinflammatory medication with ultrasound.

NEEDLING THERAPY

The regional pain associated with MPS stems from tight bands in the muscle called MTrPs. Dry needling and TPI are treatments that directly target MTrPs. Ordinarily, stretching and exercise are the foundation for pain reduction in MPS, but in the case of persistent MTrPs, providers can offer needling therapy.[88] Dry needling or TPI are most effective when they are accompanied by manual release of MTrPs and stretching that patients can perform themselves or with physical therapy.[89]

When needle therapy is necessary, it can be performed weekly over a series of several visits. At each visit, the amount of improvement and location of trigger points should be evaluated and compared with previous visits. When needling is used in combination with other therapies, some patients may find significant relief after only a few visits, whereas others may have recalcitrant areas that require more treatment. In general, TPI is performed as a series of injections. Patients need to be educated that there may be local soreness after injection, which should resolve, and that several treatments may be needed before results are noticeable.[3]

The hallmark of needling therapy is the production of a local twitch response in the targeted muscle. It is theorized that the needle mechanically disrupts and stops the dysfunctional activity of the motor end plate of the skeletal muscle motor neuron. Hong[90] described a fast-in–fast-out needling technique, which may be beneficial in eliciting maximal number of local twitch responses. In this technique, the needle penetrates the taut muscle band, is withdrawn to the superficial tissue, and then redirected to another area without coming out of the skin. Anesthetic can be injected when a twitch response is felt.

Dry needling is a low-risk intervention that is minimally invasive and inexpensive but requires training to achieve competence.[91,92] A prospective double-blind randomized controlled trial of 39 patients with MPS in an outpatient clinic found dry needling of MTrPs significantly reduced pain compared with sham dry needling.[93] A recent meta-analysis of dry needling in MPS found 3 studies in which dry needling improved pain in the cervicothoracic region both immediately and 4 weeks after treatment.[94]

Dry needling can be performed either superficially or deep. The technique of superficial dry needling is believed to deactivate MTrPs by stimulation of cutaneous A δ fibers without producing a muscle twitch response.[95] Conversely, deep dry needling targets muscular afferents and has been shown to produce greater pain reduction.[96] In a systematic review by Annaswamy and colleagues,[43] deep dry needling was found to be more effective than superficial dry needling for relief of pain from MTrPs. However, if there is a risk for damaging deep structures such as the lung or vasculature, the superficial method is preferred and is still efficacious. A preinjection block can be performed in the region or muscle of interest to allow more thorough and extensive needling with less patient discomfort. Preinjection blocks are also believed to block central sensitization and decrease any neurogenic component of the trigger point.[97]

TPI targets MTrPs by needle stimulation and treatment with anesthetics, steroids, or botulinum toxin. Shorter-acting and lower concentration anesthetic such as 0.25% lidocaine has shown to be less myotoxic than long-acting anesthetics like bupivacaine and less painful to inject than higher concentrations such as 1% lidocaine.[98,99] Although inflammation does play a role in MPS, the role of steroids in TPI is limited. A study of 45 patients with headache and MPS[100] found that steroid injection plus lidocaine produced a greater reduction of postinjection sensitivity than dry needling or lidocaine alone, but was no better at improving overall pain or cervical range of motion at 12 weeks.

Multiple systematic reviews, randomized controlled trials, and a Cochrane review have found no substantial evidence that injection provides more effective pain relief than dry needling alone.[85,100,101] Despite its limited evidence, anesthetic injection is still used in clinical practice. Because needling of MTrPs can cause local pain, the immediate antinociceptive effect of lidocaine and reduced latent soreness can improve the treatment experience overall. A single blinded randomized controlled trial of 29 patients with cervical MTrPs found TPI to be better than dry needling,[100] and Hong and colleagues[102] found that injection with lidocaine produced less postinjection soreness than dry needling alone. In addition, third-party payers in the United States reimburse for TPI but do not cover dry needling. Dry needling is an out-of-pocket expense for many patients, giving some preference to TPI. In the absence of significant adverse effect and recognizing the patient's cost burden, TPI may prove a useful treatment strategy. However, more research is needed to show the benefits of injection over dry needling.

Overall, there is no conclusive evidence that 1 needling technique is more effective than another. In their systemic literature review, Cummings and White concluded "because no technique is better than any other, we recommend that the method safest and most comfortable for the patient should be used."[101] Moreover, these techniques are based on the ability to accurately palpate and identify trigger points and discern them from other pain generators. In 1997, Gerwin[103] established that, with specialized training, interrater reliability in trigger point identification is good, but without training, localizing MTrPs and discerning twitch response during treatment is poor. Thus, using the technique that is most comfortable for the patient and with which the examiner is most proficient is likely to yield the best results.

Botulinum Toxin Injection

Botulinum toxin type A is a neurotoxic substance that is believed to act both centrally and peripherally to decrease pain. At the neuromuscular junction, it blocks the release of acetylcholine to prevent muscle hyperactivity and spasm. Its action at the neuromuscular junction allows it to target MTrPs, reducing local ischemia within muscles, and freeing entrapped nerve endings.[104] It has antinociceptive properties, preventing release of pain neurotransmitters at primary sensory neurons.[105] It also may act centrally, at the spinal and supraspinal levels,[106] and in the somatic and autonomic nervous system.[104] Botulinum toxin has an off-label use in myofascial pain and chronic musculoskeletal pain. Its multiple sites of action may prove beneficial not only to release tight MTrPs but also to disrupt nociceptive pain and treat associated autonomic symptoms.

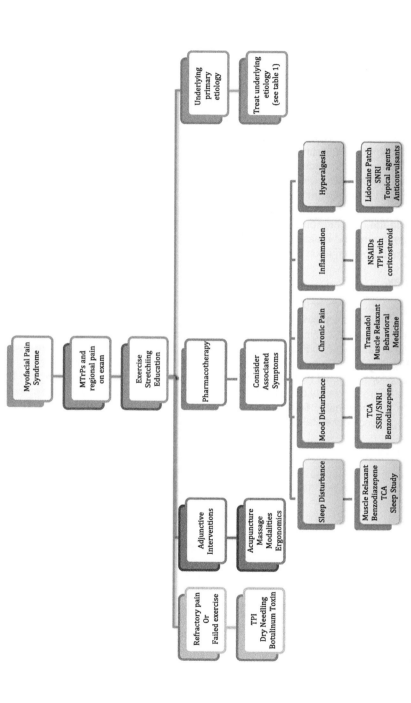

Fig. 1. MPS treatment summary. NSAIDs, nonsteroidal antiinflammatory drugs; SNRI, serotonin norepinephrine reuptake inhibitor; SSRI, selective serotonin reuptake inhibitor; TCA, tricyclic antidepressant; TPI, trigger point injection.

Studies on the efficacy of botulinum toxin in MPS are mixed. A 2012 Cochrane review[107] of botulinum toxin in MPS of the body (excluding the head and neck), evaluated 4 studies, including 233 patients, and found insufficient evidence for its use. Similarly, Ferrante and colleagues[108] conducted a randomized controlled trial of botulinum toxin for neck and shoulder pain and found it no better than placebo. Wheeler and colleagues[109] had similar results in the treatment of refractory cervicothoracic myofascial pain. However, other studies of MPS have found botulinum toxin to be beneficial.[110–114] In a multicenter randomized placebo-controlled trial of 145 patients with back and shoulder myofascial pain, Gobel and colleagues[115] found significant improvement in pain with botulinum toxin injection. Still other literature endorses that botulinum toxin may be best used in refractory cases of pain, taking advantage of its antinociceptive and muscular effects.[116]

Variations in study outcomes make the use of botulinum toxin difficult to endorse over other conservative, proven interventions. In a recent review by Gerwin,[117] the potential pitfalls of botulinum toxin studies were explored and an explanation offered for results variability. These pitfalls include a robust response to placebo, confounding variable in the control groups, incomplete treatments, and inappropriate periods between treatment and reassessment. More studies are required to better understand the role of botulinum toxin treatment in MPS.

SUMMARY

MPS is common in musculoskeletal practice, either as a primary or secondary pain disorder. As well as causing local muscle pain and limiting function, it can be associated with sympathetic dysfunction, emotional stressors, postural malalignment, and sleep disturbance. It is critically important to take a multifaceted approach to treatment (**Fig. 1**). Patient education and engagement in active training and exercise are necessary for functional restoration. Pharmacotherapy and needling therapy can be added to address primary complaints and comorbid symptoms. With a variety of tools available for treatment, MPS continues to be one of the most challenging yet rewarding musculoskeletal pain conditions to treat.

REFERENCES

1. Simons D, Travell J, Simons L. Myofascial Pain and Dysfunction: The Trigger Point Manual, Vol. 1. Upper Half of Body. Baltimore (MD): Williams & Wilkins; 1999.
2. Borg-Stein J, Simons DG. Focused review: myofascial pain. Arch Phys Med Rehabil 2002;83(3 Suppl 1):S40–7, S48–9.
3. Borg-Stein J. Treatment of fibromyalgia, myofascial pain, and related disorders. Phys Med Rehabil Clin N Am 2006;17(2):491–510, viii.
4. Fleckenstein J, Zaps D, Ruger LJ, et al. Discrepancy between prevalence and perceived effectiveness of treatment methods in myofascial pain syndrome: results of a cross-sectional, nationwide survey. BMC Musculoskelet Disord 2010; 11:32.
5. Gerwin RD. Classification, epidemiology, and natural history of myofascial pain syndrome. Curr Pain Headache Rep 2001;5(5):412–20.
6. Rollman GB, Lautenbacher S. Sex differences in musculoskeletal pain. Clin J Pain 2001;17(1):20–4.
7. Fricton JR, Kroening R, Haley D, et al. Myofascial pain syndrome of the head and neck: a review of clinical characteristics of 164 patients. Oral Surg Oral Med Oral Pathol 1985;60(6):615–23.

8. Krabak BJ, Borg-Stein J, Oas JA. Chronic cervical myofascial pain syndrome: improvement in dizziness and pain with a multidisciplinary rehabilitation program. A pilot study. J Back Musculoskelet Rehabil 2000;15(2):83–7.
9. Altindag O, Gur A, Altindag A. The relationship between clinical parameters and depression level in patients with myofascial pain syndrome. Pain Med 2008;9(2): 161–5.
10. Dohrenwend BP, Raphael KG, Marbach JJ, et al. Why is depression comorbid with chronic myofascial face pain? A family study test of alternative hypotheses. Pain 1999;83(2):183–92.
11. Schwartz RA, Greene CS, Laskin DM. Personality characteristics of patients with myofascial pain-dysfunction (MPD) syndrome unresponsive to conventional therapy. J Dent Res 1979;58(5):1435–9.
12. Hong C. Muscle pain syndromes. In: Braddom R, editor. Physical medicine and rehabilitation. Philadelphia: WB Saunders; 2011. p. 971–1002.
13. Bron C, Dommerholt J, Stegenga B, et al. High prevalence of shoulder girdle muscles with myofascial trigger points in patients with shoulder pain. BMC Musculoskelet Disord 2011;12:139.
14. Couppe C, Torelli P, Fuglsang-Frederiksen A, et al. Myofascial trigger points are very prevalent in patients with chronic tension-type headache: a double-blinded controlled study. Clin J Pain 2007;23(1):23–7.
15. Fernandez-Carnero J, Fernandez-de-Las-Penas C, de la Llave-Rincon AI, et al. Prevalence of and referred pain from myofascial trigger points in the forearm muscles in patients with lateral epicondylalgia. Clin J Pain 2007;23(4):353–60.
16. Rashiq S, Galer BS. Proximal myofascial dysfunction in complex regional pain syndrome: a retrospective prevalence study. Clin J Pain 1999;15(2):151–3.
17. Itza F, Zarza D, Serra L, et al. Myofascial pain syndrome in the pelvic floor: a common urological condition. Actas Urol Esp 2010;34(4):318–26.
18. Qerama E, Kasch H, Fuglsang-Frederiksen A. Occurrence of myofascial pain in patients with possible carpal tunnel syndrome–a single-blinded study. Eur J Pain 2009;13(6):588–91.
19. Diaz JH, Gould HJ 3rd. Management of post-thoracotomy pseudoangina and myofascial pain with botulinum toxin. Anesthesiology 1999;91(3):877–9.
20. Fernandez-Lao C, Cantarero-Villanueva I, Fernandez-de-Las-Penas C, et al. Development of active myofascial trigger points in neck and shoulder musculature is similar after lumpectomy or mastectomy surgery for breast cancer. J Bodyw Mov Ther 2012;16(2):183–90.
21. Hamada H, Moriwaki K, Shiroyama K, et al. Myofascial pain in patients with post-thoracotomy pain syndrome. Reg Anesth Pain Med 2000;25(3):302–5.
22. Karmakar MK, Ho AM. Postthoracotomy pain syndrome. Thorac Surg Clin 2004; 14(3):345–52.
23. Goldenberg DL, Felson DT, Dinerman H. A randomized, controlled trial of amitriptyline and naproxen in the treatment of patients with fibromyalgia. Arthritis Rheum 1986;29(11):1371–7.
24. Fossaluzza V, De Vita S. Combined therapy with cyclobenzaprine and ibuprofen in primary fibromyalgia syndrome. Int J Clin Pharmacol Res 1992; 12(2):99–102.
25. Russell IJ, Fletcher EM, Michalek JE, et al. Treatment of primary fibrositis/fibromyalgia syndrome with ibuprofen and alprazolam. A double-blind, placebo-controlled study. Arthritis Rheum 1991;34(5):552–60.
26. Singer E, Dionne R. A controlled evaluation of ibuprofen and diazepam for chronic orofacial muscle pain. J Orofac Pain 1997;11(2):139–46.

27. Castelnuovo E, Cross P, Mt-Isa S, et al. Cost-effectiveness of advising the use of topical or oral ibuprofen for knee pain; the TOIB study [ISRCTN: 79353052]. Rheumatology (Oxford) 2008;47(7):1077–81.

28. Hsieh LF, Hong CZ, Chern SH, et al. Efficacy and side effects of diclofenac patch in treatment of patients with myofascial pain syndrome of the upper trapezius. J Pain Symptom Manage 2010;39(1):116–25.

29. Frontera W, DeLisa J, Gans B, et al. Delisa's physical medicine and rehabilitation principles and practice. Philadelphia: Lippincott Williams & Wilkins; 2010.

30. Herman CR, Schiffman EL, Look JO, et al. The effectiveness of adding pharmacologic treatment with clonazepam or cyclobenzaprine to patient education and self-care for the treatment of jaw pain upon awakening: a randomized clinical trial. J Orofac Pain 2002;16(1):64–70.

31. Leite FM, Atallah AN, El Dib R, et al. Cyclobenzaprine for the treatment of myofascial pain in adults. Cochrane Database Syst Rev 2009;(3):CD006830.

32. Ono H, Mishima A, Ono S, et al. Inhibitory effects of clonidine and tizanidine on release of substance P from slices of rat spinal cord and antagonism by alpha-adrenergic receptor antagonists. Neuropharmacology 1991;30(6):585–9.

33. Hirata K, Koyama N, Minami T. The effects of clonidine and tizanidine on responses of nociceptive neurons in nucleus ventralis posterolateralis of the cat thalamus. Anesth Analg 1995;81(2):259–64.

34. Davies J. Selective depression of synaptic transmission of spinal neurones in the cat by a new centrally acting muscle relaxant, 5-chloro-4-(2-imidazolin-2-yl-amino)-2, 1, 3-benzothiodazole (DS103-282). Br J Pharmacol 1982;76(3):473–81.

35. Malanga GA, Gwynn MW, Smith R, et al. Tizanidine is effective in the treatment of myofascial pain syndrome. Pain Physician 2002;5(4):422–32.

36. Berry H, Hutchinson DR. A multicentre placebo-controlled study in general practice to evaluate the efficacy and safety of tizanidine in acute low-back pain. J Int Med Res 1988;16(2):75–82.

37. Berry H, Hutchinson DR. Tizanidine and ibuprofen in acute low-back pain: results of a double-blind multicentre study in general practice. J Int Med Res 1988;16(2):83–91.

38. Manfredini D, Landi N, Tognini F, et al. Muscle relaxants in the treatment of myofascial face pain. A literature review. Minerva Stomatol 2004;53(6):305–13.

39. Fishbain DA, Cutler RB, Rosomoff HL, et al. Clonazepam open clinical treatment trial for myofascial syndrome associated chronic pain. Pain Med 2000;1(4):332–9.

40. Harkins S, Linford J, Cohen J, et al. Administration of clonazepam in the treatment of TMD and associated myofascial pain: a double-blind pilot study. J Craniomandib Disord 1991;5(3):179–86.

41. Bendtsen L, Jensen R. Amitriptyline reduces myofascial tenderness in patients with chronic tension-type headache. Cephalalgia 2000;20(6):603–10.

42. Plesh O, Curtis D, Levine J, et al. Amitriptyline treatment of chronic pain in patients with temporomandibular disorders. J Oral Rehabil 2000;27(10):834–41.

43. Annaswamy TM, De Luigi AJ, O'Neill BJ, et al. Emerging concepts in the treatment of myofascial pain: a review of medications, modalities, and needle-based interventions. PM R 2011;3(10):940–61.

44. Arnold LM, Lu Y, Crofford LJ, et al. A double-blind, multicenter trial comparing duloxetine with placebo in the treatment of fibromyalgia patients with or without major depressive disorder. Arthritis Rheum 2004;50(9):2974–84.

45. Offenbaecher M, Ackenheil M. Current trends in neuropathic pain treatments with special reference to fibromyalgia. CNS Spectr 2005;10(4): 285–97.
46. Sayar K, Aksu G, Ak I, et al. Venlafaxine treatment of fibromyalgia. Ann Pharmacother 2003;37(11):1561–5.
47. Khatun S, Huq MZ, Islam MA, et al. Clinical outcomes of management of myofacial pain dysfunction syndrome. Mymensingh Med J 2012;21(2):281–5.
48. Rosenberg MT. The role of tramadol ER in the treatment of chronic pain. Int J Clin Pract 2009;63(10):1531–43.
49. Kean WF, Bouchard S, Roderich Gossen E. Women with pain due to osteoarthritis: the efficacy and safety of a once-daily formulation of tramadol. Pain Med 2009;10(6):1001–11.
50. Schnitzer TJ, Gray WL, Paster RZ, et al. Efficacy of tramadol in treatment of chronic low back pain. J Rheumatol 2000;27(3):772–8.
51. Wilder-Smith CH, Hill L, Spargo K, et al. Treatment of severe pain from osteoarthritis with slow-release tramadol or dihydrocodeine in combination with NSAID's: a randomised study comparing analgesia, antinociception and gastrointestinal effects. Pain 2001;91(1–2):23–31.
52. Affaitati G, Fabrizio A, Savini A, et al. A randomized, controlled study comparing a lidocaine patch, a placebo patch, and anesthetic injection for treatment of trigger points in patients with myofascial pain syndrome: evaluation of pain and somatic pain thresholds. Clin Ther 2009;31(4):705–20.
53. Lin SY, Neoh CA, Huang YT, et al. Educational program for myofascial pain syndrome. J Altern Complement Med 2010;16(6):633–40.
54. Treaster D, Marras WS, Burr D, et al. Myofascial trigger point development from visual and postural stressors during computer work. J Electromyogr Kinesiol 2006;16(2):115–24.
55. Edwards RH. Hypotheses of peripheral and central mechanisms underlying occupational muscle pain and injury. Eur J Appl Physiol Occup Physiol 1988; 57(3):275–81.
56. Madeleine P. On functional motor adaptations: from the quantification of motor strategies to the prevention of musculoskeletal disorders in the neck-shoulder region. Acta Physiol (Oxf) 2010;199(Suppl 679):1–46.
57. Hoyle JA, Marras WS, Sheedy JE, et al. Effects of postural and visual stressors on myofascial trigger point development and motor unit rotation during computer work. J Electromyogr Kinesiol 2011;21(1):41–8.
58. Bhatnager V, Drury CG, Schiro SG. Posture, postural discomfort, and performance. Hum Factors 1985;27(2):189–99.
59. Rota E, Evangelista A, Ciccone G, et al. Effectiveness of an educational and physical program in reducing accompanying symptoms in subjects with head and neck pain: a workplace controlled trial. J Headache Pain 2011;12(3): 339–45.
60. Komiyama O, Kawara M, Arai M, et al. Posture correction as part of behavioural therapy in treatment of myofascial pain with limited opening. J Oral Rehabil 1999;26(5):428–35.
61. McNulty WH, Gevirtz RN, Hubbard DR, et al. Needle electromyographic evaluation of trigger point response to a psychological stressor. Psychophysiology 1994;31(3):313–6.
62. Crockett DJ, Foreman ME, Alden L, et al. A comparison of treatment modes in the management of myofascial pain dysfunction syndrome. Biofeedback Self Regul 1986;11(4):279–91.

63. Turner JA, Mancl L, Aaron LA. Short- and long-term efficacy of brief cognitive-behavioral therapy for patients with chronic temporomandibular disorder pain: a randomized, controlled trial. Pain 2006;121(3):181–94.

64. Ferraccioli G, Ghirelli L, Scita F, et al. EMG-biofeedback training in fibromyalgia syndrome. J Rheumatol 1987;14(4):820–5.

65. Grossman P, Tiefenthaler-Gilmer U, Raysz A, et al. Mindfulness training as an intervention for fibromyalgia: evidence of postintervention and 3-year follow-up benefits in well-being. Psychother Psychosom 2007;76(4):226–33.

66. Kaplan KH, Goldenberg DL, Galvin-Nadeau M. The impact of a meditation-based stress reduction program on fibromyalgia. Gen Hosp Psychiatry 1993; 15(5):284–9.

67. Furlan AD, van Tulder M, Cherkin D, et al. Acupuncture and dry-needling for low back pain: an updated systematic review within the framework of the Cochrane Collaboration. Spine (Phila Pa 1976) 2005;30(8):944–63.

68. Peloso P, Gross A, Haines T, et al. Medicinal and injection therapies for mechanical neck disorders. Cochrane Database Syst Rev 2007;(3):CD000319.

69. Birch S, Jamison RN. Controlled trial of Japanese acupuncture for chronic myofascial neck pain: assessment of specific and nonspecific effects of treatment. Clin J Pain 1998;14(3):248–55.

70. Irnich D, Behrens N, Molzen H, et al. Randomised trial of acupuncture compared with conventional massage and "sham" laser acupuncture for treatment of chronic neck pain. BMJ 2001;322(7302):1574–8.

71. Ga H, Choi JH, Park CH, et al. Acupuncture needling versus lidocaine injection of trigger points in myofascial pain syndrome in elderly patients–a randomised trial. Acupunct Med 2007;25(4):130–6.

72. Zhang JF, Wu YC, Mi YQ. Observation on therapeutic effect of acupuncture at pain points for treatment of myofascial pain syndrome. Zhongguo Zhen Jiu 2009;29(9):717–20.

73. Melzack R, Stillwell DM, Fox EJ. Trigger points and acupuncture points for pain: correlations and implications. Pain 1977;3(1):3–23.

74. Trampas A, Kitsios A, Sykaras E, et al. Clinical massage and modified proprioceptive neuromuscular facilitation stretching in males with latent myofascial trigger points. Phys Ther Sport 2010;11(3):91–8.

75. Gam AN, Warming S, Larsen LH, et al. Treatment of myofascial trigger-points with ultrasound combined with massage and exercise–a randomised controlled trial. Pain 1998;77(1):73–9.

76. Ardic F, Sarhus M, Topuz O. Comparison of two different techniques of electrotherapy on myofascial pain. J Back Musculoskelet Rehabil 2002;16(1):11–6.

77. Graff-Radford SB, Reeves JL, Baker RL, et al. Effects of transcutaneous electrical nerve stimulation on myofascial pain and trigger point sensitivity. Pain 1989; 37(1):1–5.

78. Smania N, Corato E, Fiaschi A, et al. Repetitive magnetic stimulation: a novel therapeutic approach for myofascial pain syndrome. J Neurol 2005;252(3):307–14.

79. Farina S, Casarotto M, Benelle M, et al. A randomized controlled study on the effect of two different treatments (FREMS AND TENS) in myofascial pain syndrome. Eura Medicophys 2004;40(4):293–301.

80. Chu J, Schwartz I. eToims twitch relief method in chronic refractory myofascial pain (CRMP). Electromyogr Clin Neurophysiol 2008;48(6–7):311–20.

81. Chu J, Takehara I, Li TC, et al. Electrical twitch obtaining intramuscular stimulation (ETOIMS) for myofascial pain syndrome in a football player. Br J Sports Med 2004;38(5):E25.

82. Chu J, Yuen KF, Wang BH, et al. Electrical twitch-obtaining intramuscular stimulation in lower back pain: a pilot study. Am J Phys Med Rehabil 2004;83(2): 104–11.

83. Majlesi J, Unalan H. High-power pain threshold ultrasound technique in the treatment of active myofascial trigger points: a randomized, double-blind, case-control study. Arch Phys Med Rehabil 2004;85(5):833–6.

84. Srbely JZ, Dickey JP. Randomized controlled study of the antinociceptive effect of ultrasound on trigger point sensitivity: novel applications in myofascial therapy? Clin Rehabil 2007;21(5):411–7.

85. Ay S, Evcik D, Tur BS. Comparison of injection methods in myofascial pain syndrome: a randomized controlled trial. Clin Rheumatol 2010;29(1): 19–23.

86. Draper DO, Mahaffey C, Kaiser D, et al. Thermal ultrasound decreases tissue stiffness of trigger points in upper trapezius muscles. Physiother Theory Pract 2010;26(3):167–72.

87. Shin SM, Choi JK. Effect of indomethacin phonophoresis on the relief of temporomandibular joint pain. Cranio 1997;15(4):345–8.

88. Graff-Radford SB, Reeves JL, Jaeger B. Management of chronic head and neck pain: effectiveness of altering factors perpetuating myofascial pain. Headache 1987;27(4):186–90.

89. Edwards J, Knowles N. Superficial dry needling and active stretching in the treatment of myofascial pain–a randomised controlled trial. Acupunct Med 2003;21(3):80–6.

90. Hong CZ. Considerations and recommendations regarding myofascial trigger point injection. J Muscoskel Pain 1994;2(1):29–54.

91. Kalichman L, Vulfsons S. Dry needling in the management of musculoskeletal pain. J Am Board Fam Med 2010;23(5):640–6.

92. Tsai CT, Hsieh LF, Kuan TS, et al. Remote effects of dry needling on the irritability of the myofascial trigger point in the upper trapezius muscle. Am J Phys Med Rehabil 2010;89(2):133–40.

93. Tekin L, Akarsu S, Durmus O, et al. The effect of dry needling in the treatment of myofascial pain syndrome: a randomized double-blinded placebo-controlled trial. Clin Rheumatol 2013;32(3):309–15.

94. Kietrys DM, Palombaro KM, Azzaretto E, et al. Effectiveness of dry needling for upper quarter myofascial pain: a systematic review and meta-analysis. J Orthop Sports Phys Ther 2013;43(9):620–34.

95. Baldry P, Yunus M, Inanici F. Myofascial pain and fibromyalgia syndrome: a clinical guide to diagnosis and management. Edinburgh (United Kingdom): Churchill Livingstone; 2001.

96. Ceccherelli F, Rigoni MT, Gagliardi G, et al. Comparison of superficial and deep acupuncture in the treatment of lumbar myofascial pain: a double-blind randomized controlled study. Clin J Pain 2002;18(3):149–53.

97. Lennard T. Trigger point injections. In: Lennard T, editor. Pain procedures in clinical practice. Philadelphia: Elsevier; 2011. p. 89.

98. Iwama H, Akama Y. The superiority of water-diluted 0.25% to neat 1% lidocaine for trigger-point injections in myofascial pain syndrome: a prospective, randomized, double-blinded trial. Anesth Analg 2000;91(2):408–9.

99. Iwama H, Ohmori S, Kaneko T, et al. Water-diluted local anesthetic for trigger-point injection in chronic myofascial pain syndrome: evaluation of types of local anesthetic and concentrations in water. Reg Anesth Pain Med 2001;26(4): 333–6.

100. Venancio Rde A, Alencar FG, Zamperini C. Different substances and dry-needling injections in patients with myofascial pain and headaches. Cranio 2008;26(2):96–103.
101. Cummings TM, White AR. Needling therapies in the management of myofascial trigger point pain: a systematic review. Arch Phys Med Rehabil 2001;82(7): 986–92.
102. Hong CZ. Lidocaine injection versus dry needling to myofascial trigger point. The importance of the local twitch response. Am J Phys Med Rehabil 1994; 73(4):256–63.
103. Gerwin RD, Shannon S, Hong CZ, et al. Interrater reliability in myofascial trigger point examination. Pain 1997;69(1–2):65–73.
104. Casale R, Tugnoli V. Botulinum toxin for pain. Drugs R D 2008;9(1):11–27.
105. Aoki KR. Review of a proposed mechanism for the antinociceptive action of botulinum toxin type A. Neurotoxicology 2005;26(5):785–93.
106. Gobel H, Heinze A, Heinze-Kuhn K, et al. Botulinum toxin A for the treatment of headache disorders and pericranial pain syndromes. Nervenarzt 2001;72(4): 261–74.
107. Soares A, Andriolo RB, Atallah AN, et al. Botulinum toxin for myofascial pain syndromes in adults. Cochrane Database Syst Rev 2012;(4):CD007533.
108. Ferrante FM, Bearn L, Rothrock R, et al. Evidence against trigger point injection technique for the treatment of cervicothoracic myofascial pain with botulinum toxin type A. Anesthesiology 2005;103(2):377–83.
109. Wheeler AH, Goolkasian P, Gretz SS. A randomized, double-blind, prospective pilot study of botulinum toxin injection for refractory, unilateral, cervicothoracic, paraspinal, myofascial pain syndrome. Spine (Phila Pa 1976) 1998;23(15): 1662–6 [discussion: 1667].
110. Porta M. A comparative trial of botulinum toxin type A and methylprednisolone for the treatment of myofascial pain syndrome and pain from chronic muscle spasm. Pain 2000;85(1–2):101–5.
111. Fishman LM, Konnoth C, Rozner B. Botulinum neurotoxin type B and physical therapy in the treatment of piriformis syndrome: a dose-finding study. Am J Phys Med Rehabil 2004;83(1):42–50 [quiz: 51–3].
112. Lang AM. Botulinum toxin type B in piriformis syndrome. Am J Phys Med Rehabil 2004;83(3):198–202.
113. Fishman LM, Anderson C, Rosner B. BOTOX and physical therapy in the treatment of piriformis syndrome. Am J Phys Med Rehabil 2002;81(12):936–42.
114. Qerama E, Fuglsang-Frederiksen A, Kasch H, et al. A double-blind, controlled study of botulinum toxin A in chronic myofascial pain. Neurology 2006;67(2): 241–5.
115. Gobel H, Heinze A, Reichel G, et al. Efficacy and safety of a single botulinum type A toxin complex treatment (Dysport) for the relief of upper back myofascial pain syndrome: results from a randomized double-blind placebo-controlled multicentre study. Pain 2006;125(1–2):82–8.
116. Kamanli A, Kaya A, Ardicoglu O, et al. Comparison of lidocaine injection, botulinum toxin injection, and dry needling to trigger points in myofascial pain syndrome. Rheumatol Int 2005;25(8):604–11.
117. Gerwin R. Botulinum toxin treatment of myofascial pain: a critical review of the literature. Curr Pain Headache Rep 2012;16(5):413–22.

Opioid Syndrome
Failed Opioid Therapy for Chronic Noncancer Pain

Leonard B. Kamen, DO[a,b,*], Kristofer J. Feeko, DO[c]

KEYWORDS

- Opioids • Chronic pain • Opioid dependence • Buprenorphine • Pain management

KEY POINTS

- There is an alarming incidence of reported chronic noncancer pain (CNCP) in the United States despite a significant expansion of opioid therapy over the past 2 decades.
- Failed opioid therapy in CNCP is characterized by high-dose use without perceived improvement in function, quality of life, or pain reduction.
- Chronic opioid therapy (COT) produces dependence behaviors in medically compromised CNCP similar to recreational opioid substance use disorders.
- Buprenorphine has partial agonist endorphin effect on mu receptors and antagonist effects on dynorphin-biased kappa receptors when used in the treatment of opioid dependence (OD) maintenance in CNCP.
- Comprehensive CNCP management may require balanced low-dose opioids in a continuum of a biopsychosocial care environment oriented toward engaging patients in self-directed care of a chronic disease.

Opioid syndrome is a descriptive term for failed opioid therapy in CNCP, when treatment becomes a problem more than a solution.

DEMOGRAPHICS

Progressive incorporation of high-dose opioids (HDOs) (>100 mg/d of morphine equivalents) evolving in the United States over the past 20 years for the treatment of CNCP have failed to stem the rising tide of patients identifying themselves as having chronic pain. CNCP is deemed a major disease demographic by the Centers for Disease Control and Prevention (CDC) affecting more Americans than diabetes, heart disease, and cancer combined. The CDC survey identifies up to 30% of the population or over 100 million people in the United States with CNCP.[1] Physicians who declare an interest

[a] MossRehab Outpatient Center, Albert Einstein Healthcare Network, 9880 Bustleton Avenue, Suite 309, Philadelphia, PA 19115, USA; [b] Department of Physical Medicine and Rehabilitation, Temple University Hospital, Philadelphia, PA, USA; [c] Department of Rehabilitation Medicine, Jefferson Medical College, Thomas Jefferson University, Philadelphia, PA, USA
* Corresponding author. MossRehab Outpatient Center, 9880 Bustleton Avenue, Suite 309, Philadelphia, PA 19115.
E-mail address: lkamen@einstein.edu

Phys Med Rehabil Clin N Am 25 (2014) 375–395
http://dx.doi.org/10.1016/j.pmr.2014.01.005
1047-9651/14/$ – see front matter © 2014 Elsevier Inc. All rights reserved.

in addressing this complex problem are saddled with a staggering number of people who have failed to achieve satisfactory subjective pain relief with the use of even staggering high doses of opioids. To many practitioners, this dichotomous, failed, relationship between opioids and chronic pain has become more of a problem than an efficient solution. Fortunately, the CDC report also deems chronic pain as one of the 9 potentially better treatable conditions deserving additional research attention. Enhancing CNCP treatment will require a significant shift in our medical effort to harness current and future opioid and nonopioid medications and nonmedical interventions. Recognition of chronic pain as a physiologic impairment of the brain, the central nervous system (CNS), the neuromusculoskeletal system and psychosocial environment will be a critical factor in this novel approach to address the epidemic impact of CNCP. The "quick fix" model of opioid treatment of CNCP needs a conceptual shift as well by practitioners and consumers in our current medical culture. This article serves to (1) identify the source of some of the many potential pitfalls of HDO therapy, (2) help the pain practitioner construct a motivational interview to foster patients' self-introspection regarding the sustainability and value of HDOs, and (3) provide perspective on opioid pharmacology to begin the process of restructuring treatment options.

OPIOID SYNDROME CONCEPT

Opioid syndrome (OS) may be constructed as a constellation of signs of a failed therapeutic medical intervention falling into identifiable clinical domains and presentation patterns (**Table 1**). Patients taking medically prescribed opioids for more than 3 months are likely to be on these medications for more than 2 years, or longer when on high doses, often exhibiting aberrant behaviors.[2] Opioids, when administered long term, are associated with expected (on part of the treating physician) or desired (on part of the patient) and unwanted effects (**Table 2**).[3] Long-term use of HDOs may also be associated with the development of abnormal sensitivity to pain or hyperalgesia. Ballyntyne[4] in her review of opioid therapy for CNCP states that opioid dose escalation may be the result of "pharmacologic opioid tolerance, opioid-induced abnormal pain sensitivity, or disease progression". Data regarding the long-term morbidity and mortality of long-term opioids prescribed for CNCP are primarily limited to hard endpoints, including death from use or abuse. The CONSORT study (Consortium to Study Opioid Risks and Trends) studied opioid use for CNCP from 1997 to 2005 and included adult members of 2 health plans serving over 1% of the US population. Patients prescribed 100 mg/d or more had an 8.9-fold (confidence interval 4.0–19.7) increase over the 0.2% rate for 1–20 mg Morphine Equivalent Dose/day (MED/d) in overdose risk (1.8% annual overdose rate).[5] Functional data were not reported in this study. Despite a paucity of credible long-term analysis of COT,[6] the medical management of chronic painful conditions has trended to the right in the pendulum swing from underprescribing to overprescribing (**Fig. 1**). From 1999 to 2010, the sales of opioid analgesics increased 4-fold. During this same period, the average amount of analgesic consumed for pain relief has increased disproportionately: in 1997, the average MED/d consumed was 96 mg, and this increased to more than 710 MED/d in 2010.[6] Aggressive use of opioid management for CNCP has been fueled by many factors. Well-intentioned primary care practitioners (PCPs) and a growing cadre of pain specialists, orthopedic surgeons, and dentists, fueled by pharmaceutical marketing may represent an unanticipated medical source of OS.[7] Coupled with illegal procurement through friends, family, and felons, the flames of a societal epidemic of opioid abuse have been ignited. This phenomenon has recently been acknowledged by Portnoy who advanced the concepts of COT in the 1990s for CNCP.[8] Some of the most outspoken proponents

Table 1
Opioid syndrome: domains, clinical presentations, relative clinical application, and observed frequency of occurrence of failed opioid therapy in CNCP

Domain	Typical Presentations	Contribution/Frequency	Additional Common Presentations
Somatic symptoms	Diffuse myalgias Arthralgias Neuralgias	Limited specificity ++++	Sleep-wake activity cycle disorders
Physical signs	Impairments in mobility/physical capacity	Perceived greater than demonstrated Subjective > objective +++	Kinesiophobic dyskinetic motions (eg, lumbopelvic, scapulohumeral dyskinesias) Deconditioning
Imaging	Incidental inconsequential/or mild-to-moderate degeneration	Anatomic degeneration but not specific to individual symptoms/+++	Limited insight as to the value of imaging in dx and tx
Psychological issues	Depressed/anxious/PTSD/amotivational/somatization/preoccupation with minutia	Lacking and/or rejection of mental health support/+++	Prone to catastrophizing Pathologizing benign medical elements; loss of locus of control
Medical comorbidities	Multiple treaters, treatments	List of providers Polypharmacy/+++	Diabetic neuropathy + peripheral entrapments, CRPS + contracture
SA concerns	Prior or current SA including tobacco	Denial of SA or neglect of SA services/+++	Tobacco and/or alcohol abuse with+ family history of the same
Social patterns	Dysfunctional or limited social interactions/nonsupported/impairment enabled	Critical loss of self-esteem or codependency on disability status/++	Codependent/enabled by secondary gain (compensation) or anger issues (seeking retribution)
Functional performance/pain (VAS) levels	Unchanged by opioid use, disproportionate to examination and diagnostic data	Critical to justification of continued use Requires temporal reassessment/+++	Dependent on exogenous substance to perform tasks/limited insight as relationship of medication to function
Vocational directions	Employed with restrictions/unemployed limited transferable skills On compensation—work or disability related	Societal implications reproductivity/costs of downtime/++	Unable to actuate lateral or horizontal change in vocational directions

Abbreviations: CRPS, Complex Regional Pain Syndrome; PTSD, post traumatic stress disorder; SA, substance abuse.
Key: +, occasionally; ++, frequently; +++, v frequently; ++++, commonly.
[a]Authors' clinical experience.

Table 2
Predictable positive and negative symptoms of opioid use

Therapeutic Positive Values	Positive Symptoms	Negative/Adverse Symptoms	Additional Negative Consequences
Analgesia	Pain relief	Dependence	Cognitive dysfunction
		Addiction behavior	Psychomotor slowing
Anxiolytic	Sedative	Euphoria	Mood changes
		Tolerance	Hallucinations
		Pruritis	Delirium
Antidyspnea	Used in acute myocardial and trauma conditions	Respiratory depression	Sleep disturbance Myoclonus Hyperhidrosis
Antigastrointestinal hypermotility	Decreased transit time in diarrheal disorders	Nausea Vomiting/ constipation/ obstruction	Dry mouth Periodontal disease Loss of Teeth
Antisalivation	Used to dry excessive oral salivary activity	Endocrine disorders Immune system dysfunction	Hyperalgesia Allodynia Hypesthesia

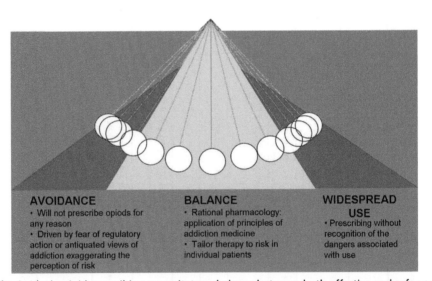

Fig. 1. Ideal opioid prescribing necessitates a balance between both effective and safe use of opioid medications in the treatment of the CNCP. Selection of the specific agent and quantity of medication must be weighed against the individual risk profile and level of function (both vocational and avocational) for each patient. Furthermore, selection and prescription cannot occur without adequate and continued consideration for the long-term medical risk and complication with continued use as well as the potential societal impact for continued use.

of COT for CNCP in the 1990s and early 2000s have readdressed the issue and concluded that there is a lot of reeducation required for the phalanx of physicians who have adopted aggressive opioid prescribing (**Box 1**).[9]

OPIOID DEPENDENCE IN THE MEDICALLY COMPROMISED CNCP POPULATION

The phenomena of OD and tolerance have been aptly defined and redefined in the pain and psychiatric literature. Controversy ensues when discussing opioid use disorders in the medically involved CNCP population when bias is perceived in crafting these definitions referring primarily to the recreational user. Dependence is a physiologic response, resulting in adaptation, whereby long-term use of opioids results in well-recognized and enumerated withdrawal symptoms (ie, Clinical Opiate Withdrawal Scale)[10] on discontinuation of use (conceived as recreational). Tolerance falls into the lines of either adaptive or associative tolerance. Adaptive tolerance refers to physiologic changes in receptor and transmitter makeup (recreational or CNCP related). Associative tolerance relates to environmental and social cues. Associative tolerance is the common explanation for overdose in which experienced recreational abusers died when using the same drug outside of their familiar environment. Classical definitions of OD and tolerance do not encompass what pain clinicians frequently encounter. The HDO user exhibits associative tolerance and OD in the context of an unrelenting perception of physical and/or social stress while being prescribed opioids for CNCP (**Table 3**). Dopaminergic reward behavior is being satiated without an improvement in the anatomic (ie, spinal or muscle pain) pathology. A vicious cycle effect is put into play with no expectation that the opioid will fix any problem other than the dependence it creates, which may represent both an adaptive and an analogous associative dependence.

Chronic pain is a disease state with an aberrant sensory (both peripheral and central) and psychologically modulated perception along with physiologic changes subject to adaptation and association. Treatment of CNCP with opioids that cross boundaries of adaptation, dependence, and tolerance with demonstrated physiologic responses in the glial cells and dorsal horn of the spinal cord cannot be held to definitions designed for the recreational user seeking a transient altered perception or engrossed in self-destructive behaviors.[11] Therefore, in the context of CNCP compared to recreational use, dependence and addiction require redefinition. The original intention of these terms did not account for or encompass the CNCP user. Application of the current Diagnostic and Statistical Manual of Mental Disorders (Fourth Edition) (DSM-IV) definition of OD outside of the context of recreational use is not sensitive to the unique adaptive pharmacology of opioids. There is significant potential for false-negative interpretation in identifying OD, tolerance, and abuse, when using only recreationally derived inclusion parameters for patients with CNCP. Substance abuse disorders are complex behaviors with multiple neurotransmitter-mediated, genetically

---

Box 1
Pain practitioners' thinking on opioid use, safety, and efficacy should be rethought as there is still relative lack of data for efficacy in CNCP

We overshot our mark, all well-intended, I believe... we certainly have a lot of reverse education that needs to occur.

—Lynn Webster, MD

From Fauber J. Chronic pain fuels boom in opioids. Milwaukee Journal Sentinel/MedPage Feb 19, 2012.

Table 3
Contrasting the recreational opioid-dependent user from the CNCP medical opioid user

Opioid Dependent—Recreational	Opioid Dependent—Chronic Pain
Compulsion	Unresolved pain focus
Difficulty controlling use	Frequent use of breakthrough pain medications
Withdrawal symptoms	Withdrawal symptoms interpreted as return of primary pain
Tolerance	Tolerant to high-potency opioid medications/and or hyperalgesic
Neglect of alternative pleasures	Altered social/occupational interactions
Persist in use despite known harm	Altered insight and judgment as to benefit/harm of medications

programmed behaviors and environmental triggers requiring an evolving fine-tuning of our current system of definition (eg, evolution of DSM-I through V).

CLINICIAN'S ROLE IN THE EVOLUTION OF HDO THERAPY AND THE OS

Clinicians are expected to identify and curtail malicious use of opioids by means of Opioid Risk Tool (ORT), (**Table 4**) urine drug screening, pill counts, monitoring of aberrant behaviors, and in some states, electronic prescription drug monitoring.

Table 4
Examples of validated clinical opioid abuse and aberrant behavior risk tools

Tool	Format	Administration/Scoring
Opioid Risk Tool	A 5-item self-report measure to assist in predicting the probability of aberrant drug-related behaviors when prescribed opioids for pain	Each risk factor is composed of one or more items, with the entire measure consisting of 10 items; items are scores with a possible total score range from 0 to 26
SOAPP	A 24-item self-report questionnaire to assist in determining potential risk of abuse when prescribing opioids for pain	SOAPP items were summed to address a range of variables that may increase risk factors for aberrant drug-related behavior, including family history of substance use, mood swings, legal problems, etc. Scored on a Likert scale from 0 (never) to 4 (very often); total scores can range from 0 to 56
DIRE	Clinician-rated measure designed to predict efficacy of analgesia and patient compliance with long-term opioid analgesic treatment	Four subcategories, including psychological, chemical health, reliability, and social support Scores on each category range from 1 to 3 (4–12 for risk), with total scores ranging from 7 to 21, with lower scores indicating greater risk

Abbreviations: DIRE, Diagnosis, Intractability, Risk, and Efficacy Inventory; SOAPP, Screener and Opioid Assessment for Patients with Pain.
From Moore TM, Jones T, Browder JH, et al. A comparison of common screening methods for predicting aberrant drug-related behaviors among patients receiving opioids for chronic pain management. Pain Med 2009;10(8):1426–33; with permission.

The policing aspect of care consumes significant resources for clinicians in time, paperwork, and staffing that may be in conflict with the additional medical care needs of the outpatient clinic population. If office staff is overwhelmed with the logistics of prescribing, evaluating, rewriting, and monitoring opioid therapy, the practitioner is at great risk of medication and compliance errors that jeopardize patient and public safety as well as licensure requirements. Pressurized office schedules and inadequate staffing conditions often result in escalation of opioids in CNCP because this is the path of least resistance when confronting challenging subjective perceptions of flaring pain symptoms. Decisions to increase opioid dose are filtered into a clinician's matrix of knowledge regarding a sometimes nebulous diagnosis, as is often the case in chronic pain. Frequently, there is no observed active shift or objective anatomic derangement that fully accounts for the fluctuation of pain perception of the HDO patient's exacerbation (ie, radiculopathy, arthritic or myofascial pain). Rather, pain can be potentiated and maintained by certain physiologic challenges (hyperalgesia), psychological challenges (ie, depression, stress, manic behavior), and/or functional overuse.[4] Upward dose titration is made against a subjective more than objective analysis of these conditions. The clinician must also consider factors other than the patient, such as the intrinsic properties of the opioid being selected. The unique properties of opioid receptors (**Fig. 2**), cytochrome P450 (CYP450) enzyme systems, as well as "drug likability" remain critical factors in dosing.[12,13] Personalities of both opioid users and physician prescribers themselves in a busy outpatient office abound in various forms of calculating manipulation, neediness, and likability as well. This scheme plays out everyday in a pain management practice, factoring into the complex

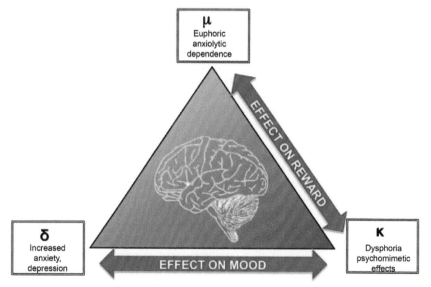

Fig. 2. Opioid receptor physiology and influence on mood, behavior, and abuse. Opioid agonists and antagonists have different receptor affinities. Mu receptors interact with the endorphin system, influencing analgesia, euphoria, anxiety, and dopaminergic-reward-related mesolimbic, prefrontal-cortex-driven behaviors. Kappa receptor agonists interact with a bias toward the dynorphin system, mediating dysphoric mood, opioid craving, and negative psychomimetic effects. Delta receptors, less-frequently clinically active, generally can lead to dysphoria, hallucinations, and strong vasomotor effects. μ, mu; κ, kappa; δ, delta.

biopsychosocial environment that has contributed to an abundance of opioid pre-scriptions in the United States.

GAP IN EXPECTATION AND UNDERSTANDING CHRONIC PAIN

A cataclysmic gap remains between the societal expectation of a rapid ablation of pain and the current neuroscience model of chronic pain as a complex, multifactorial neurosensory and emotional phenomena. Within this deep trench may be the seed and soil on which CNCP and subsequent OS has escalated out of control. The growth of quick fix pain clinics in the United States over the past decade has created an iatrogenic-induced, pathologic, pain treatment thinking process. Expectation is frequently discordant from real outcomes in chronic pain. Spinal injection therapy alone for chronic back pain has not met acceptable benchmarks for enhanced out-comes for chronic low-back pain. However, this has not curbed the enthusiasm or popularity of these interventional therapies.[14–16] The practice of fluoroscopically guided interventional procedures has increased by 159% between 2000 and 2010 alone.[17] Clinics focused on procedural interventions only, and/or opioid dispensing, providing only a narrow spectrum of medical and behavioral support for the treatment of complex CNCP have fanned the flames of many seeking immediate gratification in pursuit of instant pain relief. This type of flawed thinking on behalf of patients and prac-titioners can lead the patient with CNCP to perceive that extrinsic or passive therapeu-tics, in the form of a procedure or a medication, have greater potential to heal, or fix what is likely thought of as broken, than intrinsic or lasting means. Self-actualization of change and acceptance of the limitations in correcting altered anatomy through well-directed physical, emotional, and cognitive behavioral adaptations may be the cornerstone of chronic pain rehabilitation.

THIRD-PARTY COMPLICITY

Third-party insurers and financially strapped state and federal government payers often restrict access to a greater spectrum of medical management choices. Annual budgets may impose constraints on quality-controlled comprehensive care programs for this chronic condition that has no fixed chronologic endpoint. Limits on prescription of novel pharmaceuticals and nonmedical therapies that may be less physiologically and socially harmful are imposed on the patients often most in need of these alternative pathways. Third parties often sanction first-line treatment of CNCP with high-potency opioids generically produced despite high risk of abuse and diversion (ie, oxycodone, hydrocodone, and methadone). Short-acting opioids (SAOs) are encouraged in step edits, which may contribute to operant conditioning with frequent dosing, reinforcing continued and perhaps escalating use in some patients. No conclusive studies have demonstrated the risk of abuse in the use of SAOs versus long-acting opioids.[18] Comprehensive outpatient or intensive inpatient care of CNCP may be costly, but the outcomes projected by early studies on comprehensive pain clinics clearly point to efficiencies to be gained not only financially but also in productivity, quality of life, and social and vocational stabilization seen in properly selected, directed, and moti-vated patients with CNCP.[19] However, insurance coverage for comprehensive pain management with mental, emotional, physical, and medical alternative therapies is challenging and often rejected, despite positive data to support the efficacy of multidis-ciplinary multimodal approaches to pain.[20] Managed care capitation networks may prevent use of physical, occupational, and psychological therapies in an outpatient setting, further fracturing or making it more difficult to render the much needed cohesive care in an ambulatory comprehensive rehabilitation clinic setting.

CATASTROPHIC THINKING AND OVERMEDICALIZATION

Overmedicalization of incidental diagnostic findings or what may often be a transient mechanical and psychosocial overload or overuse syndrome to an at-risk individual creates catastrophic thinking. Catastrophizing is defined as "an exaggerated negative mental set brought to bear during an actual or anticipated painful experience."[21] Measurement of catastrophizing is recognized as a key element of cognitive behavioral treatment and has been quantified and scored by use of the Pain Catastrophizing Scale[21] with the components listed in **Fig. 3**.

Gracely and colleagues[22] demonstrated the critical role that pain catastrophizing plays in the brain through functional magnetic resonance imaging (MRI) studies. This phenomenon is said to be uniquely located in the areas of attention to pain, emotion, and motor activity. Persons who catastrophize have difficulty shifting their attention away from the pain experience, which in turn becomes a threatening, fearful experience for some, creating hypervigilance. Overmedicalization of what may be an inconsequential disk desiccation on imaging studies is frequently demonstrated by limited insight and extreme responses on pain indices (see **Table 1**). Nevertheless, despite availability of validated screening tools as simple as the ORT (see **Table 4**), which consists of only 5 brief questions, there seem to be countless inappropriately selected patients for opioid therapy.

Recent analysis of almost 24,000 physician visits from 1999 to 2010 for acute low-back pain showed a dramatic increase in use of narcotics from 19.3% to 29.1% despite publication of several guidelines over this span of time discouraging this practice.[23] Meta-analysis of studies incorporating opioids for chronic back pain illustrated limited efficacy with high rates of substance abuse (43%) and aberrant behaviors (24%) among back pain cases prescribed opioids.[23]

<u>Subscales:</u>

- **Rumination** (*I can't stop thinking about it*),
- Sum of items: 8, 9, 10, 11.
- Score: (mean 10.1 / SD 4.3)

- **Magnification** (*I know something terrible is about to happen*)
- Sum of items: 6,7,13.
- Score: (mean 4.8 / SD 2.8)

- **Helplessness** (*I feel awful and I am overwhelmed*)
- Sum of items: 1, 2, 3, 4, 5, 12.
- Score: (mean 13.3 / SD 4.3)

When I am in pain...
0 – not at all, 1- to a slight degree, 2- to a moderate degree, 3 - to a great degree, 4 – all the time

❑ 1. I worry all the time whether the pain will end.
❑ 2. I feel I can't go on.
❑ 3. It's terrible and I think it's never going to end.
❑ 4. It's awful and I feel that it overwhelms me.
❑ 5. I feel I can't stand it anymore.
❑ 6. I become afraid that the pain will get worse.
❑ 7. I keep thinking of other painful events.
❑ 8. I anxiously want the pain to go away.
❑ 9. I can't seem to keep it out of my mind.
❑ 10. I keep thinking of how much it hurts.
❑ 11. I keep thinking about how badly I want the pain to stop.
❑ 12. There's nothing I can do to reduce the intensity of the pain.
❑ 13. I wonder whether something serious may happen.

Fig. 3. The pain catastrophizing scale (Sullivan) can be used to rate affect in CNCP. Subscales isolate affective focus. SD, standard deviation. Key to scoring: higher score = greater catastrophic thinking. Total score = 52. (*Adapted from* Sullivan MJL, Bishop S, Pivik J. The pain catastrophizing scale: development and validation. Psychol Assess 1995;7: 524–32.)

MEDICAL MANAGEMENT OF OS WITHIN THE BIOPSYCHOSOCIAL MODEL OF CHRONIC PAIN

When considering medical management of the patient with criteria for OS, chronic pain is best conceived as a biopsychosocial problem.[24] The biology of chronic pain is recognized as the complex perpetuation of peripheral nociception that is neuro-transmitter dependent and behaviorally driven. This model of CNCP opens potent channels for pharmaceutical intervention well beyond the mu opioid receptor. Targeting multiple synaptic transmission pathways, cognitive perceptual reception, and modulation capacity makes for a considerably more sophisticated and rational pharmacotherapy of pain. Nociceptive signals are not perceived as pain until the brain is engaged in a neuromatrix of CNS structural areas relaying the peripheral signals to perceptual and functional areas geared to execute a response.[25] The neuromatrix, as conceived by Melzac and others, represents the web of the sensory, affective, and cognitive elements of the CNS involved in interpretation of our internal and external environment. Psychological processes are equally complex based on multiple variables including genetics, gender, prior trauma, and supportive or enabling environments to identify a few well-studied key elements. The disconcerting societal impact of CNCP and opioids is exhibited by the fact that deaths from prescription opioid use and abuse exceeded deaths from motor vehicle accidents in 2010.[26] Neglecting this biopsychosocial model of CNCP has contributed to an inadequate, insatiate medical response to a growing epidemic.

MESOLIMBIC INFLUENCE OF OPIOID DEPENDENCY IN CHRONIC PAIN

The emotional, affective component of chronic pain, as previously discussed, is equally at the core of OS. Receptor sites for opioid agonists are replete in the mesolimbic neuromatrix responsible for perception, interpretation, and relay to the prefrontal cortex to take executive action (**Fig. 4**). Opioid pharmacology (dependence and tolerance) dictates pursuit of continual dosing and escalation of use in those individuals with a limited emotional wherewithal. Patients with CNCP who are emotionally strained and are exposed to potent opioids early in their treatment are strongly drawn

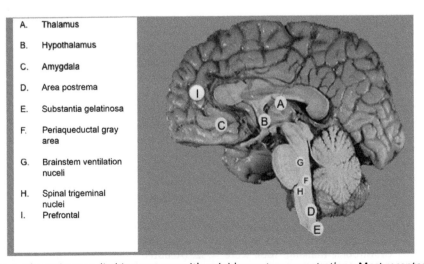

A.   Thalamus

B.   Hypothalamus

C.   Amygdala

D.   Area postrema

E.   Substantia gelatinosa

F.   Periaqueductal gray area

G.   Brainstem ventilation nuceli

H.   Spinal trigeminal nuclei

I.   Prefrontal

Fig. 4. The major mesolimbic structures with opioid receptor concentrations. Most receptors are located throughout the midbrain, pontine, and medullary structures.

to continuation and dosage escalation. This condition may represent a psychological retreat from daunting physical challenges or a particularly susceptible time to form mesolimbic-system-driven opioid dependency. Opioid therapy can worsen depression that may already be part and parcel of CNCP.[27] Withdrawal from opioids and reduction in serum levels between doses or fluctuations dependent on competition with other drugs or food on the CYP450 metabolic processing system in the liver is manifested by worsening anxiety. Misinterpretation of anxiety symptoms as a crescendo of somatic or neuropathic pain is not uncommon but difficult for CNCP opioid users to sort out or interpret as a transient nonmedical source of pain.

OPTIONS TO OPIOIDS IN THE PATIENT WITH CNCP

Where do we turn when asked to treat chronic pain, when one views the solution, in opioid medications, as more the problem than the solution? Recognition of this skew in the fine balance point is more easily identified by the astute clinician and not the consumer. Engaging the HDO user in this enlightenment and turning the wheel of change (**Fig. 5**)[28] is not accomplished without considerable effort and skill in employing the arts of reflective listening and motivational interviewing (**Boxes 2 and 3**).[29,30] Options to opioids that are equianalgesic for the management of CNCP are not abundant. Introducing new or alternative medication to a COT patient is not a simple substitution process. The list of viable nonopioid analgesics has shrunk with the elimination of nonsteroidal antiinflammatory drugs as safe and sustainable. Adjunctive agents from the classes of antidepressants known to modulate the descending inhibitory pathways of pain are primarily norepinephrine reuptake inhibitors. Antiepileptic drugs that block sodium and additional ionic channels may be helpful in neuropathic and fibromyalgic pain symptoms. Antispasmodic muscle relaxants and anxiolytic agents exert a sedative role but offer limited analgesia. Topicals, compounded by a growing array of small and larger pharmacies, offer arrays of

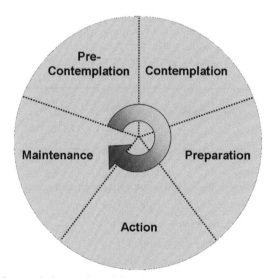

Fig. 5. Stages of change: behavioral model utilized in addiction medicine, applicable to the CNCP population on HDOs with an inclination to change treatment strategies. Generally, one stage must be completed before moving on to the next stage. The process begins with precontemplation and moves sequentially, concluding with the maintenance stage.

Box 2
Reflective listening techniques

Let patient know you are **listening**

Responding to what is **personal** rather than to what is **impersonal**...

Restating and **clarifying** what the other has said...

... understand the **feelings** contained in what the other is saying, not just the facts or ideas.

... develop the best possible sense of the **other's frame of reference** ... avoiding the temptation to respond from the listener's frame of reference.

Responding with **acceptance and empathy**...

Adapted from Charon R. Narrative medicine: a model for empathy, reflection, profession and trust. JAMA 2001;286(15):1897–902.

---

combinations of agents that have positive anecdotal responses without rigorous studies to isolate which component, vehicle, or tactile method may work best.

BUPRENORPHINE: MEDICALLY ASSISTED MAINTENANCE OF OD IN CNCP

Buprenorphine and buprenorphine-naloxone (BP-N) are unique opioid receptor models designated to be used as OD maintenance medication. The Drug Addiction and Treatment Act of 2000 allowed for a congressional waiver for specific use of BP-N for qualified physicians for office-based treatment of addiction on a limited basis.[31] The product is specifically approved for OD maintenance with strict oversight and policing of adherence by the Drug Enforcement Agency (DEA). However, buprenorphine alone as a potent mixed partial agonist-antagonist opioid is also approved for the treatment of chronic moderate to severe pain in the form of a transdermal patch in the United States and in worldwide distribution. In the United States, transdermal buprenorphine is a schedule III, long-acting analgesic.

Buprenorphine is a partial agonist with a strong affinity for the mu opioid receptor sites but only partial biologic activity (**Fig. 6**).[32] A pharmacokinetic plateau in mu opioid effects is demonstrated including limited respiratory depression and euphoria at a

---

Box 3
Key elements of motivational interviewing technique

Expressing empathy
- Conveying a real, ie, informed understanding of the person's predicament

Avoiding argument
- Encourage patients to hear themselves say why they want to change

Support self-efficacy
- Belief in one's ability to make a change and stick to it

Developing discrepancy (cognitive dissonance)
- When appropriate goals are established, then the therapist can start to *identify the difference between the current and ideal situation*

Roll with resistance
- Skillfully challenge the thought processes that underlie the behavior one wants to change

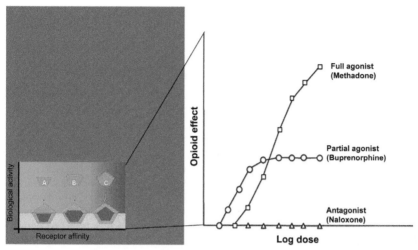

Fig. 6. Relationship of opioid receptor binding affinity and physiologic activity. Inset shows the relationship between receptor and ligand affinity by how well the ligand (A, B, and C) fits with the receptor site, where A is antagonist, B is partial agonist, and C is full agonist. Affinity is across the x-axis; with A having the least affinity and C having the greatest affinity. The biologic activity is represented by the magnitude of the overlap of the ligand into the green area, again with ligand A having the lowest activity and C having the greatest. Pharmacologic agents with opioid activity—either agonist or antagonist—will be determined by the combination of affinity for the receptor and the biologic activity. An effective antagonist, for example, naloxone, has a very high receptor affinity and very low biologic activity.

saturation point of approximately 16 mg/d. Kappa antagonism is demonstrated with implications for blocking dynorphin effects. Dynorphins play a role in craving and may stimulate pain, drug tolerance, and withdrawal symptoms in experimental models.[33]

Recognizing and documenting opioid dependence in patients with CNCP in whom use of HDOs has failed is a critical factor in using BP-N as an effective exit strategy. The criteria used for OD[34] should be unequivocal as the primary disorder with full disclosure to the patient and family of the medical priorities being set. Induction and titration of BP-N must proceed as indicated in the training process required by the DEA to administer this medication.[35] Adherence to requirements for documentation of medical necessity and perhaps most importantly, a comprehensive behavioral and medical management of OD and addiction, must be fulfilled, including appropriate referrals to drug counseling and/or mental health providers. Gratifying results are frequently achieved in this population of patients with CNCP who have come to realize the overwhelming nature of OD because of long-term exposure to prescriptions for high-potency HDOs that have been influencing and dictating day-to-day and moment-to-moment activities in their lives often for years on end.[36]

Adaptation to impairment often begins when dopaminergic pathways driving OD are satiated and behavioral as well as physical adjustments to chronic pain are now plausible. Technically, BP-N is medically assisted maintenance treatment that will not meet criteria for abstinence therapy. The terminology and phenomenology of harm reduction may apply.[37,38] Nevertheless, BP-N management of OD in patients with chronic pain on HDOs with failure to achieve reasonable life goals may be gratifying to the patients and practitioners. Many opioid substance abusers were initiated in the process because of chronic pain and have demonstrated benefit from transition to BP-N therapy.

CLINICAL SCENARIOS
Assessment: Adapting the Motivational Interview for CNCP in the HDO User

After years (now decades) of escalating opioid use for CNCP, there is a common phenomena in pain practices of patients presenting to the specialist with HDO use and low yield function. This referral group may best characterize the OS as previously described, seeking either confirmation of continued use or a takeover of opioid prescription writing from their beleaguered PCPs. Engaging the patient with CNCP on HDO in an interactive dialogue from the outset of a clinical assessment is a key component of addressing the OS once this is revealed early in the initial evaluation of this growing cadre of patient referrals. Reflective listening and motivational techniques (see **Boxes 2** and **3**) used in addiction medicine may facilitate a meaningful interview with better understanding of how HDO treatment has failed to solve any problem and may be the single most important problem to be solved.

More information may be gained from taking a careful history, examination, and observing the interactions of the accompanying person than may be gleaned from the diagnostic and consultative reports. Pathologic anatomy may blatantly exist on images but is poorly correlated on expert physical medicine/physiatric physical examination of the spinal axis and neuromuscular skeletal system. Pain character and intensity is vividly presented on pain drawings hatched and circled in dark ink blurring outlines of entire limbs, torso, head, and neck like storm clouds. Visual analog indicators shift sharply to the right, sometimes beyond linear boundaries (**Fig. 7**). There may be a well-rehearsed dialogue with catastrophic descriptors of limited tolerance for normal functions. Coaxing out details of mechanical or neuropathic qualities requires a skilled interview despite years of experience by both the patient and the practitioner.

Pain treatment may be viewed as an entitlement; once established, forever an unalienable right. This situation is said to be especially problematic with SAOs with immediate gratification however limited in longevity.[39] SAOs have been implicated as potent triggers of the brain's dopaminergic reward system. Triggering this pathway is said to "hijack" the prefrontal cortex executive decision-making function, perpetuating dependence in those susceptible individuals. No longer can these patients rationalize what may be the most beneficial survival tactic for a real, threatened, or perceived damaged anatomy. Quick fixes, albeit short lived, dominate the thinking process of these patients often accompanied by fear of being cutoff from their opioid of choice driven by memories of withdrawal experiences.

Based on the soon to be implemented DSM-V, the term opioid use disorder better characterizes the spectrum and diminishes the distinction between the recreational and the CNCP opioid consumer (**Box 4**).[40] In an effort to correct abuse trends, guidelines on opioid dosing in Washington State employing risk assessment calculations suggest an allowance of 120 mg MED/d. Greater MED without substantial improvement in pain and function requires a referral to a pain specialist. Tapering schemes or discontinuation of opioid paradigms are outlined.[41]

Management Strategies for Opioid Users with OS

Clinical Vignette 1: Evaluation and management (E&M) alternative strategies for abandoned HDO patient with back pain seeking new pain prescriber.

When challenged, the HDO patient who meets criteria for OS (see **Table 1**) responds with terms frequently repeated. "I cannot perform the tasks demanded of me without

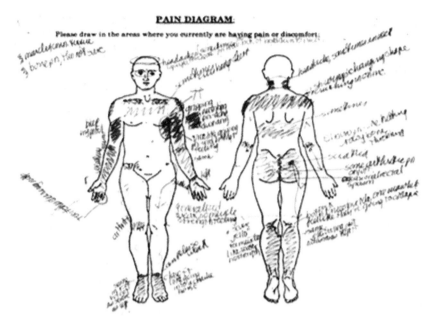

Fig. 7. Common pain diagrams for patients with CNCP. Usually the extent of painful area is discordant to the extent of original injury. In the case of escalating doses, the phenomenon of hyperalgesia may occur. Opioid-induced hyperalgesia or opioid-induced abnormal pain sensitivity has been described most commonly after long-term use of opioids; however, it has also been described after only a single high dose. Individuals may develop an increasing sensitivity to noxious stimuli and may develop a pain response to previously nonpainful stimulation (allodynia).

my HDO pain medications." Those tasks may run range from couch potato to home-making to construction work. The dialogue shifts from an analysis of medical findings that may or often may not substantiate the need for COT to a plea for a mercy opioid prescription. Available diagnostic examinations (MRI, electromyogram, X-rays) may illustrate degenerative disks or neural canal stenosis. However, careful objective clinical and neurologic assessment often fails to reveal a focal nerve root disruption or physiologic source of pain that would demand HDOs, quantitative risk tools, pain index's and functional performance scales may provide concrete baselines that could influence treatment changes and families to intercede. The findings of high opioid risk behaviors and lack of functional gains are minimized in the light of individuals' perception and plea for prescriptions so that they may maintain a marginal facade of functionality. Fear of abandonment may govern the conversation, placing the new patient in an offensive posture. Incorporation of reflective listening, and hands-on well-guided, physical and neurologic examination to gain patient confidence in the practitioner may set the stage for a shift in treatment direction. Motivational interviewing techniques, cognitive behavioral reframing, and decatastrophizing may plant the seeds of pursuing a detoxification strategy followed by psychological support and BP-N therapy (**Table 5**). Community-based counseling and physical activity programs paced to individuals' tolerance should be promoted as a responsibility of adults living with a chronic impairment over a continuum of their lives.

Clinical Vignette 2: HDO user showing minimal to no functional benefit, overwhelmed by burden of multiple somatic pain complaints despite medications.

Box 4
The new DSM-V criteria for opioid use disorder

Opioid use disorder

Problematic pattern of opioid use leading to clinically significant impairment or distress, as manifested by at least 2 of the following, occurring within a *12-month period*:

- Escalating dose and duration than was intended
- Persistent desire for the opioid
- Engaging in unsuccessful efforts to cut down or control opioid use
- Inordinate time and effort to obtain, use, or recover from the effects of the opioid
- Craving, or a strong desire or urge to use opioids
- Use that results in failure to fulfill major role obligations at work, school, or home

Continuing use despite persistent or recurrent social or interpersonal problems

- Giving up or reducing important social, occupational, or recreational activities
- Use despite physical hazards
- Use despite physical or psychological problems that are caused or exacerbated by the substance
- Tolerance, as defined by either a need for markedly increased amounts of opioids to achieve intoxications or desired effect, or a markedly diminished effect with continued use of the same amount of an opioid
- Withdrawal, as manifested by either the characteristic opioid withdrawal syndrome, or taking opioids to relieve or avoid withdrawal symptoms

---

Clinical vignette: postlaminectomy fusion HDO users for more than 5 years with chronic pain complaints reported in the realm of 8–10/10 on VAS, claiming that without HDO they may be in even further distress. Opioid therapy had escalated over the course of years. Previous physician or physicians performed testing (never reviewed with patients directly). Failed interventional injections and trials of spinal cord stimulation. Clinical examination exhibits marked guarding of lumbar paraspinal musculature above the fusion site with profoundly restricted trunk motion. Gait stance and swing is asymmetric with no assistive device. Motor strength, sensory, and reflex examination is nonfocal with guarding and inconsistent sensory levels. Similar assessment and interviewing techniques apply in this case scenario as in clinical vignette 1. When patients are engaged in a novel introspective process with an equally engaged physician, they may become unexpected stakeholders in the continuum of change (see **Fig. 5**). Additional comments are listed in the decision matrix of **Table 6** referring to clinical vignette 2.

DISCUSSION

CNCP is an isolating multidimensional sensory and emotional experience with no absolute objectification. Nevertheless, this sensory, affective, and cognitive complex drift to a disease state of chronic pain demands expert medical attention and management if outcomes are going to improve. Our current medical model has created an illusion of efficient and effective pharmaceutical treatment of acute to chronic

Table 5
Clinical vignette 1: Evaluation and management pathways for abandoned HDO-CNCP-seeking new prescriber

Rationale to Continue to Prescribe HDOs	Optional/Alternative Response	Comments
There is significant (possibly missed) pathologic condition to justify complaints and medication	Gather objective analysis of perceived pathologic condition to the extent reasonably possible; recognize sensitivity, specificity, and value of incidental findings	Order new diagnostics only if gap in physical assessment and available data do not match
HDO prescription kept the patients in their life roles	Review wanted and unwanted effects of opioids (table)	Discuss COT and sustainability of lifestyle on HDOs
Aberrant behavior, if identified, was only a minor infraction	Complete opioid treatment agreements Perform and discuss risk screening tools Obtain UDS, review prior UDS reports	Recognize hierarchy, context, and weight of aberrant behaviors before judgment
Disenfranchising patients from their fully vested belief system and current HDO regimen is time intensive	Purposeful and thorough physical examination with detailed review of diagnostics is a critical advantage for the PMR specialist in redirecting mistaken views	Respect for the clinician who listens, examines, and educates is a potent tool in the process of enhanced self-awareness and becoming an informed stakeholder in treatment
Intolerance to previous physical therapies with aggravation and exacerbation of pain leaves no other viable options	Responsibility on individual to develop self-paced continuity of care to an independent physical restoration program in community setting	Insufficient vs limited motivation or capacity to engage in meaningful physical restoration program (table)
Alternatives are limited by availability of a comprehensive pain treatment program, expense/coverage and +/− efficacy	Schedule psychological, substance abuse and mental health wellness programming within insurance or municipal mental health agencies Medical management may continue on contingent basis to ratchet down dosing/rotation to alternative opioid at 50%–75% potency in morphine equivalents Introduce concepts of alternatives to opioids Determine criteria for opioid dependence and introduce topic of buprenorphine-assisted detoxification and maintenance	Community resources may be available out of health systems' payment agreements Coordination of services may require enhanced communication efforts (phone calls, letters, e-mail)

Abbreviations: PMR, physical medicine and rehabilitation; UDS, urine drug screening.

Table 6
Decision matrix: clinical scenario 2: HDO user with no functional benefit

Rationale for: Do Not Accept for Opioid Treatment	Accept and Modify Opioid/Chronic Pain Therapy	Comments
Failed all reasonable therapies	Quality of treatments suspect Displays misinformation recondition; responsive to reflective listening	Room for improvement if motivation is instilled
Belief system is negatively entrenched	Identify untreated psychopathology and instigate therapy	Cognitive behavioral restructuring requires investment over time
Opioid dependence is evident	Recognition and acceptance of adverse consequences promoted with structured support	Requires counseling from physician and dedicated staff (psychology, D&A counselors, etc.)
Motivation for change lacking	MI techniques show efficacy	Skilled MI intervention can promote progression of change in healthcare
Little or no knowledge/or interest in alternative care	Promote acceptance, adaptation, self-efficacy, and value of self-directed community-based activities	Physical engagement is critical to address deconditioning, sleep cycle disruption, and repair of endorphin response
Suspect hyperalgesia to opioids (illustrates heightened pain levels despite escalating HDOs)	Educate as to strategic failure of COT and predictable diminished response Discuss percentage weaning or rotation techniques	Plant seeds to nurture interest in pursuing options in follow-up visits
Rejects all adjunctive medication/buprenorphine or any other medical MAT	Introduce concepts of buprenorphine for MAT of OD Review response and efficacy to prior agents	Provide literature to support concepts of OD and value of buprenorphine for MAT in the context of OD in CNCP

Abbreviations: D&A, drug and alcohol; MAT, maintenance-assisted therapies; MI, motivational interview.

pain often culminating in chronic exposure to opioids. HDOs over many years have not been shown to be either effective or safe. High-dose morphine equivalents greater than 100 mg/24 h are associated with greater rates of death and lower levels of productivity.[42,43] When confronted by the HDO user with CNCP, clinicians are required to discern when self-election of continuing use is based on efficacy or pharmacologic and psychological dependency. Our current terminology of OD is largely based on the recreational opioid user and does not seem inclusive of the patient with CNCP with years of seemingly unrelenting pain despite creeping doses of both long-acting opioids and SAOs. When these long-term users of medically prescribed HDOs are included into the definition of opioid dependent, the role that the opioid molecule receptor site plays in the CNS in regard to both pain and addiction must be inherently recognized. Recognition of how long-term HDO therapy itself may influence the perpetuation of the sensory and emotional experience of chronic pain is essential to further therapeutic decisions.

SUMMARY

Reversing a long history of HDO use for CNCP, divesting catastrophic concepts of pain, as well as tapering a highly influencing drug and initiating change in associated behavior is not a simple task. Construction of a deeper self-perspective of the multi-dimensional factors in each individual that contributes to chronic pain requires practiced interviewing and physical examination skills. Contemplation and initiation of change is most effective when patients with CNCP are drawn to consideration of the physical, cognitive, and affective dimensions of chronic pain as a chronic disease state itself, with physical and emotional impairments involved. Engaging a long-term opioid user to become a stakeholder in the process of participation in a combined physical, medical, and behavioral new direction requires motivational skills of pain practitioners. Educating patients with CNCP as to the identified adverse effects, risk elements of COT, and societal concerns about opioid abuse is a dimension of the problem that may facilitate introspection and the need to address this issue more realistically over the long term. Cognitive insights, restructuring the elements of contributing problems, and reframing the singular role of pathologic anatomic changes that has previously occupied the spotlight for many patients with CNCP is essential to pushing the conversation forward. Providing alternatives including the use of medication-assisted treatment with buprenorphine may be a potent inducer to change if the patient fits the criteria for OD. Planting the seeds of these viable options may be the beginning of this process. Passion for achievement of a broader spectrum of sensory, physical, emotional, and psychosocial experiences outside of self-consuming chronic pain is a cinder that may be rekindled with self-initiative when the opiate reward pathway is tampered or extinguished.

REFERENCES

1. Institute of Medicine. Living well with chronic illness: a call for public health action. Washington, DC: The National Academies Press; 2012.
2. Martin BC, Fan MY, Edlund MJ, et al. Long-term chronic opioid therapy discontinuation rates from the TROUP study. J Gen Intern Med 2011;26:1450–7. PMID: 21751058.
3. Eriksen J, Sjøgren P, Bruera E, et al. Critical issues on opioids in chronic non-cancer pain: an epidemiological study. Pain 2006;125(1–2):172–9. PMID: 16842922.
4. Ballantyne JC, Mao J. Opioid therapy for chronic pain. N Engl J Med 2003;349:1943–53. PMID: 14614170.
5. Dunn KM, Saunders KW, Rutter CM, et al. Opioid prescriptions for chronic pain and overdose: a cohort study. Ann Intern Med 2010;152(2):85–92. PMID: 20083827. Available at: http://www.ncbi.nlm.nih.gov/entrez/eutils/elink.fcgi?dbfrom=pubmed&retmode=ref&cmd=prlinks&id=20083827.
6. Centers for Disease Control and Prevention (CDC). CDC grand rounds: prescription drug overdoses – a U.S. epidemic. MMWR Morb Mortal Wkly Rep 2012;61(1):10–3. PMID: 22237030.
7. Manchikanti L, Helm S, Fellows B, et al. Opioid epidemic in United States. Pain Physician 2012;15(Suppl 3):ES9–38. PMID: 22786464.
8. Catan T, Perez C. A pain-drug champion has second thoughts. Wall Street Journal. December 15, 2012;A1.
9. Webster LR, Webster RM. Predicting aberrant behaviors in opioid-treated patients: preliminary validation of the Opioid Risk Tool. Pain Med 2005;6(6):432–42.
10. Wesson DR, Ling W. The clinical opiate withdrawal scale (COWS). J Psychoactive Drugs 2003;35(2):253–9.

11. Watkins LR, Hutchinson MR, Ledeboer A, et al. Norma Cousins Lecture. Glial as the "bad guys": implications for improving clinical pain control and the clinical utility of opioids. Brain Behav Immun 2007;21(2):131–46. PMID: 17175134.
12. Chu Sin Chung P, Kieffer BL. Delta opioid receptors in brain function and diseases. Pharmacol Ther 2013;140(1):112–20.
13. Van't Veer A, Carlezon WA Jr. Role of kappa-opioid receptors in stress and anxiety-related behavior. Psychopharmacology 2013;229(3):435–52.
14. Mafi JN, McCarthy EP, Davis RB, et al. Worsening trends in the management and treatment of back pain. JAMA Intern Med 2013;173(17):1573–81. http://dx.doi.org/10.1001/jamainternmed.2013.8992. PMID: 23896698.
15. Chou R, Qaseem A, Snow V, et al. Diagnosis and treatment of low back pain: a joint clinical practice guideline from the American College of Physicians and the American Pain Society. Diagnosis and treatment of low back pain: a joint clinical practice. Ann Intern Med 2007;147:478–91.
16. Staal JB, Nelemans PJ, de Bie RA. Spinal injection therapy for low back pain. JAMA 2013;309(23):2439–40. PMID: 23681274.
17. Armstrong D. Epidurals linked to paralysis seen with $300 billion pain market. Bloomberg News 2011. Available at: http://www.bloomberg.com/news/2011-12-28/epidurals-linked-to-paralysis-seen-with-300-billion-pain-market.html. Accessed August 28, 2013.
18. Manchikanti L, Manchukonda R, Pampati V, et al. Evaluation of abuse of prescription and illicit drugs in chronic pain patients receiving short-acting (hydrocodone) or long-acting (methadone) opioids. Pain Physician 2005;8(3):257–61.
19. Gatchel RJ, Okifuji A. Evidence-based scientific data documenting the treatment and cost-effectiveness of comprehensive pain programs for chronic nonmalignant pain. J Pain 2006;7(11):779–93.
20. Flor H, Fydrich T, Turk DC. Efficacy of multidisciplinary pain treatment centers: a meta-analytic review. Pain 1992;49(2):221–30.
21. Sullivan MJL, Bishop S, Pivik J. The pain catastrophizing scale: development and validation. Psychol Assess 1995;7:524–32.
22. Gracely RH, Geisser ME, Giesecke T. Pain catastrophizing and neural responses to pain among persons with fibromyalgia. Brain 2004;127:835–43.
23. Martell BA, O'Connor PG, Kerns RD, et al. Systematic review: opioid treatment for chronic back pain: prevalence, efficacy and association with addiction. Ann Intern Med 2007;146(2):116–27.
24. Turk DC, Monarch ES. Biopsychosocial perspective on chronic pain. In: Turk DC, Gatchel RJ, editors. Psychological approaches to pain management: a practitioner's handbook. New York: Guilford; 2002. p. 3–30.
25. Moseley GL, Nicholas MK, Hodges PW. A randomized controlled trial of intensive neurophysiology education in chronic low back pain. Clin J Pain 2004;20(5):324–30.
26. Paulozzi LJ, Jones CM, Mack KA, et al. Vital signs: overdoses of prescription opioid pain relievers – United States, 1999-2008. MMWR Morb Mortal Wkly Rep 2011;60(43):1487–92.
27. Harden RN. Chronic opioid therapy: another reappraisal. APS Bulletin 2002; 12(1).
28. Prochaska JO, Velicer WF. The transtheoretical model of health behavior change. Am J Health Promot 1997;12(1):38–48.
29. Charon R. Narrative medicine: a model for empathy, reflection, profession and trust. JAMA 2001;286(15):1897–902.
30. Bundy C. Changing behavior: using motivational interviewing techniques. J R Soc Med 2004;97(Suppl 44):43–7.

31. Drug Addiction Treatment Act of 2000. Pub. L. No. 106-310, 106th Congress.
32. Jaffe J, Martin W. Opioid analgesics and antagonists. In: Goodman L, Gilman A, editors. Pharmacological basis of therapeutics. New York: MacGraw-Hill Publishing; 2011. p. 512–3.
33. Lai J, Luo MC, Chen Q, et al. Dynorphin A activates bradykinin receptors to maintain neuropathic pain. Nat Neurosci 2006;9(12):1534–40.
34. American Psychiatric Association. Diagnostic and statistical manual of mental disorders. 4th edition. Washington, DC: American Psychiatric Association; 2000. p. 197.
35. Center for Substance Abuse Treatment. Clinical guidelines for the use of buprenorphine in the treatment of opioid addiction. Treatment Improvement Protocol (TIP) Series 40. DHHS Publication No. (SMA) 04–3939. Rockville (MD): Substance Abuse and Mental Health Services Administration; 2004.
36. Heit HA, Gourlay DL. Buprenorphine. New tricks for an old molecule for pain management. Clin J Pain 2008;24:93–7.
37. Marlatt GA. Highlights of harm reduction. In: Marlatt GA, Larimer ME, Witkiewitz K, editors. Harm reduction: pragmatic strategies for managing high-risk behaviors. New York: Guilford Press; 2002. p. 3.
38. Harmreduction.org [Internet]. New York: Harmreduction.org. Available at: http://harmreduction.org. Accessed August 1, 2013.
39. Rauck RL. What is the case for prescribing long-acting opioids over short-acting opioids for patients with chronic pain? A critical review. Pain Pract 2009;9(6):468–79.
40. American Psychological Association. Diagnostic and statistical manual of mental disorders. 5th edition. Arlington (VA): American Psychiatric Association; 2013. p. 541–6.
41. Interagency guideline on opioid dosing for chronic non-cancer pain: an educational aid to improve care and safety with opioid therapy. 2010. Available at: http://www.agencymeddirectors.wa.gov/. Accessed August 28, 2013.
42. Dunn KM, Saunders KW, Rutter CM. Overdose and prescribed opioids: associations among chronic non-cancer pain patients. Ann Intern Med 2010;152(2):85–92.
43. Von Korff M, Saunders K, Ray GT. Defacto long-term opioid therapy for non-cancer pain. Clin J Pain 2008;24(6):521–7.

Spinal Cord Injury Pain

Michael Saulino, MD, PhD[a,b,*]

KEYWORDS

- Spinal cord injury • Musculoskeletal pain • Neuropathic pain • Spasticity

KEY POINTS

- Spinal cord injury (SCI)-associated pain has a specific classification approach that assists in guiding treatment strategies.
- SCI-related pain seems to be prevalent, but there is considerable variability in the epidemiology of this condition.
- Evaluation of SCI-associated pain relies heavily on history and is supplemented by a neuromusculoskeletal examination and judicious use of laboratory and radiologic testing.
- Relatively few treatments for SCI-associated pain have been extensively studied.

INTRODUCTION

Although traumatic SCI results in a number of serious impairments including paralysis, sensory loss, and neurogenic bowel/bladder function, perhaps no SCI-associated condition is more vexing to the treating physiatrist than chronic pain. Some of these SCI-related impairments can be accommodated with compensatory strategies, whereas chronic pain, especially neuropathic pain associated with injury to the spinal cord, remains quite recalcitrant. In addition to the expected challenges in treating any chronic pain condition, treatment of SCI-related pain has the difficulty of disruption of normal neural pathways that subserve pain transmission and attenuation. This article attempts to describe the classification, epidemiology, evaluation methods, and treatment strategies for this serious pain syndrome.

CLASSIFICATION

Before 2000, there was no consistent approach to the classification of SCI-related chronic pain. This variability was described by Hicken and colleagues[1] during a review in 2002 in which 29 distinct schemes were described with potentially confusing and inconsistent terminology. By 2008, 3 classifications systems emerged as the leading systems based on their utility, comprehensiveness, validity, and reliability. These schemes included the Cardenas classification,[2] the taxonomy of the International

[a] MossRehab, 60 Township Line Road, Elkins Park, PA 19027, USA; [b] Department of Rehabilitation Medicine, Jefferson Medical College, Thomas Jefferson University, Philadelphia, PA, USA
* MossRehab, 60 Township Line Road, Elkins Park, PA 19027.
E-mail address: saulinom@einstein.edu

Phys Med Rehabil Clin N Am 25 (2014) 397–410
http://dx.doi.org/10.1016/j.pmr.2014.01.002
1047-9651/14/$ – see front matter © 2014 Elsevier Inc. All rights reserved.

Association for the Study of Pain,[3] and the Bryce-Ragnarsson classification.[4] Through the leadership of Bryce, a unified system was created and published in 2011. The International Spinal Cord Injury Pain Classification (ISCIP) has been adopted by many leading SCI and pain professional associations throughout the world.[5] This classification is visually depicted in **Fig. 1**.

Given the probable ubiquity of the ISCIP classification, some commentary on this approach is warranted. The first tier of this system is divided into nociceptive, neuropathic, other, and unknown categories. The distinction between the nociceptive and neuropathic categories is certainly approximate because the treatment approaches to these syndromes are often vastly different. As discussed later in this article, nociceptive pain can often be addressed by classic physiatric techniques (in the case of musculoskeletal pain) or other medical interventions (in visceral and other nociceptive pain). This fact is in contradistinction to neuropathic pain in which many treatment approaches are either pharmacologic or interventional. The ISCIP classification also demonstrates the continued difficulties of even expert clinicians and scientists to categorize every single pain condition associated with the SCI population, as demonstrated by the other and unknown categorizations. The reliability of the ISCIP

Tier 1: pain type	Tier 2: pain subtype	Tier 3: primary pain source and/or pathology (write or type in)
☐ Nociceptive pain	☐ Musculoskeletal pain	☐ _____ e.g., glenohumeral arthritis, lateral epicondylitis, comminuted femur fracture, quadratus lumborum muscle spasm
	☐ Visceral pain	☐ _____ e.g., myocardial infarction, abdominal pain due to bowel impaction, cholecystitis
	☐ Other nociceptive pain	☐ _____ e.g., autonomic dysreflexia headache, migraine headache, surgical skin incision
☐ Neuropathic pain	☐ At-level SCI pain	☐ _____ e.g., spinal cord compression, nerve root compression, cauda equina compression
	☐ Below-level SCI pain	☐ _____ e.g., spinal cord ischemia, spinal cord compression
	☐ Other neuropathic pain	☐ _____ e.g., carpal tunnel syndrome, trigeminal neuralgia, diabetic polyneuropathy
☐ Other pain		☐ _____ e.g., fibromyalgia, complex regional pain syndrome type I, interstitial cystitis, irritable bowel syndrome
☐ Unknown pain		☐ _____

Fig. 1. The International Spinal Cord Injury Pain Classification (ISCIP). (*From* Bryce TN, Biering-Sorensen F, Finnerup NB, et al. International spinal cord injury pain classification: part I. Background and description. March 6–7, 2009. Spinal Cord 2012;50(6):415; with permission.)

classification has undergone initial testing using a clinical vignette approach by clinicians experienced with SCI who received minimal training in use of the system. The correctness levels varied from 65% to 85% based on the degree of correlation strictness for the various responses.[6] This result confirms the difficulty in assessment and classification of SCI-associated pain.

The relationship of spasticity to pain is complex. Spasticity can limit the range of motion about a joint and result in musculoskeletal pain. Reduction of spasticity may reduce the pain associated with biomechanical pain. However, as noted above, SCI can also produce neuropathic pain. Modulation of spasticity may not be effective in reducing neuropathic pain.[7] It is also relevant to note that some interventions to treat spasticity may also modulate the pain transmission pathways. In addition, the sensory loss in many patients with SCI, especially those with American Spinal Injury Association impairment scale A neurologic levels, may eliminate or substantially reduce the pain responses associated with noxious events. Increased spasticity may be the only harbinger of these events.[8]

EPIDEMIOLOGY

Given the classification ambiguity of chronic SCI-related pain described above, attempts at epidemiology can be problematic. Other potential confounders include oversampling because patients may have more than one pain syndrome, adequate pain description, criteria used for chronicity and severity, traumatic versus nontraumatic differentiation, and appropriate inclusion/exclusion criteria. Dijkers and colleagues[9] executed a review consisting of 42 articles that described the epidemiology of this clinical problem. A wide variance was noted in the literature, with prevalence of SCI-associated pain in the literature varying from 26% to 96% without an apparent clustering around any group of percentages. The quality of the individual study did not seem to significantly influence the reported prevalence rate. More detailed analysis failed to demonstrate appreciable difference in SCI-associated pain prevalence related to gender, injury completeness, or paraplegia versus tetraplegia. Some individual studies have reported trends for these demographic items, but when viewed from the perspective of the entirety of the medical literature, these trends disappear. Pain conditions among individuals with SCI are generally stable over time. Emergence or dramatic change in a chronic pain condition is worthy of new evaluative approach.

EVALUATION

The approach to SCI pain should commence in a manner similar to all chronic pain conditions—history, physical examination, and judicious use of diagnostic testing. Information should be obtained regarding the patient's initial SCI including date, mechanism of injury, associated injuries such as long bone and visceral trauma, description of vertebral column stabilization procedures, and comorbidities of the acute hospitalization and rehabilitation phase of injury. Descriptors should be attained regarding pain history, including time of onset from initial injury, time course, pain location, intensity and quantity, alleviating and aggravating factors, past evaluations, treatments (including effectiveness), and pharmacologic assessment. Inquiry into the presence or change in upper motor neuron signs, such as clonus or spasticity, is reasonable. Functional, occupational, and recreational history should be acquired for 2 reasons. First, these activities may contribute to the development of pain (eg, development of shoulder pain in a wheelchair athlete). Second, the degree of pain interference with these activities will allow the clinician to judge the functional impact of the patient's pain condition. Some degree of psychological assessment is warranted with exploration into possible depression, anxiety, personality disorders, concomitant brain injury, substance use, and cognitive impairment. In selected cases, a more formal psychological assessment, including psychometric testing, by either a psychologist or a psychiatrist may be appropriate. Last, the patient should be queried as to what diagnostic tests have been undertaken previously.

Although not an absolute "red flag," emergence of below-level pain after years or even decades from the initial SCI should be viewed as a concerning sign. For above-level pain syndromes, the typical elements of history should be queried as for the non-SCI patient with added elements that are pertinent to the patient with SCI. A reasonable example of this approach is a patient with SCI who presents with a suspected carpal tunnel syndrome. The patient should be asked questions about sensory symptoms and their distribution with the added elements of wheelchair, crutch, or cane use because use of these devices could be a contributing factor to a suspected median neuropathy. Particular attention should be paid to treatment failures. Some patients may have been exposed to a particular agent but were not given sufficient time or dose that would reasonably be expected to result in a therapeutic response. Other patients may have discontinued use of a medication because of intolerable adverse effects. If these 2 scenarios are present, insufficient response might be overcome with either a rechallenge of prior medications or use of adjuvant therapies to manage side effects.

Pain assessment should have a component of patient self-report. These measures supplement information obtained during the clinical interview and provide a means of evaluating success or failure of treatment strategies. The most commonly used measure of pain, for all types of pain, is the numerical rating scale (NRS). An NRS includes a range of numbers, generally starting from 0 (eg, 0–10 or 0–100), which is anchored to descriptors, for example, no pain at the lowest extreme of the range and worst pain imaginable at the highest extreme. Several studies have established the NRS as a reliable measure of pain intensity.[10] Another typical measure of pain intensity is a visual analog scale, which consists of a line (horizontal or vertical) anchored at either extremes with no pain on one end and another extreme (eg, worst pain imaginable) on the other end. Respondents are instructed to draw a small line that intersects with the scale at the point that represents their pain intensity. The measured distance (eg, in millimeters) from the no pain anchor to the recorded mark represents the subject's pain intensity. Typically, a clinically meaningful change in pain intensity is approximately a 33% decrement in visual analog score (VAS).[11]

Beyond pain intensity, it is reasonable to attempt assessment of pain according to daily activities. Of note, the Initiative on Methods, Measurement, and Pain Assessment in Clinical Trials (IMMPACT) group recommended that measures of pain severity, physical functioning, and emotional functioning be included in all clinical trials of chronic pain interventions.[12] The impact of pain on physical functioning may be obtained through a number by pain interference scales such as the Graded Chronic Pain Disability scale, the Brief Pain Inventory, and the Multidimensional Pain Inventory. These scales have demonstrated reasonable reliability and validity in SCI populations.[13]

Many patients with chronic pain disorders and SCI have comorbid psychological disorders including depression, anxiety, anger, psychosis, eating disorders, substance dependence, cognitive impairment, and personality disorders. The physician should inquire about the existence and severity of these behavioral problems. Cotreatment with mental health professionals is often warranted for more in-depth neuropsychological assessments. Examples of standardized psychological assessments used in these populations include the Beck Depression Inventory and the Patient Health Questionnaire. The latter has demonstrated validity in the SCI population.[14]

The physical examination of the individual with SCI-associated pain should start with the International Standards for Neurologic Classification of Spinal Cord Injury neurologic evaluation.[15] This examination is supplemented by further neurologic testing including reflex testing, assessment of other sensory abnormalities (allodynia, hyperalgesia, and hyperpathia), and evaluation of muscle overactivity (spasms, spasticity, and clonus). Focal examination of a particular pain area would then proceed as a neuromusculoskeletal approach used for pain complaints in all populations. Items to be included are inspection, palpation, active and passive range of motion, and provocative maneuvers. Observation of wheelchair propulsion, posture, and gait may be appropriate in selected patients. Appropriate comfort and fit of assistive devices (cane, walker, and crutch) and orthotic devices should be undertaken if these equipment seem to contribute to the pain syndrome. A survey of mood, behavior, personality, and cognition is certainly reasonable.

Regarding diagnostic testing, above-level syndromes can be evaluated in a manner parallel to the non-SCI patient. Conditions associated with at-level and below-level lesions are more challenging. Imaging of the site of initial spinal region should be considered in these circumstances. Potential examples of pain generators that might be detected include segmental instability or compression about the site of injury, spinal nerve impingement, orthopedic hardware loosening, fluid collections, and syringomyelia. Discussion with the interpreting radiologist is recommended to assist with the choice of imaging modalities. Potential discussion points could include interference of hardware, the need for radiographic contrast (intravenous gadolinium for magnetic resonance imaging [MRI], subarachnoid ionic contrast for computed tomographic [CT] myelogram, etc), and the differentiation of acute from chronic changes. Given the possible unreliability of abdominal/pelvic examinations in an insensate patient, imaging may also be warranted if visceral pain is suspected. In addition to the traditional MRI and CT modalities, specialized techniques may be warranted for potential pain generator relative to neurogenic bowel and bladder (ie, colonoscopy, cystoscopy, urodynamics testing, etc). Triple-phase bone scanning could be appropriate for evaluation of unsuspected fractures or complex regional pain syndrome.[16]

Judicious use of laboratory testing follows a parallel pathway for above-level syndromes and a surveillance approach for at-level and below-level syndromes. Care must be taken with regard to interpretation so as not to "over read" the importance of particular abnormality. An example of this pitfall would be to attribute asymptomatic urinary bacterial colonization as the sole cause of visceral pain. Potential laboratory tests in this population might include a complete blood cell count, erythrocyte sedimentation rate/C-reactive protein levels (to trend an inflammatory process such as abscess), and hormonal assessment (including pregnancy testing). Subtherapeutic vitamin B_{12}[17] and Vitamin D levels[18] have been implicated in neuronal dysfunction in SCI and represent potentially reversible abnormalities.

MANAGEMENT
Nonpharmacologic

A generalized exercise program in the form of global strength training, cardiovascular training, or recreational physical activities has the potential to be beneficial for several SCI-related conditions (eg, spasticity, muscle atrophy, bone health), but its effect on global pain in this population has not been greatly satisfactory. Animal studies have suggested that antinociceptive behaviors can be reduced with weeks of exercise training.[19,20] Extrapolation from these experiments to the human condition has not been straightforward. Some human trials suggest that a long-term exercise program can attenuate global pain complaints,[21] but these effects may not persist if regular exercise is discontinued.[22] More targeted exercise programs for specific pain complaints have a much higher likelihood of success. The best example of this approach is seen with shoulder pain in paraplegic individuals.[23–25]

In addition to generalized and specified exercise programs, referral to physical or occupational therapy may be appropriate for the patient with SCI with musculoskeletal pain in an effort to address biomechanical abnormalities that can be associated with mobility aids. Modification of orthotics, canes, walkers, crutches, and wheelchairs has the potential to influence detrimental ergonomics. Perhaps the best example of this intervention is adjustment of rear wheel of a manual wheelchair in an effort to modify the forces about the shoulder that can occur as a result of wheelchair propulsion.[26]

Acupuncture is popular for both the general and SCI populations. In 1997, a report from the National Institutes of Health supported the use of acupuncture for certain conditions, including pain.[27] Survey assessments have reported that between 15% and 35% of individuals with SCI have tried acupuncture for pain relief with a variable degree of effectiveness. One retrospective review reported that two-thirds of patients treated with acupuncture for below-level neuropathic pain found it effective.[28] Support for acupuncture from prospective studies is limited. Nayak and colleagues[29] reported that approximately half of the patients who received 15 sessions of this modality experienced a clinically meaningful reduction in pain. This study suggested that acupuncture may be more effective in individuals with incomplete injuries or musculoskeletal pain when compared with complete injuries or neuropathic pain. Dyson and colleagues[30] reported that both acupuncture and sham acupuncture groups had reductions in pain ratings when exposed in a double-blind manner.

Pharmacologic

At present, there is only one medication that currently has US Food and Drug Administration (FDA) indication for SCI-associated pain. Pregabalin is a structural derivative of the inhibitory neurotransmitter γ-aminobutyric acid. Pregabalin is an alpha-2-delta ligand that has analgesic, anticonvulsant, anxiolytic, and sleep-modulating activities. Pregabalin binds potently to the alpha-2-delta subunit of voltage-gated calcium channels. It is hypothesized that this binding reduces the influx of calcium into hyperexcited neuron, which in turn results in a reduction in the release of several neurotransmitters, including glutamate, noradrenaline, serotonin, dopamine, and substance P.[31] Siddall and colleagues[32] randomized 137 patients with SCI to either placebo (67 patients) or flexible dosing of pregabalin (70 patients). Roughly half of the patients had complete injuries. The dosing ranged from 150 to 600 mg/d in 2 divided doses. The mean baseline pain score was 6.54 in the pregabalin group and 6.73 in the placebo group. The mean endpoint pain score was lower in the active treatment group (4.62) compared with that in the placebo group (6.27; $P<.001$), with efficacy observed as early as week 1 and maintained for the duration of the study (12 weeks). The average pregabalin dose after the 3-week stabilization phase was 460 mg/d. During this trial, pregabalin was associated with improvements in disturbed sleep and anxiety. The most common adverse events were mild or moderate, typically transient, somnolence and dizziness. Edema was reported in 20% of the pregabalin patients, which resulted in 3 discontinuance episodes, compared to 6% in the placebo group, which resulted in 2 discontinuance episodes. Cardenas and colleagues[33] executed a similar study with 230 patients with 108 patients receiving active drug and 112 patients receiving placebo. This study had a longer duration (16 weeks). Approximately half of the patients had complete injuries. Pregabalin-treated patients experienced a nearly 2-point improvement on a 10-point NRS scale in the intensity of SCI-related pain during the previous 24 hours compared to baseline levels. Similarly, the patients experienced an improvement in disturbed sleep and sleep interference. The average daily dose of pregabalin was 410 mg/d during the dose maintenance period and 357 mg/d over the full treatment period. The most frequent treatment-related adverse effects included somnolence, dizziness, edema, dry mouth, fatigue, and blurred vision. Most adverse effects were mild to moderate in severity and transient in nature. Treatment-emergent peripheral edema was reported in 13.4% of pregabalin-treated patients in this study, resulting in 1 discontinuation. The incidence of edema in this study, as well as the previous study, was comparable with the reported incidence of other neuropathic pain conditions including diabetic peripheral neuropathy and postherpetic neuralgia. Thus, patients with SCI do not seem more susceptible to developing peripheral edema in response to pregabalin than patients with other neuropathic pain conditions.

Before pregabalin release and also at present, gabapentin remains commonly used. Similar to pregabalin, gabapentin is active at voltage-gated calcium channels. This agent has been considered effective in SCI-associated neuropathic pain in several smaller studies. Levendoglu and colleagues[34] reported that gabapentin was more effective than placebo in a crossover study involving 20 patients with paraplegia with neuropathic pain that had been present for more than 6 months. Tai and colleagues[35] conducted a prospective, randomized, double-blind, crossover study on 7 patients who had for more than 30 days postinjury SCI-related pain. This study found a significant reduction in "unpleasant feelings" with gabapentin compared to placebo. Reduction in pain intensity and burning pain trended toward significance, whereas no differences were observed for other pain descriptors. To and colleagues[36] performed a retrospective chart review of 44 patients with SCI-related neuropathic pain examining the effectiveness of gabapentin. About 76% of these subjects reported a reduction in pain intensity. The mean pretreatment VAS was 8.86, which decreased to 4.13 after 6 months of treatment. Last, Putzke and colleagues[37] examined the use of gabapentin in this population with a longitudinal observational study on 27 patients. This group observed a relatively high discontinuance rate (6/27 or 22%). Of the remaining 21 patients, 14 (67%) reported a greater than 2-point reduction in VAS at 6 months. It is reasonable to conclude that gabapentin can be effective in neuropathic pain in SCI-associated neuropathic pain. A recent study of intrathecal gabapentin failed to demonstrate any benefit in an unselected chronic pain population despite promising results from animal data, particularly with neuropathic pain.[38] Although pregabalin has US FDA approval for SCI-related pain, there is no head-to-head trial comparing the effectiveness of gabapentin with that of pregabalin. The affordability of gabapentin may make it the more desirable choice. Many insurers require a trial of gabapentin before approving pregabalin.

The use of antidepressants for below-level neuropathic pain SCI pain has a long-standing tradition. The substantial benefit of tricyclic antidepressants (TCAs) in neuropathic pain has led to this use.[39] Perhaps the most commonly used agent is amitriptyline. There are conflicting results in the medical literature with some studies demonstrating efficacy[40] and other studies demonstrating descriptive minimal efficacy[41] in SCI-associated pain. One comparison trial described a therapeutic benefit of amitriptyline over gabapentin.[40] The so-called second-generation TCAs (ie, secondary amines such as nortriptyline, desipramine, and protriptyline) are preferred because analgesic efficacy is equivalent and tolerability is better compared to those of first-generation TCAs (ie, tertiary amines such as amitriptyline, clomipramine, and doxepin). All TCAs are considered to have a ceiling effect. Thus, once a therapeutic effect is achieved, further dosing increases should be avoided in order to minimize adverse effects.[42]

The most recent additions to antidepressant use for chronic pain are the dual serotonin and norepinephrine reuptake inhibitors. Medications in this class include duloxetine, milnacipran, and desvenlafaxine. Pain modulation seems to be independent of their antidepressant properties. Duloxetine, the first medication approved for use in the United States within this class, has FDA indication for chronic musculoskeletal pain, fibromyalgia, and diabetic neuropathy. A small trial of duloxetine for central neuropathic pain caused by either stroke or SCI failed to show a reduction in pain intensity but did demonstrate changes in other aspects of these chronic pain syndromes, including allodynia.[43] There are no reports of using either milnacipran or venlafaxine for chronic SCI-associated pain. Several serotonin-norepinephrine reuptake inhibitors are in various stages of clinical development for a wide variety of indications.[44]

Opioid medications have been suggested as reasonable options for chronic nociceptive and perhaps neuropathic pain. Perhaps, no other decision in medicine causes more anxiety than prescribing opiates for patients with chronic, noncancer pain. Concerns over diversion, misuse, dependence, addiction, monitoring, and cost can make the analysis of using chronic opiate therapy troublesome for even experienced clinicians.[45] In the patient with SCI, concerns over the potential exacerbation of neurogenic bowel because of opioid-related constipation makes this decision even more challenging. There are several new strategies for the management of opioid-related constipation including peripheral opioid receptor antagonists and prokinetic agents.[46] A review of the use of opioids in neuropathic pain suggested clinical efficacy of this medication class for long-term use. It is relevant to note that this review has a large preponderance of peripheral-based neuropathic pain (diabetic neuropathy or postherpetic neuropathy), but some subjects with SCI were included.[47] There are several developments within the opioid class medications that may be of specific interest to physiatrists treating SCI-related pain. Tapentadol is a centrally acting analgesic with dual mechanisms of action—agonist activity at the mu opioid receptor and inhibition of norepinephrine reuptake. A potential therapeutic advantage of this agent is its utility in neuropathic pain. This benefit has been observed with both low–back pain with a neuropathic pain component as well as diabetic peripheral neuropathy.[48,49] There are no specific reports on the use of this agent in SCI. In addition, this medication may also have therapeutic advantages over other opiates including a lower incidence of withdrawal symptoms as well as decreased frequency of gastrointestinal side effects. However, because of the activity that this agent has with monoamine metabolism, there is a potential to exacerbate or precipitate serotonin syndrome.[50] Another dual-acting product is tramadol, which is a combination of a serotonin and noradrenaline reuptake inhibitor and a mu opioid agonist. This medication is noteworthy because its mechanism of action is distinct from those of other opioids. Tramadol has been shown to demonstrate benefit in osteoarthritis, fibromyalgia, and neuropathic pain; however, there is insufficient evidence to definitely define tramadol as more effective compared with other opioids.[51] A small, randomized controlled trial in SCI-related neuropathic pain demonstrated a positive response to this medication.[52]

The relationship between pain and spasticity is complex. Reduction of spasticity may reduce the pain associated with biomechanical pain. Modulation of spasticity may not be effective in reducing neuropathic pain.[7] There are several oral medications that can accomplish spasticity reduction including baclofen, tizanidine, diazepam, and dantrolene. Of particular interest, tizanidine has a dual mechanism of action: an

α_2-adrenergic agonism at the spinal level and an influence on descending noradrenergic pathways. It is this latter mechanism that may be of particular interest in the management of SCI-related pain.[53] Similarly, botulinum toxins have the potential to reduce muscle overactivity in a focally directed manner. Abobotulinum toxin A has formal FDA indication for adult, upper extremity spasticity after stroke and brain injury, although there are ongoing clinical trials for the other preparations and indications. Over and above their antispasticity activities, botulinum toxins have the capacity to be antinociceptive.[54] However, there are no formal studies examining the effects of botulinum toxin on SCI-related pain independent of their spasticity reduction properties.

Medicinal marijuana and synthetic cannabinoids represent intriguing pharmacologic choices for the management of SCI-associated pain. Cannabis contains 60 or more cannabinoids, the most abundant of which are delta-9-tetrahydrocannabinol (THC) and cannabidiol (CBD). Rintala and colleagues[55] executed a small study with dronabinol on SCI-related neuropathic pain. This agent is a pure isomer of THC. This investigation failed to demonstrate a significant difference in pain intensity compared with an active control. Sativex is a cannabis extract that contains THC + CBD in a fixed ratio, delivered as an oromucosal spray. Sativex has indication for multiple-sclerosis-related spasticity in several countries but not in the United States.[56] A recent study of neuropathic pain associated with multiple sclerosis failed to demonstrate significant differences during the double-blind phase of this trial.[57] There are no specific reports on the use of this agent in SCI-associated pain. There is an ongoing clinical trial examining the use of vaporized cannabis in SCI pain. There are no formal studies examining the use of medicinal marijuana in this patient population despite Cardenas and Jensen[58] reporting that up to 37% of patients with SCI have used marijuana for pain reduction purposes.

Nicotine has been reported to exacerbate SCI-related pain with abstinence resulting in relief. One recent study examined the effect of nicotine in a randomized, placebo-controlled crossover design on the subtypes of SCI-related pain (neuropathic, musculoskeletal, and mixed pain) among smokers and nonsmokers. This study involved 42 subjects of whom two-thirds had paraplegia. Nonsmokers with SCI showed a reduction in mixed forms of pain after nicotine exposure, whereas smokers with SCI reported increase in pain for both mixed and neuropathic pain. This study suggests differential effects on SCI-related pain for smokers and nonsmokers. This observation potentially offers some insight into the mechanisms of SCI-associated pain as well as supports the suggestion of smoking cessation in some patients with SCI.[59]

Interventional

Spinal cord stimulation is defined as posterior epidural stimulation of the dorsal columns. The proposed mechanisms of action of this therapy involve the gate theory of pain, enhancement of parasympathetic activity, inhibition of sympathetic activity, upregulation of descending inhibitory pathways, and downregulation of ascending pain pathways. There have been many case reports documenting both success and failure of this technology for this pain syndrome. Shaw[60] has presented a meeting abstract in which 12 patients with SCI received dorsal column stimulation for treatment of pain. The patients with complete injuries had variable success; however, none of them experienced paresthesias at stimulation above their injury. In the incompletely injured patients, paresthesias were experienced at varying levels of stimulation intensity. The patients with incomplete SCI had a higher degree of pain relief than those with complete SCI; however, 1 patient with complete SCI, who had been injured for less than 2 years, had complete relief of pain.[60] Lagauche and colleagues[61] executed a review of this modality in SCI-related pain and failed to find a consistently positive therapeutic effect.

Intrathecal drug delivery provides direct administration of therapeutic agents to the subarachnoid space where they have enhanced access to receptor sites. Intrathecal baclofen is a well-established technique for reduction of spasticity associated with SCI.[62,63] To the extent that spasticity is related to musculoskeletal pain, this technique has the capacity to attenuate pain in this population. However, the use of intrathecal baclofen as a pure pain-modulating agent is limited.[64] The utility of more traditional intrathecal analgesic agents has not been overwhelmingly successful. Combination therapy with baclofen and clonidine,[65] morphine and clonidine,[66] baclofen and morphine,[67] baclofen and ziconotide,[68] as well as hydromorphone and ziconotide[69] have resulted in varying degrees of success. Intrathecal gabapentin failed to demonstrate a therapeutic effect in a generalized pain population.[38]

A particularly interesting, albeit experimental, neuromodulation approach to SCI-associated pain is oscillating field stimulation. A human trial of a low-voltage, alternating polarity device was undertaken to assess the possibility of this therapy, causing substantive neurologic recovery as suspected from animal studies. Pain was assessed during this trial to insure that this device did not cause pain. Somewhat surprisingly, use of this device was associated with a rather dramatic reduction in pain. After the 15-week treatment phase, VAS scores improved from a mean of 8 to a mean of 2 six months after treatment had been discontinued. No neuropathic pain was reported in any patient. The status of this device is uncertain until a larger, multicenter trial is undertaken.[70]

SUMMARY

SCI pain is clearly a challenging pain syndrome. Each element of this review (classification, epidemiology, evaluation, and management) has demonstrated limitations. Further investigation by clinicians and researchers in both the SCI and pain communities is warranted in an effort to further delineate the nature of this problem and create more effective treatment strategies. Physiatrists are uniquely positioned to participate in this process and should engage in this endeavor whenever possible.

REFERENCES

1. Hicken BL, Putzke JD, Richards JS. Classification of pain following spinal cord injury: literature review and future directions. In: Burchiel K, Yezierski RP, editors. Spinal cord injury pain: assessment, mechanisms, management. Seattle (WA): International Association for the Study of Pain Press; 2002. p. 25–38.
2. Cardenas DD, Turner JA, Warms CA, et al. Classification of chronic pain associated with spinal cord injuries. Arch Phys Med Rehabil 2002;83(12):1708–14.
3. Siddall P, Yezierski RP, Loeser JD. Pain following spinal cord injury: clinical features, prevalence and taxonomy. International Association for the Study of Pain 2000;3:3–7.
4. Bryce TN, Dijkers MP, Ragnarsson KT, et al. Reliability of the Bryce/Ragnarsson spinal cord injury pain taxonomy. J Spinal Cord Med 2006;29(2):118–32.
5. Bryce TN, Biering-Sorensen F, Finnerup NB, et al. International spinal cord injury pain classification: part I. Background and description. March 6–7, 2009. Spinal Cord 2012;50(6):413–7.
6. Bryce TN, Biering-Sorensen F, Finnerup NB, et al. International spinal cord injury pain (ISCIP) classification: part 2. Initial validation using vignettes. Spinal Cord 2012;50(6):404–12.

7. Ward AB, Kadies M. The management of pain in spasticity. Disabil Rehabil 2002;24(8):443–53.

8. Phadke CP, Balasubramanian CK, Ismail F, et al. Revisiting physiologic and psychologic triggers that increase spasticity. Am J Phys Med Rehabil 2013;92(4): 357–69.

9. Dijkers M, Bryce T, Zanca J. Prevalence of chronic pain after traumatic spinal cord injury: a systematic review. J Rehabil R D 2009;46(1):13–29.

10. Jensen MP, Turner JA, Romano JM, et al. Comparative reliability and validity of chronic pain intensity measures. Pain 1999;83(2):157–62.

11. Hanley MA, Jensen MP, Ehde DM, et al. Clinically significant change in pain intensity ratings in persons with spinal cord injury or amputation. Clin J Pain 2006; 22(1):25–31.

12. Dworkin RH, Turk DC, Peirce-Sandner S, et al. Research design considerations for confirmatory chronic pain clinical trials: IMMPACT recommendations. Pain 2010;149(2):177–93.

13. Bryce TN, Budh CN, Cardenas DD, et al. Pain after spinal cord injury: an evidence-based review for clinical practice and research. Report of the national institute on disability and rehabilitation research spinal cord injury measures meeting. J Spinal Cord Med 2007;30(5):421–40.

14. Bombardier CH, Richards JS, Krause JS, et al. Symptoms of major depression in people with spinal cord injury: implications for screening. Arch Phys Med Rehabil 2004;85(11):1749–56.

15. Kirshblum SC, Waring W, Biering-Sorensen F, et al. Reference for the 2011 revision of the international standards for neurological classification of spinal cord injury. J Spinal Cord Med 2011;34(6):547–54.

16. Le Chapelain L, Perrouin-Verbe B, Fattal C, SOFMER French Society for Physical Medicine and Rehabilitation. Chronic neuropathic pain in spinal cord injury patients: what relevant additional clinical exams should be performed? Ann Phys Rehabil Med 2009;52(2):103–10.

17. Petchkrua W, Little JW, Burns SP, et al. Vitamin B12 deficiency in spinal cord injury: a retrospective study. J Spinal Cord Med 2003;26(2):116–21.

18. Hummel K, Craven BC, Giangregorio L. Serum 25(OH)D, PTH and correlates of suboptimal 25(OH)D levels in persons with chronic spinal cord injury. Spinal Cord 2012;50(11):812–6.

19. Hutchinson KJ, Gomez-Pinilla F, Crowe MJ, et al. Three exercise paradigms differentially improve sensory recovery after spinal cord contusion in rats. Brain 2004;127(Pt 6):1403–14.

20. Kuphal KE, Fibuch EE, Taylor BK. Extended swimming exercise reduces inflammatory and peripheral neuropathic pain in rodents. J Pain 2007;8(12): 989–97.

21. Hicks AL, Martin KA, Ditor DS, et al. Long-term exercise training in persons with spinal cord injury: effects on strength, arm ergometry performance and psychological well-being. Spinal Cord 2003;41(1):34–43.

22. Ditor DS, Latimer AE, Ginis KA, et al. Maintenance of exercise participation in individuals with spinal cord injury: effects on quality of life, stress and pain. Spinal Cord 2003;41(8):446–50.

23. Curtis KA, Tyner TM, Zachary L, et al. Effect of a standard exercise protocol on shoulder pain in long-term wheelchair users. Spinal Cord 1999;37(6): 421–9.

24. Nawoczenski DA, Ritter-Soronen JM, Wilson CM, et al. Clinical trial of exercise for shoulder pain in chronic spinal injury. Phys Ther 2006;86(12):1604–18.

25. Mulroy SJ, Thompson L, Kemp B, et al. Strengthening and optimal movements for painful shoulders (STOMPS) in chronic spinal cord injury: a randomized controlled trial. Phys Ther 2011;91(3):305–24.

26. Katalinic OM, Harvey LA, Herbert RD. Effectiveness of stretch for the treatment and prevention of contractures in people with neurological conditions: a systematic review. Phys Ther 2011;91(1):11–24.

27. NIH consensus conference. Acupuncture. JAMA 1998;280(17):1518–24.

28. Rapson LM, Wells N, Pepper J, et al. Acupuncture as a promising treatment for below-level central neuropathic pain: a retrospective study. J Spinal Cord Med 2003;26(1):21–6.

29. Nayak S, Shiflett SC, Schoenberger NE, et al. Is acupuncture effective in treating chronic pain after spinal cord injury? Arch Phys Med Rehabil 2001;82(11): 1578–86.

30. Dyson-Hudson TA, Kadar P, LaFountaine M, et al. Acupuncture for chronic shoulder pain in persons with spinal cord injury: a small-scale clinical trial. Arch Phys Med Rehabil 2007;88(10):1276–83.

31. Gajraj NM. Pregabalin: its pharmacology and use in pain management. Anesth Analg 2007;105(6):1805–15.

32. Siddall PJ, Cousins MJ, Otte A, et al. Pregabalin in central neuropathic pain associated with spinal cord injury: a placebo-controlled trial. Neurology 2006; 67(10):1792–800.

33. Cardenas DD, Nieshoff EC, Suda K, et al. A randomized trial of pregabalin in patients with neuropathic pain due to spinal cord injury. Neurology 2013; 80(6):533–9.

34. Levendoglu F, Ogun CO, Ozerbil O, et al. Gabapentin is a first line drug for the treatment of neuropathic pain in spinal cord injury. Spine (Phila Pa 1976) 2004; 29(7):743–51.

35. Tai Q, Kirshblum S, Chen B, et al. Gabapentin in the treatment of neuropathic pain after spinal cord injury: a prospective, randomized, double-blind, crossover trial. J Spinal Cord Med 2002;25(2):100–5.

36. To TP, Lim TC, Hill ST, et al. Gabapentin for neuropathic pain following spinal cord injury. Spinal Cord 2002;40(6):282–5.

37. Putzke JD, Richards JS, Kezar L, et al. Long-term use of gabapentin for treatment of pain after traumatic spinal cord injury. Clin J Pain 2002;18(2): 116–21.

38. Rauck R, Coffey RJ, Schultz DM, et al. Intrathecal gabapentin to treat chronic intractable noncancer pain. Anesthesiology 2013;119(3):675–86.

39. Sindrup SH, Jensen TS. Efficacy of pharmacological treatments of neuropathic pain: an update and effect related to mechanism of drug action. Pain 1999; 83(3):389–400.

40. Rintala DH, Holmes SA, Courtade D, et al. Comparison of the effectiveness of amitriptyline and gabapentin on chronic neuropathic pain in persons with spinal cord injury. Arch Phys Med Rehabil 2007;88(12):1547–60.

41. Cardenas DD, Warms CA, Turner JA, et al. Efficacy of amitriptyline for relief of pain in spinal cord injury: results of a randomized controlled trial. Pain 2002; 96(3):365–73.

42. Mico JA, Ardid D, Berrocoso E, et al. Antidepressants and pain. Trends Pharmacol Sci 2006;27(7):348–54.

43. Vranken JH, Hollmann MW, van der Vegt MH, et al. Duloxetine in patients with central neuropathic pain caused by spinal cord injury or stroke: a randomized, double-blind, placebo-controlled trial. Pain 2011;152(2):267–73.

44. Stahl SM, Grady MM, Moret C, et al. SNRIs: their pharmacology, clinical efficacy, and tolerability in comparison with other classes of antidepressants. CNS Spectr 2005;10(9):732–47.

45. Hallinan R, Osborn M, Cohen M, et al. Increasing the benefits and reducing the harms of prescription opioid analgesics. Drug Alcohol Rev 2011;30(3): 315–23.

46. Walters JB, Montagnini M. Current concepts in the management of opioid-induced constipation. J Opioid Manag 2010;6(6):435–44.

47. Eisenberg E, McNicol E, Carr DB. Opioids for neuropathic pain. Cochrane Database Syst Rev 2006;(3):CD006146.

48. Steigerwald I, Muller M, Davies A, et al. Effectiveness and safety of tapentadol prolonged release for severe, chronic low back pain with or without a neuropathic pain component: results of an open-label, phase 3b study. Curr Med Res Opin 2012;28(6):911–36.

49. Schwartz S, Etropolski M, Shapiro DY, et al. Safety and efficacy of tapentadol ER in patients with painful diabetic peripheral neuropathy: results of a randomized-withdrawal, placebo-controlled trial. Curr Med Res Opin 2011; 27(1):151–62.

50. Riemsma R, Forbes C, Harker J, et al. Systematic review of tapentadol in chronic severe pain. Curr Med Res Opin 2011;27(10):1907–30.

51. Leppert W. Tramadol as an analgesic for mild to moderate cancer pain. Pharmacol Rep 2009;61(6):978–92.

52. Norrbrink C, Lundeberg T. Tramadol in neuropathic pain after spinal cord injury: a randomized, double-blind, placebo-controlled trial. Clin J Pain 2009;25(3): 177–84.

53. Kamen L, Henney HR 3rd, Runyan JD. A practical overview of tizanidine use for spasticity secondary to multiple sclerosis, stroke, and spinal cord injury. Curr Med Res Opin 2008;24(2):425–39.

54. Wheeler A, Smith HS. Botulinum toxins: mechanisms of action, antinociception and clinical applications. Toxicology 2013;306:124–46.

55. Rintala DH, Fiess RN, Tan G, et al. Effect of dronabinol on central neuropathic pain after spinal cord injury: a pilot study. Am J Phys Med Rehabil 2010; 89(10):840–8.

56. Notcutt W, Langford R, Davies P, et al. A placebo-controlled, parallel-group, randomized withdrawal study of subjects with symptoms of spasticity due to multiple sclerosis who are receiving long-term Sativex(R) (nabiximols). Mult Scler 2012;18(2):219–28.

57. Langford RM, Mares J, Novotna A, et al. A double-blind, randomized, placebo-controlled, parallel-group study of THC/CBD oromucosal spray in combination with the existing treatment regimen, in the relief of central neuropathic pain in patients with multiple sclerosis. J Neurol 2013;260(4):984–97.

58. Cardenas DD, Jensen MP. Treatments for chronic pain in persons with spinal cord injury: a survey study. J Spinal Cord Med 2006;29(2):109–17.

59. Richardson EJ, Richards JS, Stewart CC, et al. Effects of nicotine on spinal cord injury pain: a randomized, double-blind, placebo controlled crossover trial. Top Spinal Cord Inj Rehabil 2012;18(2):101–5.

60. Shaw E. Clinical outcomes of Spinal cord stimulation (SCS) in patients with chronic spinal cord injury. Neuromoduation 2011;14(5):444–84. [Abstract].

61. Lagauche D, Facione J, Albert T, et al. The chronic neuropathic pain of spinal cord injury: which efficiency of neuropathic stimulation? Ann Phys Rehabil Med 2009;52(2):180–7.

62. Coffey JR, Cahill D, Steers W, et al. Intrathecal baclofen for intractable spasticity of spinal origin: results of a long-term multicenter study. J Neurosurg 1993;78(2): 226–32.

63. Ordia JI, Fischer E, Adamski E, et al. Continuous intrathecal baclofen infusion by a programmable pump in 131 consecutive patients with severe spasticity of spinal origin. Neuromodulation 2002;5(1):16–24.

64. Saulino M. The use of intrathecal baclofen in pain management. Pain Manag 2013;2(6):603–8.

65. Middleton JW, Siddall PJ, Walker S, et al. Intrathecal clonidine and baclofen in the management of spasticity and neuropathic pain following spinal cord injury: a case study. Arch Phys Med Rehabil 1996;77(8):824–6.

66. Siddall PJ, Molloy AR, Walker S, et al. The efficacy of intrathecal morphine and clonidine in the treatment of pain after spinal cord injury. Anesth Analg 2000; 91(6):1493–8.

67. Saulino M. Simultaneous treatment of intractable pain and spasticity: observations of combined intrathecal baclofen-morphine therapy over a 10-year clinical experience. Eur J Phys Rehabil Med 2011;48(1):39–45.

68. Saulino M, Burton AW, Danyo DA, et al. Intrathecal ziconotide and baclofen provide pain relief in seven patients with neuropathic pain and spasticity: case reports. Eur J Phys Rehabil Med 2009;45(1):61–7.

69. Saulino M. Successful reduction of neuropathic pain associated with spinal cord injury via of a combination of intrathecal hydromorphone and ziconotide: a case report. Spinal Cord 2007;45(11):749–52.

70. Walters BC. Oscillating field stimulation in the treatment of spinal cord injury. PM R 2010;2(12 Suppl 2):S286–91.

Hemiplegic Shoulder Pain
An Approach to Diagnosis and Management

John M. Vasudevan, MD[a],*, Barbara J. Browne, MD[b]

KEYWORDS

- Hemiplegic shoulder pain • Poststroke shoulder pain • Stroke rehabilitation
- Shoulder subluxation

KEY POINTS

- Hemiplegic shoulder pain (HSP) occurs in most patients with hemiplegia, and has an adverse effect on functional outcomes.
- Evaluation and management is challenging, as HSP remains a clinical diagnosis, and many of the available treatments for HSP lack sufficient or robust support in the medical literature.
- The pathogenesis of HSP is multifactorial and includes neurologic and mechanical factors, often in combination, which vary among those affected.
- The systematic approach discussed in this article is intended help practitioners to accurately identify the factors contributing to each patient's pain, and to prescribe the most effective treatment based on the available evidence.

INTRODUCTION

Stroke, or cerebrovascular accident, is the third leading cause of death and the leading cause of adult long-term disability in the United States. Impairments from stroke vary widely, but one of the most common is hemiplegic shoulder pain (HSP). Pain and loss of function in the upper limb is a significant detriment to quality of life. HSP is a challenge to patients and their health care providers, as it reduces participation in rehabilitation, discourages motion, hinders recovery, and adversely affects function. The causes of HSP are multifactorial, have neurologic and mechanical causes, and can be generated peripherally in the limb or centrally within the brain.

Although HSP has been recognized and discussed in the medical community for decades, the evidence in the medical literature lacks sufficient quantity and quality, and

Disclosures: None.

[a] Physical Medicine & Rehabilitation, University of Pennsylvania, 1800 Lombard Street, 1st Floor, Philadelphia, PA 19146, USA; [b] Rehabilitation Medicine, Magee Rehabilitation Hospital, Jefferson Medical College, Thomas Jefferson University, 1513 Race Street, Philadelphia, PA 19102, USA
* Corresponding author.
E-mail address: john.vasudevan@uphs.upenn.edu

is inconsistent in its conclusions. It can be confusing to manage HSP when each of its components has its own controversies in treatment. For example, even if adhesive capsulitis is identified as a contributor to HSP, debate remains regarding the best treatment practice for adhesive capsulitis itself. The purpose of this article is to assist the reader in developing a strategy for the management of HSP. No patient is exactly the same, so a one-size-fits-all treatment is unlikely to be effective. Instead, the focus should be on a consistent approach to ensure that all components of the diagnosis are addressed appropriately.

SCOPE AND SIGNIFICANCE

Every year in the United States 795,000 people suffer a new or recurrent stroke: 1 stroke every 40 seconds. More than 7 million Americans older than 20 years have had a stroke. Stroke is the third leading cause of death and the leading cause of long-term disability, costing the United States $18.8 billion annually, and with a lifetime cost of $140,000 per patient with ischemic stroke.[1] Of those who survive a stroke, approximately half have hemiplegia. Although 70% of those with hemiplegia will achieve ambulatory status, half are left with a nonfunctional arm.[2] The incidence of HSP is widely reported in previous literature, ranging from 16% to 84% but most commonly reported as near 70%.[3]

It is not only pain but associated psychological distress that limits a patient's participation in the rehabilitation process. The presence of HSP is strongly correlated with a prolonged hospital stay and lower Barthel functional score in the first 12 weeks after stroke.[4] Of patients who had a Barthel Index score of less than 15, 59% experienced shoulder pain during their hospital stay, compared with 25% of patients with a Barthel Index score greater than 15.[5] Patients with HSP are less likely to return to their home.[6] Conversely, improvement of upper limb function within the first 5 weeks after a stroke can result in improved use of the affected limb in functional tasks.[7]

PREDICTORS AND PROGNOSIS IN HEMIPLEGIC SHOULDER PAIN

HSP has a significant impact on function both during and after rehabilitation. A meta-analysis of 58 studies assessed outcomes of overall upper limb recovery according to age, sex, lesion site, initial motor impairment, motor-evoked potentials, and somatosensory-evoked potentials.[8] Only initial measures of impairment and function predicted long-term outcome. Age in itself is not clearly a risk factor on its own, but those of older age are more likely to have preexisting abnormality that affects impairment. Additional risk factors for developing shoulder pain within the first 6 months after stroke include impaired voluntary motor control, diminished proprioception, tactile extinction, abnormal sensation, spasticity of the elbow flexor muscles, restricted range of motion (ROM) for both shoulder abduction and shoulder external rotation trophic changes, and type 2 diabetes mellitus.[9] Barlak and colleagues[10] found a significant correlation between HSP and adhesive capsulitis and complex regional pain syndrome, but none between HSP and grade of subluxation, spasticity, impingement syndrome, or thalamic pain.

In addition to new impairments following a stroke, the practitioner must also consider the likelihood of pre-existing abnormality, whether symptomatic or not, which may contribute to pain in the shoulder. Shoulder pain is a common musculo-skeletal complaint made to primary care physicians and a reason for referral to a musculoskeletal specialist. Rotator cuff disorders are the most common source of such pain. Partial tears of the rotator cuff are frequently seen as early as age 50 years, with the risk of severe injury increasing in the 60s and 70s age groups.[11] Degeneration of articular surfaces may reduce ROM, and damage to soft tissue can increase joint laxity.[12] Further complicating a proper diagnosis are data that suggest a poor correlation between symptoms and findings on physical examination. Dromerick and colleagues[13] found that examination findings consistent with injury to the supraspinatus and long head of the biceps are more consistently associated with early onset of HSP, regardless of whether the patient reported pain.

SHOULDER ANATOMY

The human shoulder is a complex ball-and-socket joint that allows multidirectional reach. This agility comes at the sacrifice of stability.[14] The extensive ROM is due largely to the shallow depth of the glenoid fossa, with only 25% of the humeral head coming into contact with the glenoid. This agility is necessary to properly position the hands for a large variety of functional tasks. The only true joint directly connecting the entire upper quarter to the trunk is the sternoclavicular joint. Stability of movement, therefore, depends on both static and dynamic stabilizers (**Fig. 1**). Stability is provided by the surrounding muscles and ligaments. The glenohumeral ligaments serve as the primary static stabilizers and include the superior, middle, and inferior

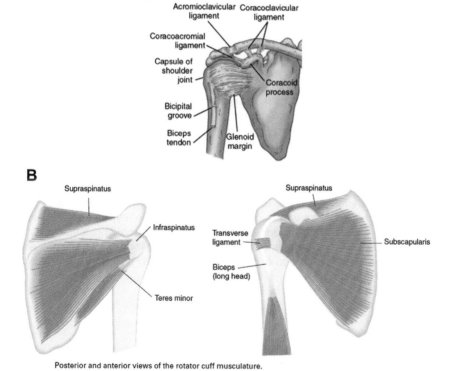

Fig. 1. Static (*A*) and dynamic (*B*) stabilizers of the shoulder. Image *B* shows the posterior (*left*) and anterior (*right*) views of the rotator cuff musculature. (*From* [A] O'Donoghue DH. Treatment of injuries to athletes, 4th ed. Philadelphia: Saunders, 1984; with permission; and [B] DeLee JC, Drez D, Miller MD. DeLee and Drez's Orthopaedic Sports Medicine, 3rd Ed. Philadelphia: Saunders, 2009, p. 989; with permission.)

glenohumeral ligaments. The primary dynamic stabilizers are the rotator cuff muscles, whose attachments form a cuff around the head of the humerus.

The glenohumeral joint derives passive support from a cartilaginous labrum, glenohumeral ligaments, and joint capsule. Functional movements require coordinated movements of dynamic stabilizers. The deltoid and rotator cuff muscles (supraspinatus, infraspinatus, teres minor, and subscapularis) act on the humerus, and the position of the scapula is primarily controlled by the trapezius, serratus, and latissimus dorsi. The subscapularis rotates the humerus internally, whereas the infraspinatus and teres minor are external rotators. Abduction is primarily achieved by the deltoid and is aided by the supraspinatus. The rotator cuff muscles compress the humeral head in the glenoid fossa, thereby stabilizing the joint and providing a counterbalance to opposing forces on the humerus. Overhead activity requires simultaneous abduction by the deltoid and external rotation by the infraspinatus. Movements in a single anatomic plane, such as abduction, can only be accomplished with a predictable ratio of movement termed scapulohumeral rhythm.[15] Impairment of rotator cuff action can lead to superior subluxation of the humeral head, predisposing to impingement of the supraspinatus between the greater tubercle of the humerus and the acromion.

MECHANISMS OF INJURY

Although many mechanisms for HSP have been proposed, pinpointing the cause in individual patients can be elusive. The etiology may be multifactorial, relating to disruption of the biomechanical balance of the shoulder caused by stroke-induced weakness, spasticity, and sensory impairment. Several systems for categorizing HSP exist. A model by Ryerson and Levit identified 4 major sources of pain in patients with HSP.[16] Joint pain resulting from instability can cause sharp pain with passive or active movement. Atrophic or spastic muscle can result in a "pulling" pain with movement. Abnormal pain sensitivity can arise from inappropriate central nervous system modulation of the pain, which can vary from diffuse and achy to sharp and lancinating. Complex regional pain syndrome, though less common, is characterized by reduced ROM, dysesthesia, and trophic changes.

The difficulty in interpreting this and other descriptions of HSP is the absence of any pathognomonic relationship to any particular subtype of pain. Achy pain emanating from muscle or tendon impingement can just as likely result from an upper motor neuron disorder such as spasticity. Sharp pain, allodynia, or hyperpathia caused by a lower motor neuron disorder, such as axillary neuropathy, could present with similar symptoms associated with central causes of pain and altered sensation. To avoid such confusion, the classification of HSP is more accurately based on etiology rather than symptoms alone.

APPROACH TO DIFFERENTIAL DIAGNOSIS

To more effectively determine the factors that contribute to hemiplegic shoulder pain, the authors suggest that factors affecting HSP should be divided into 2 categories: neurologic and mechanical (**Box 1**). Neurologic factors include spasticity, brachial plexus injury, complex regional pain syndrome (CRPS), and central sensitization. Mechanical factors include shoulder subluxation, rotator cuff injury, glenohumeral joint disorders, adhesive capsulitis, and direct trauma. It is important to appreciate that the cause of pain may involve a combination of neurologic and mechanical factors.

Box 1
Components of hemiplegic shoulder pain

Neurologic Factors

  Upper motor neuron neurologic factors

    Paralysis, spasticity, central poststroke pain, central sensitization

  Lower motor neuron neurologic factors

    Peripheral neuropathy, brachial plexus injury, complex regional pain syndrome

Mechanical Factors

  Shoulder subluxation, rotator cuff injury, glenohumeral joint disorders, adhesive capsulitis, myofascial pain, direct trauma

---

Neurologic Factors

Weakness

Weakness of the muscles supporting the shoulder joint is a commonly seen after a stroke and often persists chronically. Weakness disrupts the stabilizers of the shoulder joint and often precedes subsequent development of spasticity. It is an underlying factor common to both neurologic and mechanical factors. Weakness of the trunk muscles and the muscles stabilizing the head is also common after stroke and frequently affects posture, most commonly creating a forward flexed and stooped posture, which can further lead to anterior subluxation of the shoulder and further exacerbate rotator cuff impingement and traction on the joint capsule.

Spasticity

Muscle spasticity is commonly defined as a velocity-dependent resistance to passive stretch. It is a consequence of an upper motor neuron disorder, creating an imbalance between agonist-antagonist muscle pairs. The result in hemiplegia is typical posturing with a dominant flexor tone in the upper limbs. Overactivity of the pectoralis and subscapularis is most predominant about the shoulder, resulting in excessive humeral flexion, adduction, and internal rotation. Combined with increased activity of teres major and latissimus dorsi, spasticity inhibits active and passive abduction, extension, and external rotation at the shoulder. The consequence is inability to achieve desired ROM for activities of daily living (ADLs), and predisposition to mechanical injury (eg, rotator cuff impingement).

Of patients with HSP, approximately 85% with spastic hemiplegia experienced pain, compared with 18% in those with a flaccid hemiplegia.[17] Patients with reduced external rotation experience more pain, and use of a subscapular nerve block to a spastic subscapularis muscle has been demonstrated to reduce pain.[18] Preservation of joint mobility in patients with spasticity and prevention of contracture in those with flaccid hemiplegia are intended to reduce the incidence of HSP.

Brachial plexus and peripheral nerve injury

The brachial plexus is derived from C5-T1 roots, and arises at the lower aspect of the neck. It runs behind scalenes proximally, and behind the clavicle and pectoralis muscles distally. Injury to the plexus can be traumatic or atraumatic. In the setting of hemiplegia, the cause is most likely a traction injury caused by improper handling of the flaccid hemiplegic limb, such as pulling on the arm during transfers and repositioning.[19,20] One study based on needle electromyography (EMG) reported that 75% of supraspinatus and deltoid muscles in hemiplegic arms had neuropathic responses.[21]

The upper trunk of the plexus is most susceptible to injury. The most common isolated peripheral nerve injury in HSP is axillary neuropathy, thought to be subsequent to downward displacement of the humeral head in shoulder subluxation.[22,23] However, other studies have failed to reveal significant evidence of plexus or peripheral nerve injuries associated with HSP.[24,25] Given the conflicting evidence, it is not possible to ascertain whether plexopathy or mononeuropathy plays a substantial role in HSP. However, if a plexus or peripheral nerve injury occurs it may contribute to a cycle of pain, weakness, and progressive subluxation.

Complex regional pain syndrome

Type 1 CRPS, previously termed reflex sympathetic dystrophy or shoulder-hand syndrome, and Type 2 CRPS, previously termed causalgia, are characterized by pain that is out of proportion to the pathologic condition, peripheral and/or central autonomic abnormalities, and dystrophic changes to a limb often (but not always) following a traumatic injury. CRPS can inhibit mobility by both pain that discourages motion and the associated adhesive capsulitis that restricts it. The incidence of CRPS in patients with hemiplegia has been cited to be as high as 23%.[17] However, there is considerable variability in past reported incidence, likely attributable to various diagnostic criteria. The precise mechanism of this disorder remains unclear. There are studies demonstrating an association between shoulder-hand syndrome and spasticity, confusion, and sensory loss.[26–28] Damage to the soft tissues surrounding the hemiplegic shoulder have been implicated as a cause of shoulder-hand syndrome.[29] Abnormalities in the brain itself have also been implicated. Further study is needed before a definite causality between HSP and CRPS can be confirmed.

Central poststroke pain and sensitization

Sensory disturbance and neglect can alter a patient's proprioception and perception of pain, predisposing the shoulder to injury. Central poststroke pain (CPSP) is another impairment deriving from stroke that can contribute to pain in the shoulder and elsewhere. Also termed thalamic pain syndrome, a lesion of the spinothalamocortical pathway may result in abnormal neural reorganization. The result is an improper generation of pain in the absence of injury, which can be reported as neuropathic, spastic, or musculoskeletal in quality. Central sensitization is a separate entity that can be observed in the presence of CRPS and CPSP, whereby abnormal responsiveness of nociceptive neurons results in dysesthesia. Sensitization often involves alterations in neurotransmitter levels, including serotonin and norepinephrine.[14]

Mechanical Factors

Shoulder subluxation

Shoulder subluxation refers to the static displacement of the humeral head in relation to the glenoid, and represents a common source of mechanical pain in HSP. Subluxation requires a disruption in the integrity of the glenohumeral joint. Clinical findings are a gap between the humeral head and the acromion. This gap can be measured with calipers, radiography, or ultrasonography, but is commonly described by finger breadths in the clinical setting. During the early stages following stroke the muscles in the hemiplegic arm are usually flaccid, thereby impairing joint stability and predisposing the shoulder to traction-type injury. The most common reason is an inability of the paralyzed shoulder girdle musculature to provide dynamic stability at the joint. Articular tissues (eg, the joint capsule) can become distended, particularly in the flaccid stage following stroke. This distension is also hypothesized to contribute to ischemia in the tendons of the supraspinatus and long head of the biceps.[30] Downward displacement of the humerus is most common during the flaccid stage, whereas the spastic stage often leads to anterior displacement, posterior displacement, or internal rotation.[11] Anteroposterior (AP) and oblique radiographs help diagnose and characterize shoulder subluxation. Clinical diagnosis of subluxation is often achieved by measuring arm-length discrepancy or by palpating or measuring the subacromial space.[31,32]

The association between shoulder subluxation and HSP remains controversial. Paci and colleagues[30] studied 107 patients with hemiplegia in a case-control design, and measured the presence of shoulder pain in those with shoulder subluxation and those without. Patients with shoulder subluxation had significantly greater pain at admission, discharge, and at a 30- to 40-day follow-up assessment; they also had greater impairment with ADLs and required longer hospital stays. However, other studies argue that patients without subluxation are just as likely to develop pain.[33] Comparative studies of the association between shoulder subluxation and pain are limited by sample size or methodology. However, there is enough evidence to suggest that shoulder subluxation may be a contributing factor in HSP. Proper positioning, support, and correct transfer techniques by caregivers may be helpful in prevention and alleviation of pain.

Rotator cuff injury

As discussed previously, the primary purpose of the rotator cuff is to stabilize the humeral head relative to the glenoid during shoulder movements. Rotator cuff injuries are a common source of shoulder pain in the general population. Rotator cuff tears occur in 20% to 40% of the general population, with increasing incidence with age. The incidence of rotator cuff tears in hemiplegic patients ranges from 33% to 40%.[33] It is unlikely that hemiplegia is a cause of rotator cuff injury per se, but abnormal positioning, muscle imbalance caused by weakness, and spasticity can all increase the likelihood of impingement and tearing. In addition, falls can be a common occurrence during the initial onset of the stroke itself, and may be a cause of rotator cuff tear, which may go unnoticed during the initial stages of the stroke. Improper handling of the hemiplegic arm could also cause injury to the rotator cuff tendons. Treatment of rotator cuff injuries in the plegic or paretic arm is usually conservative and supportive.

Adhesive capsulitis

The term frozen shoulder is often used to describe a shoulder with decreased ROM, but the term is nonspecific and fails to determine how much of the restriction is passive (ie, a block to motion) versus active (ie, limited by pain or weakness). Adhesive capsulitis is a more specific term that refers to a condition of uncertain origin characterized by significant restriction of both active and passive shoulder motion that occurs in the absence of a known intrinsic shoulder disorder.[34] A painful shoulder may develop adhesive capsulitis because of pain inhibition of mobility, leading to subsequent disuse atrophy and contracture. The pain of adhesive capsulitis is also theorized to lead to increased immobility.[35] The decreased ROM can lead to inflammation, muscle atrophy, and contracture resulting from adhesions.[36] The prognosis of adhesive capsulitis is favorable, but requires diligence to preserve available ROM and strength. Increased immobilization from spasticity can increase the likelihood of developing adhesions.[11]

Myofascial pain

A more complete discussion of myofascial pain and trigger-point theory can be found in other articles by Dr Gerwin and by Dr Borg-Stein and Iaccarino elsewhere in this issue. As with most musculoskeletal disorders, it is important for the clinician to consider the contribution of muscle-generated pain from muscles about the shoulder girdle, and the contribution to posture and muscle balance on the level of myofascial pain. Although there is a larger body of data regarding the impact of myofascial pain on shoulder pain in the general population, there is only one published study specifically studying myofascial pain in HSP, which demonstrated improvement of pain with dry needling of trigger points when combined with standard rehabilitation.[37]

DIAGNOSIS OF HEMIPLEGIC SHOULDER PAIN

There are no clear or widely accepted criteria for diagnosing HSP. Therefore, the authors recommend confirming the diagnosis following the same approach of dividing the workup according to suspected neurologic and mechanical factors (**Box 2**).

Neurologic Factors

History and physical examination
A proper history and physical examination are paramount, especially when symptoms can be explained by multiple causes. Important information to elicit during history taking includes preexisting shoulder pain and use of analgesics, limited functional use of the arm, prior trauma, and surgery. Regardless of the diagnosis, the key steps in the physical examination include observation (for asymmetry, deformity, and erythema), ROM, palpation, sensation, reflexes, strength, and special tests. The patient should demonstrate maximum active range of motion (AROM) before the examiner assesses full passive range of motion (PROM). Pain is most often the limiting factor in AROM, followed by weakness. If there is reduced PROM, contracture or anatomic block should be suspected. A goniometer can provide more objective monitoring of changes to ROM. Palpation is performed to assess for muscle bulk, abnormal contour or masses, or areas of tenderness. Key targets of palpation should include rotator cuff, deltoid, periscapular muscles, long head biceps tendon, other upper quarter musculature, and acromioclavicular joint. Strength testing in the C5-T1 myotomes (graded 0–5), sensory testing in the C5-T1 dermatomes (graded 0–2+), and C5-C7 reflexes (graded 0–4+) will help to localize a neurologic lesion, whether central or peripheral.

As with any neurologic injury, careful consideration to sensation and strength are useful in determining whether the lesion is central (brain and spinal cord) or peripheral, and whether the damage is focal (as in axillary neuropathy) or diffuse (as in CRPS). Because hemiplegia is an upper motor neuron disorder, it is also important to assess the presence and severity of spasticity. Muscle spasticity is determined using the Modified Ashworth Scale (**Box 3**).

Electrodiagnosis
Electrodiagnostic testing has excellent sensitivity and specificity for nerve injury within the peripheral nervous system. Electrodiagnostic testing may have limited utility in patients with HSP. Although it may be helpful in diagnosing a peripheral neuropathy, it cannot reliably exclude shoulder pain related to centrally mediated weakness or spasticity. Nevertheless, it may be useful in situations where there is underlying or

---

Box 2
Diagnosing the causes of hemiplegic shoulder pain

History, physical examination, special tests/maneuvers

Imaging (radiography, magnetic resonance imaging, ultrasonography)

Electrodiagnosis

Diagnostic nerve blocks or injections (intramuscular, intra-articular)

Box 3
Modified Ashworth Scale

0: No increase in muscle tone

1: Slight increase in muscle tone, manifested by catch and release, or minimal resistance to the end range of motion (flexion or extension)

1+: Slight increase in muscle tone, manifested by catch and then minimal release through the remainder (less than half) of the range of motion

2: Moderate (marked) increase in muscle tone through most of the range of motion, but affected part is easily moved

3: Severe (considerable) increase in muscle tone through most of the range of motion, and affected part is difficult to move

4: Affected part is rigid in flexion or extension, little to no passive range of motion

---

concomitant possibility of brachial plexus nerve injury, peripheral mononeuropathy, or cervical radiculopathy.

Sympathetic block

A sympathetic ganglion block is a diagnostic option considered for patients with suspected CRPS. This block may assist in reducing symptoms mediated by the sympathetic nervous system, which includes alterations in skin color and temperature. These blocks will often cause a temporary Horner syndrome.

Mechanical Factors

Physical examination

The basic components of the physical examination, such as testing of strength, sensation, and reflexes, are used regardless of the cause of HSP. In addition, there are multiple specialized tests for the shoulder, but only a few most pertinent to the mechanical components of HSP (**Fig. 2**A–F).

Neer, Hawkins, and Jobe ("empty can") tests can assess for subacromial impingement. Apprehension and sulcus tests assess for glenohumeral joint instability. The apprehension test is performed by placing the patient in a supine position near the edge of the bed with the arm externally rotated, abducted, and in slight extension. Apprehension against further motion during the maneuver suggests anterior shoulder instability with 63% sensitivity. The sulcus test is performed in the sitting position with the affected arm at the patient's side. The examiner pulls the elbow inferiorly to measure the physiologic separation between the acromion and humeral head. Separation of 1 cm is scored as Grade 1, 1 to 2 cm is scored as Grade 2, and more than 2 cm is scored as Grade 3. Grade 3 separation indicates multidirectional glenohumeral instability, but the maneuver has only 28% sensitivity.[38]

The Neer test is performed by passive forward elevation of the arm with scapula stabilized. A modification of the test includes adding internal rotation of the humerus to approximate the acromion and greater tuberosity of the humerus. Positive pain using this maneuver suggests subacromial impingement with 88% sensitivity. The Hawkins test for impingement is positive if pain is produced with passive horizontal adduction and internal rotation. The Jobe (or empty can) test is positive for impingement if pain is produced when resistance is applied to arms elevated and internally rotated in the scapular plane (horizontal abduction to approximately 45°).

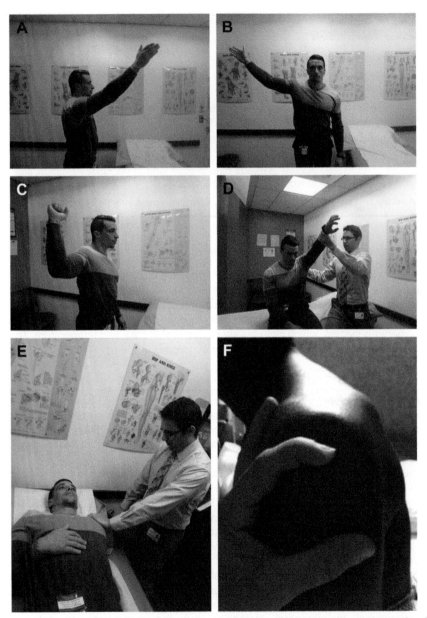

Fig. 2. Key examination maneuvers in hemiplegic shoulder pain. Examination should include active and passive flexion (*A*), abduction (*B*), and external rotation (*C*). Specialized maneuvers include Neer test modified with humeral internal rotation (*D*), apprehension test (*E*), sulcus test (*F*), hand-behind-neck (*G*), and hand-behind-back (*H*).

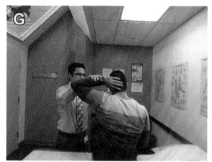
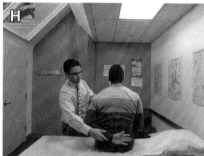

Fig. 2. (*continued*)

In stroke patients able to comply, a simple and efficient bedside screen for shoulder ROM includes the hand-behind-back (HBB) and hand-behind-neck (HBN) maneuvers. The HBB maneuver combines internal rotation and extension, and the HBN maneuver combines external rotation and abduction (see **Fig. 2**G, H). Differences or pain in passive or active external rotation of the shoulder can indicate the onset of HSP.

The value of the physical examination is often greatest when multiple maneuvers are positive, or when overall movement is asymmetric relative to the unaffected side. Rajaratnam and colleagues[38] concluded that HSP could be successfully diagnosed clinically by using only 3 of the aforementioned methods: Neer test, HBN, and a difference of greater than 10° passive external rotation at the shoulder joint. When combined with a report of at least moderate pain at rest, the sensitivity and positive predictive value for HSP was 96.7%. Another study of proprioception and kinematics of shoulder motion in patients with and without HSP found that those with HSP demonstrated increased lateral scapular rotation and decreased perception of passive movement.[39] Furthermore, patients who had a stroke were more likely to demonstrate abnormal scapular movement on the nonparetic side when compared with controls, arguing that rehabilitation must always take both sides of the body into account.

Diagnostic imaging

Ultimately the diagnosis of HSP is clinical, and does not necessitate diagnostic imaging. However, the use of imaging may be of benefit if the history and examination raise suspicion of underlying traumatic or structural abnormalities that may contribute to the patient's pain.

Radiography

Radiographic imaging is a useful starting point for evaluating suspected mechanical components of HSP. An AP view will rule out fracture and help to assess for subluxation. Adding AP views with the humerus in external rotation will bring the greater tuberosity and associated soft tissue into better view, and may help reveal calcific rotator cuff tendinopathy. Rotator cuff impingement by the acromion is best evaluated with a scapular Y view. If there is concern for shoulder instability, an axillary view will evaluate the relationship of the humerus to glenoid, and an AP view with humerus in internal rotation may reveal a Hill-Sachs lesion seen in traumatic dislocation.

Conventional and Magnetic Resonance Arthrography

Conventional x-ray arthrography is rarely used in clinical practice as an isolated method of diagnosis, but can help diagnose both adhesive capsulitis and rotator cuff tears. A normal joint will have a volume exceeding 10 mL, smooth glenohumeral capsular margin contours, and the presence of an axillary recess (a pouch of the capsule bordered by the inferior rim of the glenoid cavity and inferior portion of the humeral head). Patients with the presence of adhesive capsulitis demonstrate less than 10 mL of volume, irregular capsule margins, and a diminished or absent axillary recess. A rotator cuff injury will be demonstrated by contrast leakage from the glenohumeral joint to the subdeltoid bursa. The high sensitivity of arthrography (as high as 99%) makes this procedure the gold standard for detecting such tears.[40] However, soft tissues cannot be visualized using this method.

A 1-year study of 32 patients with HSP by Lo and colleagues[40] attempted to correlate arthrographic and clinical findings of HSP. Clinical measurements included Brunnstrom stage (**Box 4**), spasticity distribution, presence or absence of shoulder subluxation, or CRPS Type 1. Arthrographic measurements included shoulder joint volume and capsular morphology. Fifty percent of the patients had evidence of adhesive capsulitis, 44% had shoulder subluxation, 22% had rotator cuff tears, and 16% had CRPS Type 1. Disorders were often present in combination. The study determined that arthrography was useful in identifying adhesive capsulitis, and that most cases developed within 2 months of developing HSP. Most significantly, outcomes worsened the longer adhesive capsulitis remained untreated. Even when diagnostic imaging is not used, the findings emphasize the importance of initiating appropriate treatment whenever adhesive capsulitis is clinically suspected.

Magnetic resonance arthrography (MRA) has the advantage of better visualization to identify abnormality of the soft-tissue structures of the shoulder, and with little loss of sensitivity and specificity. Multiple criteria exist to diagnose adhesive capsulitis by MRA, including thickness of capsule and synovium greater than 3 mm on T2-weighted coronal sequence without fat suppression, an axillary recess diameter greater than 9.0 mm, or rotator cuff interval thickness exceeding 8.4 mm.[41,42]

A study of magnetic resonance imaging findings between stoke survivors with and without shoulder pain in the chronic stage found synovial capsule thickening, synovial capsule enhancement, and enhancement in the rotator cuff interval to be more prominent in those with shoulder pain.[43] There was no significant difference in rotator cuff tendinopathy, joint effusion, subacromial bursal fluid, acromioclavicular capsular hypertrophy, and muscle atrophy. Shoulder subluxation was not observed, and was postulated to have resolved in the more acute to subacute stages of recovery. The findings suggest that chronic mechanical limitations in HSP most closely resemble those of adhesive capsulitis.

Box 4
Brunnstrom stages of stroke recovery

1. Flaccidity (immediate after onset), no voluntary movements can be initiated
2. Spasticity appears, basic synergy patterns appear, minimal voluntary movements present
3. Increased spasticity, patient gains more voluntary control over synergies
4. Decreased spasticity, patient masters control of synergistic movement patterns
5. Further decreased spasticity, synergies lose dominance over motor acts
6. Spasticity disappears, joint movements improve, and coordination approaches normal
7. Normal function is restored

Ultrasonography

Although ultrasonography is not a new modality, there has been a recent surge in its popularity as a method of diagnosing a wide variety of musculoskeletal disorders of the shoulder. The primary advantages of ultrasonography include excellent visualization of superficial soft tissue, dynamic assessment, and lack of ionizing radiation. However, there is limited utility for some deep structures and those blocked behind bone. The pain from HSP that limits ROM may interfere with optimal positioning during ultrasonography.[44] Pathologic features easily identified by ultrasonography include rotator cuff tendinopathy, dynamic rotator cuff impingement, acromioclavicular arthrosis, and long head biceps tenosynovitis. In adhesive capsulitis, ultrasonography may reveal hypoechoic echotexture and increased vascularity within the rotator interval (triangular space bounded by superior border of the subscapularis anteriorly, anterior border of the supraspinatus tendon posteriorly, and coracoid process as base).[45]

A unique advantage to the use of ultrasonography is the ability to provide serial assessments of the shoulder throughout the course of rehabilitation. The risk of injury appears to be greatest in the early stages of recovery after stroke. Pong and colleagues[46] used ultrasonography to evaluate for soft-tissue injuries at admission and 2 weeks after completion of rehabilitation. Patients admitted at Brunnstrom stages I to III were more likely to demonstrate new or worsening injuries to the shoulder after rehabilitation in comparison with those admitted at Brunnstrom stages IV to VI. These results are consistent with those in similarly designed studies.[47,48]

MANAGEMENT OF HEMIPLEGIC SHOULDER PAIN

There are many available modalities, both pharmacologic and nonpharmacologic, for the treatment of HSP, which are outlined in **Box 5**.

Regardless of Cause

Prevention through positioning

The key to prevention of HSP is proper handling and positioning, especially in the first days after stroke. The patient depends on multiple members of the health care team to assist with positioning and transfers throughout each day. In the flaccid stage, the shoulder capsule has significant laxity and is particularly vulnerable to injury from static stabilizers. Patients who require assistance with transfers are more likely to develop shoulder pain.[5] There is no clear guideline regarding which method best reduces strain on the shoulder. However, simply raising patient and caretaker awareness of potential injuries caused by poor handling can reduce injury as a result of increased vigilance.[26]

A commonly suggested position for the shoulder is abduction, external rotation, and flexion.[33] However, there is no consensus on which position is ideal, and no one position has been proved to be significantly better in studies of the subject.[6] The aim is to achieve symmetry between the affected and unaffected shoulders, and caretakers should strive for symmetric positioning of both scapulae. Carr and Kenney[49] recommend that the shoulder be protracted, with the arm forward, wrist neutral or slightly supinated, and fingers extended. Bobath suggested a technique of positioning in a reflex-inhibiting pattern to prevent inefficient movement and maintain muscle tone.[50] The affected limb is positioned away from the direction of muscle spasticity. The precise direction varies, and depends on the muscle tone patterns of each individual. Small sample sizes in studies of positioning limit the significance of any one suggested pattern.

Box 5
Approach to treatment of hemiplegic shoulder pain

Regardless of Cause

- Prevention through positioning
- Bracing, slings, taping
- Physical therapy to optimize range of motion and strength

Neurologic Factors

- Transcutaneous electrical nerve stimulation (TENS)
- Functional electrical stimulation (FES)
- Relaxation/electromyography biofeedback
- Botulinum toxin injection
- Sympathetic blocks
- Pharmacotherapy (eg, antispasticity, neuropathic pain)

Mechanical Factors

- Pharmacotherapy (eg, anti-inflammatory)
- Corticosteroid injection
- Suprascapular nerve block
- Trigger-point injections and dry needling

Complementary and Alternative Medicine

- Acupuncture
- Aromatherapy
- Surgical treatment

Strapping and slings

Strapping is used to maintain the shoulder joint in an appropriate anatomic position to prevent or reduce subluxation. Strapping from the onset of stroke until restoration of muscle tone may prevent the incidence, or at least delay the onset, of HSP.[51,52] Taping perpendicular to a muscle inhibits activity, and taping parallel to a muscle promotes activity.[33] The exact mechanism of pain relief remains uncertain. This technique requires a trained care provider to apply the dressing, and repeat applications to prevent skin irritation. A small study comparing taping versus sham taping in patients with shoulder pain revealed decreased pain-free shoulder abduction, but no significant change in overall pain or ROM.[53] Furthermore, the study was performed without regard to specific diagnosis, and was not applied to patients with HSP. There are no high-quality studies demonstrating the benefit of taping specifically for HSP.

In addition to strapping, shoulder slings have also been used to decrease the stress on the shoulder joint and prevent subluxation by reducing the gravitational pull on the shoulder joint. However, if the arm is incorrectly positioned, or if use of a sling is not alternated with therapeutic exercise, soft-tissue contractures may occur. Such contractures can contribute to the very pain the sling is intended to prevent. Slings are recommended primarily for a flaccid upper extremity, when the patient is upright or walking, for the purpose of protection.[54] Arm troughs and lap trays are recommended for use in a wheelchair to support the limb and prevent shoulder subluxation, as well as to prevent traumatic injury. The properly positioned tray and trough can also maintain abduction and limit excessive internal and external rotation.[55] Arm slings can support the flaccid arm and are protective in ambulating patients, but because many slings hold the arm in flexion, adduction, and internal rotation, their use must be balanced with ROM exercises. Axillary supports such as the Bobath sling are less popular, as they have not been proved to reduce subluxation and can increase soft-tissue injury through lateral displacement of the humeral head.[11]

Like strapping, there is insufficient evidence to indicate the effectiveness, best type, or proper positioning for the use of slings. Some studies demonstrate a reduction in subluxation immediately after application of the sling, but do not prove that this reduction is maintained on resuming functional activities.[33] Regardless of the effect on pain or subluxation, another reason to use a sling is to promote efficiency during ambulation. Han and colleagues[56] performed a randomized crossover gait evaluation in hemiplegic patients with and without a sling, and found improvements in heart rate and gait speed, with decreased oxygen cost and oxygen rate in patients using the sling.

Physical therapy
Physical therapy is an essential component of poststroke rehabilitation, and plays a major role in the prevention and treatment of HSP. PROM exercises should be initiated as soon as the patient is medically stable. Care should be taken during passive abduction of the arm, as this may cause or aggravate a rotator cuff injury. If pain consistent with impingement is noted during the PROM exercises, the amplitude of movement should be decreased. Performing PROM exercises within such a pain-free range has been shown to reduce reports of shoulder pain by 43%.[57]

Physical therapy is directed at both improving upper extremity mechanics and reducing neurologic injury. Heat and cold therapy are used to decrease pain, increase mobility, and reduce inflammation. Slings and strapping may be used as an adjunct to minimize subluxation and reduce mechanical pain. Overhead exercise pulleys are strongly discouraged, as they can cause impingement and rotator cuff injury.[58] Rehabilitation methods include the Bobath and Brunnstrom approaches, and task-specific motor retraining. No particular technique has been proved to be more effective than another.[36]

Lynch and colleagues[59] studied the effectiveness of a continuous passive motion (CPM) device versus self-ROM group exercises in 32 hemiplegic patients. All patients received 3.5 hours of standard therapy daily, and the additional therapies were supervised by an occupational therapist. A blinded assessor evaluated joint strength and integrity at discharge. CPM was associated with greater shoulder stability, but there was no significant improvement in motor impairment, disability, pain, or tone.

Masiero and colleagues[60] used a single-blinded trial to evaluate the addition of early sensorimotor training using a robotic device in addition to standard therapy in 35 patients with acute stroke. Robotic devices are used to provide high-intensity, repetitive, interactive training of an impaired limb, and the controlled movement helps prevent injury and ensure maximal benefit to targeted muscle groups. Patients in the treatment group underwent a total of 20 hours (4 hours daily for 5 weeks) of programmed shoulder and elbow manipulation by the robotic device. Patients in the control group underwent robotic training of the unaffected limb. The treatment group experienced a significant reduction in impairment and gains in function, with effects maintained at an 8-month follow-up assessment.

Neurologic Factors

Transcutaneous electrical nerve stimulation
Transcutaneous electrical nerve stimulation (TENS) provides an external electrical stimulus to the affected limb, and is postulated to be effective based on the gate-

control theory of pain. At high intensity, the electrical impulse can also activate the muscles to maintain muscle bulk. TENS can be delivered with low intensity (just enough stimulation to be sensed on the skin) or high intensity (noticeable muscle contraction and near-painful skin sensation). High-intensity TENS may reduce HSP in comparison with low-intensity TENS or placebo.[61]

Functional electrical stimulation

Several studies suggest that functional electrical stimulation (FES) reduces HSP and shoulder subluxation, and improves functional strength and ability.[36] FES is most often directed at the supraspinatus and (to a lesser extent) the posterior deltoid muscles because of their role in maintaining dynamic shoulder stability (**Fig. 3**). Research suggests that FES may reduce, or even prevent, subluxation. Wang and colleagues[62] compared the effects of a 6-week FES program in 16 patients with acute hemiplegia (less than 21 days) and 16 with chronic hemiplegia (more than 1 year). Those with acute hemiplegia improved with treatment while those with chronic hemiplegia did not. In addition, the reduction of shoulder subluxation in the patients with acute hemiplegia was lost on withdrawal of FES treatment. A randomized controlled trial of 50 patients with HSP found that FES and therapy, compared with therapy alone, reduced shoulder subluxation on radiography, but without a significant difference in AROM, PROM, or pain in either group at completion of inpatient rehabilitation.[63] A review of 9 controlled trials of FES for HSP by Chae and colleagues[64] found only 2 demonstrating sustained improvement after completion of treatment. A Cochrane review concluded that FES benefits pain-free passive external rotation ROM and reduces subluxation, but does not improve shoulder pain or motor impairment.[65]

Chae and colleagues[66] evaluated the effectiveness of intramuscular electrical stimulation (IES) in a multicenter, single-blinded randomized clinical trial of 61 chronic stroke survivors. Rather than traditional FES, which uses externally applied pads to deliver an electrical stimulation through the skin, IES delivers the stimulation directly to the targeted muscles via a percutaneous electrode. Advantages include more direct stimulation, reduced pain, and the ability to use the device at home with more precise targeting of the intended muscles. Patients in the treatment group were given 6 weeks of 6-hour stimulations to the supraspinatus, posterior deltoid, middle deltoid, and upper trapezius. Patients in the control group were managed with a cuff-like sling for 6 weeks. Patients who underwent IES reported a significant reduction in pain when compared with controls, sustained at 1 year after treatment. There is a single case report of complete and sustained relief of pain 13 months after a 3-week course of IES into the deltoid muscle.[67] Another case study of a fully implanted peripheral nerve

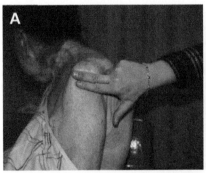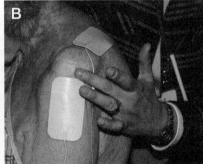

Fig. 3. Functional electrical stimulation (FES). A patient with Grade 2 shoulder subluxation (A) demonstrates reduced subluxation during use of FES (B).

stimulator targeting the axillary nerve demonstrated persistent pain relief and increased pain-free ROM, but without effects on sensation or strength.[68] IES represents a promising treatment, but is not yet widely available.

EMG biofeedback and relaxation exercises

A randomized crossover trial by Williams[69] of 20 patients with HSP who had no shoulder pain before stroke were given either 150 minutes of EMG biofeedback (30 minutes per day for 5 days) or 60 minutes of relaxation exercises (30 minutes per day for 2 days). Patients were assigned to the opposite group 1 week later. After the 2 weeks of intervention, both groups had increased ROM, increased muscle tone, and a 50% to 60% reduction in pain. Although the methodology of this study fails to distinguish the relative benefit of each therapy, the results suggest that such treatment provides patients with more psychological control over their pain.

Botulinum toxin

Botulinum toxin, a presynaptic acetylcholine inhibitor, has gained popularity for focal reduction of spasticity. Although targeted to reduce motor activity, the toxin also inhibits neurotransmitter release by sensory neurons. Several small studies have demonstrated improvement in ROM and reduction in pain in comparison with placebo.[17,70,71] Conversely, de Boer and colleagues[72] failed to find improvements in pain level or ROM after toxin injection into the subscapularis in 21 patients with HSP.

Lim and colleagues[73] compared botulinum toxin type A injected in the infraspinatus, pectoralis, and subscapularis with intra-articular triamcinolone acetonide injections in a randomized, double-blind, controlled study of 29 patients with HSP. There was a strong trend indicating that the botulinum toxin reduced pain and increased ROM when compared with intra-articular injection of triamcinolone. Of note, Ashworth scores were not significantly improved in the botulinum toxin group.

A smaller randomized controlled study of 17 stroke patients with HSP injected with botulinum toxin type A into the biceps and pectoralis major more than 3 months after stroke demonstrated a significant improvement in Ashworth scores for shoulder adduction and elbow flexion at week 4, but not at weeks 8 and 12. Shoulder pain and passive shoulder abduction ROM improved to a similar extent in the study and placebo groups.[71]

Another small, noncontrolled pilot study of 5 patients with HSP demonstrated decreased pain at 2 and 8 weeks after an intra-articular injection of botulinum toxin.[74] Despite the limitations of these case series, the results raise interest in the nociceptive properties of the toxin.

Sympathetic blocks for CRPS

A comprehensive explanation of CRPS management is discussed in a separate article by Dr Freedman and colleagues elsewhere in this issue. It is important to understand the essentials of recognizing and treating this condition as early as possible to prevent severe disability. There are 3 major components to management: pain management, rehabilitation, and psychological therapy.[75–80]

Pain is managed by many methods, but the basic concept is to reduce pain and altered sensitivity, prevent further injury, and increase mobility. Sympathetic blocks (often to the stellate ganglion) are used to interrupt abnormal sympathetic activity when other pharmacologic therapy fails.

Rehabilitation should use modalities for pain and edema control, and stress isometric and stress-loading exercises (repetitive and demanding motions with minimal joint motion such as scrubbing or carrying). PROM should be performed, but restricted to a pain-free range. Psychological therapy helps reduce fear avoidance and encourage active involvement in rehabilitation.

Mechanical Factors

Pharmacotherapy

HSP originates not only via mechanical injury but also through altered sensitivity. Patients experiencing HSP will frequently require pharmacotherapy to complement other physical treatment modalities. As with most painful conditions, simple analgesics and anti-inflammatory drugs should be tried first. Acetaminophen taken before therapies can be useful and well tolerated, with less risk of adverse drug interactions and side effects than other analgesics, and is often a good medication to start with alongside a therapy program. Topical agents such as lidocaine can be helpful, and carry little risk of side effects. Although there is insufficient evidence to support or refute the effectiveness of nonsteroidal anti-inflammatory drugs (NSAIDs) in the treatment of HSP, they are considered worth a therapeutic trial if there are no contraindications. However, care must be taken in the stroke population, as many patients are already on antiplatelet treatment and often have comorbidities such as coronary artery disease, chronic kidney disease, or peptic ulcer disease (PUD).[11] NSAIDs can interfere with antiplatelet treatment, provide an unwanted anticoagulant effect, and further impair kidney function at high or chronic doses. Chronic NSAID use can also lead to PUD, which can be of greater risk in stroke patients on anticoagulants for secondary stroke prophylaxis. Topical NSAIDs carry less risk of kidney damage and PUD because of mostly local analgesic effects with limited systemic absorption.

Antiepileptic agents may be helpful with pain that seems to be of neurogenic character, as may be seen with central poststroke shoulder pain or shoulder-hand syndrome. Likewise, tricyclic antidepressants (TCAs) may have pain-relieving properties and may also aid with sleep. Other antidepressants such as selective serotonin reuptake inhibitors (SSRIs) may also be helpful with neuropathic pain. Oral pharmacologic agents that reduce spasticity help facilitate better participation in physical therapy; their use can be limited by side effects of sedation, although a bedtime dose is often well tolerated.

Small studies have demonstrated reduction in HSP with the use of oral corticosteroids.[26,81] However, the side effects associated with chronic use must be considered.

Berthier and colleagues[82] investigated the use of donepezil (without simultaneous physical therapy) in a single patient with chronic hemiplegia and observed improved sensorimotor function in the shoulder, but this finding has not been validated.

Corticosteroid injection

Corticosteroid injections targeted to the appropriate site of abnormality, most often to the glenohumeral joint or subacromial bursa, may reduce pain in patients with HSP.[33] These injections are best suited to reduce inflammatory pain from rotator cuff tears, bicipital tendonitis, subacromial bursitis, or adhesive capsulitis. If used appropriately and coupled with therapeutic exercise, the addition of steroid injections can significantly reduce pain and increase ROM for 2 to 4 weeks.[83,84] Two studies using intra-articular corticosteroid injections both demonstrated a reduction in pain but without a significant reduction in spasticity or improved function.[85,86] Pain radiating down the lateral shoulder and into the arm may reflect subacromial bursitis, for which Joynt[35] demonstrated that 50% of patients receiving 10 mL of a 1% lidocaine solution had moderate pain relief and improved ROM. Repeated injections increase the risk of weakening soft tissues and contributing to atrophic changes in the shoulder capsule.[11] Therefore, repeated or long-term use of intra-articular steroid injections must be performed sparingly. Injections (particularly glenohumeral) are increasingly performed with fluoroscopic or ultrasound guidance, because their increased accuracy may help confirm the location of inflammatory pain, particularly if clinical suspicion remains high and there has been lack of effect after anatomic landmark-guided injection.

Suprascapular nerve block
The use of suprascapular nerve block has been studied for mechanical shoulder pain in the general population, and now with emerging studies in those with HSP. The purpose of the block is to decrease pain and allow for greater pain-free ROM, and the anesthetic medication may also be coupled with corticosteroid. A small randomized study comparing suprascapular nerve block with intra-articular injection in patients with chronic HSP found both increased ROM and decreased pain by 1 month after injection, but there was no statistical difference between the treatments.[87] Another randomized, controlled, nonblinded study comparing a block with anesthetic and corticosteroid with a placebo injection of saline in patients with HSP is currently under way.[88] A major concern with phenol motor point blocks of mixed nerves is causation of neuropathic pain. However, as reported by Chironna and Hecht,[89] the suprascapular nerve does not have a sensory component and, therefore, this risk is lower. The effect of the block varies from 3 to 9 months. Botulinum toxin can be used instead of a nerve block, although this method provides a shorter duration of action.

Complementary and alternative medicine
Acupuncture is thought to decrease myofascial pain by a neurohormonal mechanism, involving β-endorphin, dynorphin A and B, substance P, 5-hydroxytryptamine, or noradrenaline. A pilot study by Shin and Lee[90] studied the addition of acupuncture to standard rehabilitation therapy in 21 hemiplegic patients with shoulder subluxation. From the time of admission to discharge, there was significant improvement in ROM and muscle strength. A systemic review of acupuncture specifically for HSP by Lee and colleagues[91] discovered only 7 randomized controlled trials of sufficient methodology. The data suggest that acupuncture combined with therapeutic exercise is superior to either modality alone.

Aromatherapy uses plant-derived essential oils applied to the skin or inhaled through the nose to stimulate physiologic changes, including blood pressure and pulse, muscle tension, skin temperature, and blood flow. A trial comparing acupuncture with acupuncture and aromatherapy in the rehabilitation setting favored the addition of aromatherapy.[92] The limitation of this and similar studies is a failure to compare with standard rehabilitation or placebo.

Surgery
Surgical procedures are reserved only for severe shoulder pain or stiffness, most typically in the setting of adhesive capsulitis, not improved by all conservative measures. Surgery is often postponed until at least 6 months after the patient has had a stroke. Operations include release of muscle contractions, repair of rotator cuff tear, and scapular mobilization.[36] Little research has been done in this area, but a small study by Braun and colleagues[93] found that HSP was relieved in all 13 patients who had contracture release, versus no relief in patients treated without surgery. Rotator cuff repair is typically not done specifically for HSP, as it may have been present before the stroke and may offer little in the way of improvement in the plegic or paretic arm. Such repair may be more strongly considered for a traumatic rupture after stroke, but should account for the procedural risks and possibility of persistent pain from other generators of HSP.

SUGGESTED TREATMENT PROTOCOL FOR HEMIPLEGIC SHOULDER PAIN

Two things are clear regarding shoulder pain after stroke: it is a multifactorial process, and inability to prevent or treat the disorder results in poor outcomes. A review of the literature makes one thing clear: the quantity or quality of available evidence provides little guidance on how to manage this troubling complication of stroke. Until future research advances our understanding of HSP, the authors suggest a 5-step treatment approach (**Box 6**).

The first 2 steps of the protocol occur simultaneously as part of initial and subsequent evaluations of a patient with HSP. As detailed in the preceding sections, the most important part of treating a multifactorial process is to systematically consider each of the common neurologic and mechanical factors that is either present, or at risk of occurring. The treatment of a patient presenting with a flaccid upper limb after acute stroke will change as spasticity develops. Determining a history of rotator cuff tendinopathy before the cerebrovascular accident can help the clinician improve considerations for physical therapy. Once the various factors are considered, baseline measurements (eg, ROM and Modified Ashworth Scale) and appropriate diagnostic testing should be ordered to confirm diagnoses and document severity before treatment.

The third step is important at all stages of treatment, but is most pertinent during the flaccid stage after stroke and as acute rehabilitation commences. Clinicians, therapists, and family members must avoid applying excessive stress to the shoulder by reducing the effect of gravity with slings and lap trays in wheelchairs, or by reducing traction on the arm during transfers.

Only after careful examination of the shoulder and education on its proper positioning should the fourth step begin. The primary goals of rehabilitation include modalities for comfort and facilitation of movement, careful maintenance of ROM, spasticity management, and strengthening and facilitation with electrical stimulation, taping, and functional training. Only when mobility or participation in therapy is restricted by pain should the clinician introduce pharmacologic treatment for symptomatic control.

Interventional management is the fifth and final step in the treatment protocol, and is indicated when conservative measures fail. Procedures may also be considered when a patient cannot tolerate or progress through therapy because of pain, spasticity, or concern for developing CRPS.

KEY POINTS FOR TREATMENT
Positioning

- Supine: keep shoulder protracted, arm forward, wrist neutral to slightly supinated, fingers extended
- Spastic limb: keep arm abducted, externally rotated, flexed

---

Box 6
Approach to the treatment of hemiplegic shoulder pain

Step 1: Assess and diagnose neurologic factors contributing to HSP

Step 2: Assess and diagnose mechanical factors contributing to HSP

Step 3: Phase 1 of treatment: prevention through positioning

Step 4: Phase 2 of treatment: rehabilitation and symptomatic control

Step 5: Phase 3 of treatment: pathology-based intervention

Strapping/Taping

- Taping perpendicular to a muscle inhibits activity; taping parallel to a muscle promotes activity.

Slings and Supports

- Flaccid: use when sitting, ambulating, transferring for protection
- Spastic: avoid prolonged use to prevent contractures
- Sitting: use a lap board or arm trough positioned in slight abduction and external rotation
- Avoid axillary supports (can displace humeral head)

Physical Therapy and Modalities

- Strive for maximal amplitude of movement within a pain-free range
- Avoid overhead pulley exercises to reduce shoulder impingement
- TENS: may reduce pain, particularly when used at high intensity
- FES: apply to deltoid and supraspinatus; expect temporary reduction in shoulder subluxation
- EMG biofeedback: use to encourage active participation and psychological sense of control

Pharmacotherapy

- Neurologic:
  - Neuropathic pain: trials of TCAs or SSRIs for centrally mediated pain, gabapentinoids for peripherally mediated pain
  - Spasticity: trials of antispasmodics when ROM and positioning fail
- Mechanical pain:
  - Modalities, acetaminophen, and NSAIDs, if not contraindicated by a comorbid medical condition
  - Opioids may be considered for severe debilitating pain not responding to other measures
  - Oral corticosteroids are of little known benefit, but may be tried in short courses for debilitating pain not controlled by other measures

Injection Therapy

- Neurologic
  - Botulinum toxin intramuscular injections are beneficial for the focal reduction of spasticity
    - Muscles often targeted include subscapularis, pectoralis, infraspinatus, latissimus dorsi
    - There is emerging but insufficient evidence to suggest that intra-articular botulinum toxin may offer an antinociceptive benefit
  - CRPS: Stellate ganglion blocks are considered on when criteria for CRPS are met, and are most effective in early stages to treat autonomic symptoms
- Mechanical:
  - Corticosteroid injections are most beneficial when the pain-generating structure is correctly identified, and when there is an inflammatory component (eg, acute tendinitis rather than chronic tendinosis)
    - Structures most often targeted include the subacromial space and glenohumeral joint
  - Trigger-point injections and dry needling may benefit patients with myofascial pain; evaluate for altered posturing and kinematics (including unaffected limb)

Surgery

- Rarely indicated; usually performed after at least 6 months of failed nonsurgical treatment
- Neurologic: release of contractures if other methods for spasticity fail
- Mechanical: rotator cuff repair is usually only considered if pain clearly associated based on acute trauma, capsular release for adhesive capsulitis

Complementary/Alternative Medicine

- Acupuncture combined with therapeutic exercise may be superior to either treatment alone
- Aromatherapy may provide additional benefit (small pilot studies only)

SUMMARY

HSP is a common complication of stroke that can lead to poor functional outcomes. It is a multifactorial process that demands careful consideration of the contributing factors, both neurologic and mechanical. Efforts at prevention should be maintained throughout the course of treatment. The available evidence for nearly all treatments discussed in this article is conflicting and is limited by poor or variable methodology. The clinician is urged to consider the diagnostic and treatment approach presented in this article to ensure that all components of HSP are considered, and that treatments are provided in a logical manner. This method, along with constant vigilance by clinicians and properly educated caretakers, will provide the best opportunity to restore function and maximize quality of life.

REFERENCES

1. Roger VL, Go AS, Lloyd-Jones DM, et al. Heart disease and stroke statistics—2012 update. A report from the American Heart Association. Circulation 2012; 125(1):e2–220.
2. Aoyagi Y, Tsubahara A. Therapeutic orthosis and electrical stimulation for upper extremity hemiplegia after stroke: a review of effectiveness based on evidence. Top Stroke Rehabil 2004;11(3):9–15.
3. Bohannon RW, Larkin PA, Smith MB, et al. Shoulder pain in hemiplegia: statistical relationship with five variables. Arch Phys Med Rehabil 1986;67(8): 514–6.
4. Roy CW, Sands MR, Hill LD. Shoulder pain in acutely admitted hemiplegics. Clin Rehabil 1994;8(4):334–40.
5. Wanklyn P, Forster A, Young J. Hemiplegic shoulder pain (HSP): natural history and investigation of associated features. Disabil Rehabil 1996;18(10):497–501.
6. Murie-Fernández M, Carmona Iragui M, Gnanakumar V, et al. Painful hemiplegic shoulder in stroke patients: causes and management. Neurología 2012;27(4): 234–44.
7. Higgins J, Mayo NE, Desrosiers J, et al. Upper-limb function and recovery in the acute phase poststroke. J Rehabil R D 2005;42(1):65–76.
8. Coupar F, Pollock A, Rowe P, et al. Predictors of upper limb recovery after stroke: a systematic review and meta-analysis. Clin Rehabil 2012;26(4): 291–313.
9. Roosink M, Renzenbrink GJ, Buitenweg JR, et al. Persistent shoulder pain in the first 6 months after stroke: results of a prospective cohort study. Arch Phys Med Rehabil 2011;92(7):1139–45.

10. Barlak A, Unsal S, Kaya K, et al. Poststroke shoulder pain in Turkish stroke patients: relationship with clinical factors and functional outcomes. Int J Rehabil Res 2009;32(4):309–15.

11. Turner-Stokes L, Jackson D. Shoulder pain after stroke: a review of the evidence base to inform the development of an integrated care pathway. Clin Rehabil 2002;16(3):276–98.

12. Saario L. The range of movement of the shoulder joint at various ages. Acta Orthop Scand 1963;33(4):366–7.

13. Dromerick AW, Edwards DF, Kumar A. Hemiplegic shoulder pain syndrome: frequency and characteristics during inpatient stroke rehabilitation. Arch Phys Med Rehabil 2008;89(8):1589–93.

14. Kalichman L, Ratmansky M. Underlying pathology and associated factors of hemiplegic shoulder pain. Not Found In Database 2011;90(9):768–80.

15. Smith M. Management of hemiplegic shoulder pain following stroke. Nurs Stand 2012;26(44):35.

16. Ryerson S, Levit K. The shoulder in hemiplegia. Physical therapy of the shoulder. New York: Churchill Livingstone; 1987. p. 105–31.

17. Van Ouwenaller C, Laplace PM, Chantraine A. Painful shoulder in hemiplegia. Arch Phys Med Rehabil 1986;67(1):23–6.

18. Hecht JS. Subscapular nerve block in the painful hemiplegic shoulder. Arch Phys Med Rehabil 1992;73(11):1036–9.

19. Kaplan PE, Meridith J, Taft G, et al. Stroke and brachial plexus injury: a difficult problem. Arch Phys Med Rehabil 1977;58(9):415–8.

20. Moskowitz E, Porter JI. Peripheral nerve lesions in the upper extremity in hemiplegic patients. N Engl J Med 1963;269(15):776–8.

21. Chino N. Electrophysiological investigation on shoulder subluxation in hemiplegics. Scand J Rehabil Med 1980;13(1):17–21.

22. Ring H, Feder M, Berchadsky R, et al. Prevalence of pain and malalignment in the hemiplegic's shoulder at admission for rehabilitation. A preventive approach. Eur J Phys Med Rehabil 1993;3(5):199–203.

23. Tsur A. Common peroneal neuropathy in patients after first-time stroke. Isr Med Assoc J 2007;9(12):866.

24. Kingery WS, Date ES, Bocobo CR. The absence of brachial plexus injury in stroke. Am J Phys Med Rehabil 1993;72(3):127–35.

25. Alpert S, Idarraga S, Orbegozo J, et al. Absence of electromyographic evidence of lower motor neuron involvement in hemiplegic patients. Arch Phys Med Rehabil 1971;52(4):179.

26. Braus DF, Krauss JK, Strobel J. The shoulder-hand syndrome after stroke: a prospective clinical trial. Ann Neurol 1994;36(5):728–33.

27. Finch L, Harvey J. Factors associated with shoulder-hand-syndrome in hemiplegia: clinical survey. Physiother Can 1983;35(3):145–8.

28. Daviet JC, Preux PM, Salle JY, et al. Clinical factors in the prognosis of complex regional pain syndrome type I after stroke: a prospective study. Am J Phys Med Rehabil 2002;81(1):34–9.

29. Chae J. Poststroke complex regional pain syndrome. Top Stroke Rehabil 2010; 17(3):151–62.

30. Paci M, Nannetti L, Taiti P, et al. Shoulder subluxation after stroke: relationships with pain and motor recovery. Physiother Res Int 2007;12(2):95–104.

31. Hall J, Dudgeon B, Guthrie M. Validity of clinical measures of shoulder subluxation in adults with poststroke hemiplegia. Am J Occup Ther 1995;49(6): 526–33.

32. Boyd EA, Torrance GM. Clinical measures of shoulder subluxation: their reliability. Can J Public Health 1992;83:S24.
33. McKenna LB. Hemiplegic shoulder pain: defining the problem and its management. Disabil Rehabil 2001;23(16):698–705.
34. Zuckerman JD, Cuomo F, Rokito S. Definition and classification of frozen shoulder: a consensus approach. J Shoulder Elbow Surg 1994;3(1):S72.
35. Joynt RL. The source of shoulder pain in hemiplegia. Arch Phys Med Rehabil 1992;73(5):409–13.
36. Walsh K. Management of shoulder pain in patients with stroke. Postgrad Med J 2001;77(912):645–9.
37. DiLorenzo L, Traballesi M, Morelli D, et al. Hemiparetic shoulder pain syndrome treated with deep dry needling during early rehabilitation: a prospective, open-label, randomized investigation. J Muscoskel Pain 2004;12(2): 25–34.
38. Rajaratnam BS, Venketasubramanian N, Kumar PV, et al. Predictability of simple clinical tests to identify shoulder pain after stroke. Arch Phys Med Rehabil 2007; 88(8):1016–21.
39. Niessen MH, Veeger DH, Meskers CG, et al. Relationship among shoulder proprioception, kinematics, and pain after stroke. Arch Phys Med Rehab 2009; 90(9):1557–64.
40. Lo SF, Chen SY, Lin HC, et al. Arthrographic and clinical findings in patients with hemiplegic shoulder pain. Arch Phys Med Rehabil 2003;84(12):1786–91.
41. Jung JY, Jee WH, Chun HJ, et al. Adhesive capsulitis of the shoulder: evaluation with MR arthrography. Eur Radiol 2006;16(4):791–6.
42. Lefevre-Colau MM, Drapé JL, Fayad F, et al. Magnetic resonance imaging of shoulders with idiopathic adhesive capsulitis: reliability of measures. Eur Radiol 2005;15(12):2415–22.
43. Távora DG, Gama RL, Bomfim RC, et al. MRI findings in the painful hemiplegic shoulder. Clin Radiol 2010;65(10):789–94.
44. Ozcakar L, Tok F, De Muynck M, et al. Musculoskeletal ultrasonography in physical and rehabilitation medicine. J Rehabil Med 2012;44(4):310–8.
45. Lee JC, Sykes C, Saifuddin A, et al. Adhesive capsulitis: sonographic changes in the rotator cuff interval with arthroscopic correlation. Skeletal Radiol 2005; 34(9):522–7.
46. Pong YP, Wang LY, Wang L, et al. Sonography of the shoulder in hemiplegic patients undergoing rehabilitation after a recent stroke. J Clin Ultrasound 2009; 37(4):199–205.
47. Huang YC, Liang PJ, Pong YP, et al. Physical findings and sonography of hemiplegic shoulder in patients after acute stroke during rehabilitation. J Rehabil Med 2010;42(1):21–6.
48. Lee IS, Shin YB, Moon TY, et al. Sonography of patients with hemiplegic shoulder pain after stroke: correlation with motor recovery stage. Am J Roentgenol 2009;192(2):W40–4.
49. Carr EK, Kenney FD. Positioning of the stroke patient: a review of the literature. Int J Nurs Stud 1992;29(4):355–69.
50. Nepomuceno CS, Miller JM 3rd. Shoulder arthrography in hemiplegic patients. Arch Phys Med Rehabil 1974;55(2):49.
51. Ancliffe J. Strapping the shoulder in patients following a cerebrovascular accident (CVA): a pilot study. Aust J Physiother 1992;38(1):37–41.
52. McCollough NC 3rd. The role of the orthopedic surgeon in the treatment of stroke. Orthop Clin North Am 1978;9(2):305–24.

53. Thelen MD, Dauber JA, Stoneman PD. The clinical efficacy of kinesio tape for shoulder pain: a randomized, double-blinded, clinical trial. J Orthop Sports Phys Ther 2008;38(7):389.

54. Garrison SJ, Rolak LA. Rehabilitation of the stroke patient. In: Gans Bruce M, editor. Rehabilitation medicine: principles and practice, Vol. 15. Philadelphia: Lippincott; 1993. p. 801.

55. Brooke MM, De Lateur BJ, Diana-Rigby GC, et al. Shoulder subluxation in hemiplegia: effects of three different supports. Arch Phys Med Rehabil 1991;72(8): 582–6.

56. Han SH, Kim T, Jang SH, et al. The effect of an arm sling on energy consumption while walking in hemiplegic patients: a randomized comparison. Clin Rehabil 2011;25(1):36–42.

57. Caldwell CB, Wilson DJ, Braun RM. Evaluation and treatment of the upper extremity in the hemiplegic stroke patient. Clin Orthop Relat Res 1969;63:69–93.

58. Kumar R, Metter EJ, Mehta AJ, et al. Shoulder pain in hemiplegia: the role of exercise. Am J Phys Med Rehabil 1990;69(4):205–8.

59. Lynch D, Ferraro M, Krol J, et al. Continuous passive motion improves shoulder joint integrity following stroke. Clin Rehabil 2005;19(6):594–9.

60. Masiero S, Celia A, Rosati G, et al. Robotic-assisted rehabilitation of the upper limb after acute stroke. Arch Phys Med Rehabil 2007;88(2):142–9.

61. Leandri M, Parodi CI, Corrieri N, et al. Comparison of TENS treatments in hemiplegic shoulder pain. Scand J Rehabil Med 1990;22(2):69.

62. Wang RY, Chan RC, Tsai MW. Functional electrical stimulation on chronic and acute hemiplegic shoulder subluxation. Am J Phys Med Rehabil 2000;79(4): 385–94.

63. Koyuncu E, Nakipoglu-Yüzer GF, Dogan A, et al. The effectiveness of functional electrical stimulation for the treatment of shoulder subluxation and shoulder pain in hemiplegic patients: a randomized controlled trial. Disabil Rehabil 2010;32(7): 560–6.

64. Chae J, Sheffler LR, Knutson JS. Neuromuscular electrical stimulation for motor restoration in hemiplegia. Top Stroke Rehabil 2008;15(5):412–26.

65. Price CI, Pandyan AD. Electrical stimulation for preventing and treating post-stroke shoulder pain: a systematic Cochrane review. Clin Rehabil 2001;15(1):5–19.

66. Chae J, David TY, Walker ME, et al. Intramuscular electrical stimulation for hemiplegic shoulder pain: a 12-month follow-up of a multiple-center, randomized clinical trial. Am J Phys Med Rehabil 2005;84(11):832–42.

67. Wilson RD, Bennett ME, Lechman TE, et al. Single-lead percutaneous peripheral nerve stimulation for the treatment of hemiplegic shoulder pain: a case report. Arch Phys Med Rehabil 2011;92(5):837–40.

68. David TY, Friedman AS, Rosenfeld EL. Electrical stimulation for treating chronic poststroke shoulder pain using a fully implanted microstimulator with internal battery. Am J Phys Med Rehabil 2010;89(5):423–8.

69. Williams JM. Use of electromyographic biofeedback for pain reduction in the spastic hemiplegic shoulder: a pilot study. Physiother Can 1982;34(6):327–33.

70. Yelnik AP, Colle FM, Bonan IV, et al. Treatment of shoulder pain in spastic hemiplegia by reducing spasticity of the subscapular muscle: a randomised, double blind, placebo controlled study of botulinum toxin A. J Neurol Neurosurg Psychiatr 2007;78(8):845–8.

71. Kong KH, Neo JJ, Chua KS. A randomized controlled study of botulinum toxin A in the treatment of hemiplegic shoulder pain associated with spasticity. Clin Rehabil 2007;21(1):28–35.

72. De Boer KS, Arwert HJ, De Groot JH, et al. Shoulder pain and external rotation in spastic hemiplegia do not improve by injection of botulinum toxin A into the sub-scapular muscle. J Neurol Neurosurg Psychiatr 2008;79(5):581–3.

73. Lim JY, Koh JH, Paik NJ. Intramuscular botulinum toxin-A reduces hemiplegic shoulder pain: a randomized, double-blind, comparative study versus intraartic-ular triamcinolone acetonide. Stroke 2008;39(1):126–31.

74. Castiglione A, Bagnato S, Boccagni C, et al. Efficacy of intra-articular injection of botulinum toxin type A in refractory hemiplegic shoulder pain. Arch Phys Med Rehabil 2011;92(7):1034–7.

75. Bruehl S, Chung OY. Psychological and behavioral aspects of complex regional pain syndrome management. Clin J Pain 2006;22(5):430–7.

76. Harden RN, Bruehl SP. Diagnosis of complex regional pain syndrome: signs, symptoms, and new empirically derived diagnostic criteria. Clin J Pain 2006; 22(5):415–9.

77. Quisel A, Gill JM, Witherell P. Complex regional pain syndrome: which treat-ments show promise? J Fam Pract 2005;54(7):599.

78. Rowbotham MC. Pharmacologic management of complex regional pain syn-drome. Clin J Pain 2006;22(5):425–9.

79. Stanton-Hicks M. Complex regional pain syndrome. Anesthesiol Clin North America 2003;21(4):733–44.

80. Teasdall RD, Smith BP, Koman LA. Complex regional pain syndrome (reflex sympathetic dystrophy). Clin Sports Med 2004;23(1):145–55.

81. Fitzgerald-Finch OP, Gibson II. Subluxation of the shoulder in hemiplegia. Age Ageing 1975;4(1):16–8.

82. Berthier ML, Pujol J, Gironell A, et al. Beneficial effect of donepezil on sensori-motor function after stroke. Am J Phys Med Rehabil 2003;82(9):725–9.

83. Lakse E, Gunduz B, Erhan B, et al. The effect of local injections in hemiplegic shoulder pain: a prospective, randomized, controlled study. Am J Phys Med Re-habil 2009;88(10):805–11.

84. Chae J, Jedlicka L. Subacromial corticosteroid injection for poststroke shoulder pain: an exploratory prospective case series. Arch Phys Med Rehabil 2009; 90(3):501–6.

85. Dekker JH, Wagenaar RC, Lankhorst GJ, et al. The painful hemiplegic shoulder: effects of intra-articular triamcinolone acetonide1. Am J Phys Med Rehabil 1997; 76(1):43–8.

86. Snels IA, Beckerman H, Twisk JW, et al. Effect of triamcinolone acetonide injec-tions on hemiplegic shoulder pain a randomized clinical trial. Stroke 2000; 31(10):2396–401.

87. Yasar E, Vural D, Safaz I, et al. Which treatment approach is better for hemiple-gic shoulder pain in stroke patients: intra-articular steroid or suprascapular nerve block? A randomized controlled trial. Clin Rehabil 2011;25(1):60–8.

88. Allen Z, Shanahan E, Crotty M. Does suprascapular nerve block reduce shoul-der pain following stroke: a double-blind randomised controlled trial with masked outcome assessment. BMC Neurol 2010;10(1):83.

89. Chironna RL, Hecht JS. Subscapularis motor point block for the painful hemiple-gic shoulder. Arch Phys Med Rehabil 1990;71(6):428.

90. Shin BC, Lee MS. Effects of aromatherapy acupressure on hemiplegic shoulder pain and motor power in stroke patients: a pilot study. J Altern Complement Med 2007;13(2):247–52.

91. Lee JA, Park SW, Hwang PW, et al. Acupuncture for shoulder pain after stroke: a systematic review. J Altern Complement Med 2012;18(9):818–23.

92. Shin BC, Lim HJ, Lee MS. Effectiveness of combined acupuncture therapy and conventional treatment on shoulder range of motion and motor power in stroke patients with hemiplegic shoulder subluxation: a pilot study. Int J Neurosci 2007; 117(4):519–23.
93. Braun RM, West F, Mooney V, et al. Surgical treatment of the painful shoulder contracture in the stroke patient. J Bone Joint Surg Am 1971;53:1307–12.

Cancer Pain and Current Theory for Pain Control

Brian Kahan, DO, DAOCRM, DABIPP, DABPM, FIPP

KEYWORDS

- Cancer pain • Opioid therapy • NMDA antagonists
- Splanchnic nerve blocks opioid pharmacogenetic testing

KEY POINTS

- Although the diagnosis of cancer has been stereotyped as a disease to end all, treatment of pain in cancer is showing hopeful prospects.
- A strong background in anatomy and physiology is the foundation on which to approach pain in cancer patients, with multiple options accessible.
- Use of new medications geared at enhancing the descending inhibitory pathways in combination with classic pharmacologic treatment can improve a patient's quality of life and reduce side effects.
- Reducing pain has been reported to enhance patients' quality of life and has been associated with longer survival rates.
- Being diligent in the reassessment of treatment is the answer to effectively managing complicated cases of cancer pain.
- Pain is always changing and, therefore, an astute physician will know how to address the treatment of patients at any time by understanding how pain works.

INTRODUCTION

Cancer is a disease that many people prefer not to talk about. Patients with a diagnosis of cancer are met with fear and thoughts of a life-ending illness. During their treatment they suffer significant pain. Various studies have looked at the prevalence of cancer pain, with one study reporting that 50% to 60% of all patients with cancer will experience pain, and other studies reporting a range of anywhere from 19% to 95% of patients with cancer have had or are still having pain. Although studies vary in the reported prevalence of pain in patients with cancer, approximately 70% of patients who die from cancer experience unrelieved pain. Despite national efforts by the Joint Commission on Accreditation of Hospitals and health organizations in the Agency for Healthcare Research and Quality, World Health Organization, and the International Association for the Study of Pain, pain continues to be a significant problem in patients with cancer.

The author has nothing to disclose.
The Kahan Center for Pain Management, 2002 Medical Parkway, Suite 150, Annapolis, MD 21401, USA
E-mail address: bkahan@thekahancenter.com

Phys Med Rehabil Clin N Am 25 (2014) 439–456
http://dx.doi.org/10.1016/j.pmr.2014.01.013   **pmr.theclinics.com**
1047-9651/14/$ – see front matter © 2014 Elsevier Inc. All rights reserved.

In a European study, the prevalence of pain based on the type of cancer has been well documented (**Fig. 1**). The most painful cancers appear to be pancreatic, bone, and lung.

In 2011, Marcus and colleagues[1] reported the prevalence of cancer pain to be consistent, with 56% of patients in their study suffering from pain. Thirty-three percent had pain after they underwent treatment, 59% had pain during treatment, and 64% had pain secondary to metastatic disease. All patients suffered functional limitations related to their cancer pain. Patients with head and neck cancer, gynecologic cancer, gastrointestinal cancer, and breast cancer appeared to suffer the most pain. The most consistent barriers to effective treatment of pain were concerns about addiction, cost of therapy, or lack of endorsement by health care providers.[2]

This article discusses pharmacologic management, interventional treatment, and specific cancers that seem to have the highest prevalence of pain, and how interventional treatment and medications can help.

PAIN IN CANCER

Treating cancer pain needs to be systematically evaluated. The etiology of cancer pain is related to either direct neoplasm involvement, side effects of chemotherapeutic agents, or radiation-induced plexopathies. The clinician must determine whether the cause of pain is neuropathic, nociceptive, or a combination of both, after which effective treatment can be decided upon.

The OPQRSTU mnemonic will help assess a patient's pain (**Table 1**).[3]

PHARMACOLOGIC MANAGEMENT OF CANCER PAIN
Opioid Therapy

The most common medication used to treat cancer pain is opioids. Although opioids have been used for many years, their efficacy in alleviating cancer pain is questioned.[4]

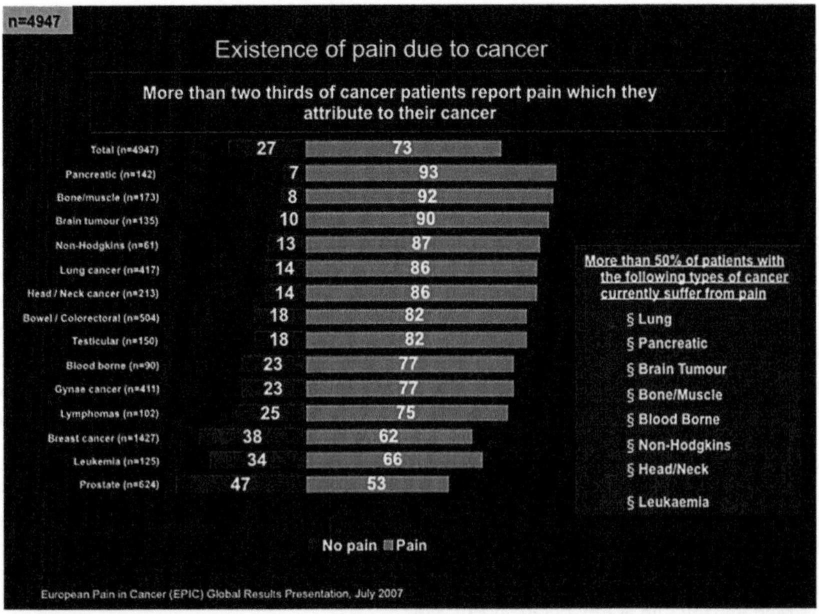

Fig. 1. Existence of pain due to cancer, reported by patients when asked "have you suffered any pain due to cancer?"

Table 1
Cancer pain assessment mnemonic

O	Onset	When did it start? Acute or gradual? Pattern since onset?
P	Provoking/palliating	What brings it on? What makes it better or worse (eg, rest, medication)?
Q	Quality	Identifying neuropathic pain (burning, tingling, numb, itchy, etc)
R	Region/radiation	Primary location(s) of pain, radiation pattern(s)
S	Severity	Use verbal description and/or 1–10 scale
T	Treatment	Current and past treatment; side effects
U	Understanding	Meaning of the pain to the sufferer, "total pain"
V	Values	Goals and expectations of management for this symptom

When opioids were discovered, medical knowledge was extremely limited with regard to how pain was transmitted. Early theories attributed pain to only an afferent pathway generating a tissue-injuring message to the spinal dorsal horn. Thus treatment of this pathway for pain consisted of pharmacologic management specific to modulation of components of this sensory message to higher centers.[5] Management consisted of opioid receptor blockers and sodium/potassium channel blockers. Although opioids demonstrated antinociception to the brainstem, forebrain, spinal cord, and the periphery, binding occurred heterogeneously, leading to inadequate treatment of pain.

Descending Pathway Inhibitors

In 1985 Fields and Heinricher[6] demonstrated the presence of a dual-projection system to be highly effective in treating pain through use of the descending pathway.

The interrelationship of major neuroanatomic components exerting descending nociceptive control is shown in **Fig. 2**. The periaqueductal gray and rostral ventral medulla are strategically located to integrate input from cerebral structures and relay processed information to the spinal dorsal horn. Noradrenergic pontine and medullary nuclei constitute a second important structure directly projecting to the dorsal horn. Presynaptic and postsynaptic mechanisms modulate nociceptive information that is transmitted from primary afferents to spinal projection neurons. Alternatively, indirect actions are exerted via inhibition or excitation of spinal interneurons. Cortical areas, the amygdala and the hypothalamus, are among the cerebral structures exerting top-down control. These structures are relevant for the modulation of pain by stress, emotion, and cognition.[7]

The discovery of a descending inhibitory pathway for pain led to the discovery of various nociceptive neurotransmitters (**Box 1**). In addition to finding more pain regulators, scientists have also determined how and where these neurotransmitters exert their affect (**Fig. 3**).

Fig. 3 illustrates that descending control of spinal nociceptive processes is exerted by multiple neurotransmitters. Transmitters contributing to inhibition of nociceptive signaling are depicted on the left while transmitters enhancing nociceptive signaling are depicted on the right. This physical separation serves didactic reasons and has no anatomic foundation. Transmitters are contained in descending pathways, in inhibitory or excitatory interneurons, and in primary afferent terminals. Only principal transmitter locations are shown, with subtypes indicated in parentheses.[7]

Neuropathic pain does not respond well to opioid therapy and tends to be more problematic. The focus of treating neuropathic pain should be blocking the ascending pathways or increasing the inhibition provided by the descending pathways.

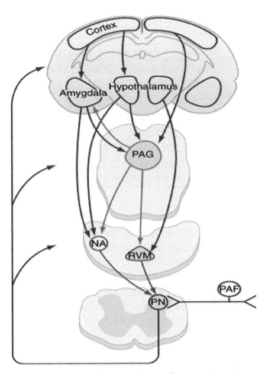

Fig. 2. Major structural components exerting descending nociceptive control. NA, noradrenergic pontine and medullary nuclei; PAF, primary afferents; PAG, periaqueductal gray; PN, spinal projection neurons; RVM, rostral ventral medulla. (*From* Ottestad E, Angst MS. Nociceptive Physiology. In: Hemmings HC, Egan TD, eds. Pharmacology and physiology for anesthesia: foundations and clinical application. Philadelphia: Saunders/Elsevier, 2013; with permission. *Modified from* Millan MJ. Descending control of pain. Prog Neurobiol 2002;66:355–474.)

It is theorized that an initiation phase of neuropathic pain is driven by activity from primary afferents, whereas the maintenance phase is mediated by central neuroplastic adaptations.[8] Treatment focused on blocking transmission to the rostral ventromedial medulla (see **Fig. 2**) through lesions or pharmacologic addition of medications that prevent upregulation of spinal dynorphin will help reduce neuropathic pain and neuropathic pain states. Newer medications attempt to work on these descending pathways, on the periphery by modulating GABAergic receptors and centrally by increasing serotonin and norepinephrine. Selective norepinephrine medications such as duloxetine (Cymbalta) are showing promise in treating various forms of pain by enhancing the descending pathways and working centrally on norepinephrine and serotonin receptors and voltage gated calcium-channel blockers such as gabapentin (Neurontin) and pregabalin (Lyrica). Today research is focusing not on opioids but on ways to block these neuropeptides.

NMDA Antagonists

Pharmacology assays in animal behavioral models of neuropathic pain suggest that the *N*-methyl-ᴅ-aspartate (NMDA) receptor is at least partially responsible for facilitated processing, augmentation of painful responses, and subsequent stimuli, but

Box 1
Nociceptive neurotransmitters
Peripheral neurotransmitters
Hydrogen ions
Norepinephrine
Bradykinin
Histamine
Potassium ions
Prostanoids
Purines
Cytokines (interleukin, tumor necrosis factor)
Serotonin (5-HT)
Neuropeptides
Substance P, calcitonin gene-related peptide, neurokinin A
Leukotrienes
Central neurotransmitters
Glutamate
Neurokinin 1
Substance P
G protein
Neurokinin A
γ-Aminobutyric acid
Calcitonin gene-related peptide
Calcium
Nitric oxide

not normal pain sensation.[9] Using NMDA-receptor antagonists such as methadone and buprenorphine can allow titration of analgesic therapy while preventing respiratory depression. Opioid tolerance results in a requirement for increasing doses to achieve a given degree of analgesia. It is thought that continued doses of an opioid will enhance levels of cyclic adenosine monophosphate, protein phosphorylation, and subsequent upregulation of the NMDA-receptor mechanisms within the dorsal horn and supraspinal sites. In addition, accumulation of morphine metabolites may antagonize the analgesic action normally produced by opioid receptor activation. Animal studies indicate that the administration of NMDA antagonists can prevent both the development of tolerance to morphine and the withdrawal syndrome in morphine-dependent rats. Therefore, coadministration of NMDA antagonists such as methadone, buprenorphine, and ketamine with opioids may attenuate the development of opioid tolerance and potentiate opioid analgesic mechanisms.[10] However, the therapeutic window needs to be improved by the use of drug combinations and more selective administration of systemic NMDA-receptor antagonists, and physicians must understand the benefits of NMDA antagonists in comparison with their current use as adjunctive medications. It is hoped that more education on the transmission

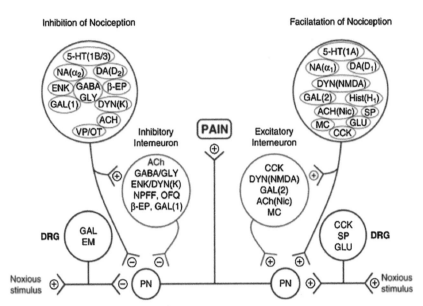

Fig. 3. Major biochemical components exerting descending nociceptive control. ACH, acetylcholine; β-EP, β-endorphin; CCK, cholecystokinin; DA, dopamine; DRG, dorsal root ganglion; DYN, dynorphin; EM, endomorphin; ENK, enkephalin; GABA, γ-hydroxybutyric acid; GAL, galanin; GLU, glutamate; GLY, glycine; Hist, histamine; MC, melanocortin; NA, noradrenaline; NMDA, N-methyl-D-aspartate; NPFF, neuropeptide FF; OFQ, orphanin FQ; OT, oxytocin; PN, projection neuron; SP, substance P; VP, vasopressin; 5-HT, serotonin. (*From* Ottestad E, Angst MS. Nociceptive Physiology. In: Hemmings HC, Egan TD, eds. Pharmacology and physiology for anesthesia: foundations and clinical application. Philadelphia: Saunders/Elsevier, 2013; with permission. *Modified from* Millan MJ. Descending control of pain. Prog Neurobiol 2002;66:355–474.)

of pain in medical school, residency, fellowship, and continuing medical education will lead to elimination of the stereotyping of NMDA antagonists.

Cannabis

Various societies are debating the efficacy of cannabinoids in treating pain. Cannabinoid receptors are found throughout the central and peripheral nervous system, and even in the immune system. CB1 receptor tends to predominate in the central nervous system, and CB2 receptors are more extensive in the peripheral and immune systems.[11] Endogenous cannabinoid compounds such as anandamide, 2-arachidonylglycerol, and palmitoylethanolamide act on the CB1 and CB2 receptors to help modulate inflammatory pain and possibly provide analgesic effects. *Cannabis sativa* L. contains 60 or more cannabinoids; the most prevalent are δ9-tetrahydrocannabinol (THC) and cannabidiol (CB). These 2 cannabinoids seem to mimic the action of endogenous cannabinoid compounds. THC seems to be a partial CB1 and CB2 receptor agonist, thus acting centrally and peripherally, and may produce more psychoactive side effects, whereas cannabidiol seems to act more centrally and produce analgesic and anti-inflammatory effects.

A systemic review of single-dose studies of dronabinol, nabilone, and levonantradol found them to be as effective as 5 to 120 mg of oral codeine.[12] There are also suggestions that cannabis can augment opioid analgesia.[13] Although there is public interest in the utilization of cannabis, more controlled, sizable studies demonstrating true effectiveness are required.

Intrathecal Administration

Intrathecal administration offers an advanced way of delivering opioid therapy with a more direct effect on supraspinal pathways. Although relatively uncommon in patients with cancer, it has some advantages. Patients undergoing intrathecal administration of opioids via an implantable pump (**Figs. 4** and **5**) will have fewer side effects than those taking oral medications. Owing to the direct effects on the supraspinal pathways, lower doses are required than if used orally. It is generally thought that the concentration ratio from oral to intrathecal is 300:1. A comprehensive review of intrathecal drug-delivery systems is beyond the scope of this article, but certain aspects are highlighted.

Using a dosage 300 times less will reduce systemic absorption and reduce the incidence of gastrointestinal and cognitive side effects. Another advantage over oral medication is once on a stable dosage of intrathecal medication, a patient will require fewer visits to a clinician. In general, patients receiving intrathecal medication will be refilled every 90 days as an outpatient procedure. In addition to supplying a continuous flow of medication, patient dosage adjustments for breakthrough pain or pain increased at night can be programmed into the pump either through flexible dosing schedules or with a patient hand-held device that communicates through telemetry to give the patient a programmed bolus based on the physician-adjusted settings. This procedure is identical to patient-controlled administration in the hospital.

Complications of intrathecal medication tend to be more technical, such as catheter dislodgment and kinking, rather than infection, granulomas, and overdosing. Pump complications tend to involve premature battery failure. However, there are reports that compounded medication can potentially cause corrosion attributable to pH levels.

Intrathecal drug-delivery systems can be used in about 10% to 20% of patients suffering from cancer pain who have failed other therapeutic measures and are eligible

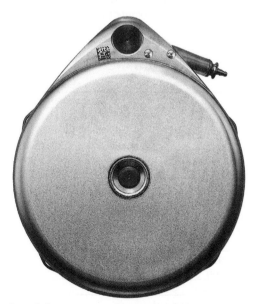

Fig. 4. Implantable drug-delivery system. (*Courtesy of* Medtronic, Minneapolis, MN; with permission.)

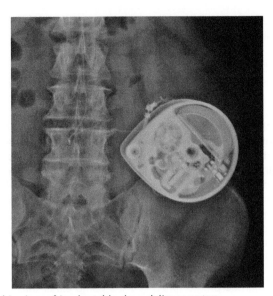

Fig. 5. Radiographic view of implantable drug-delivery system.

for an intrathecal trial. Patient selection can be subjective, but there are some definitive contraindications. **Table 2** lists some of the relevant indications and contraindications for intrathecal drug-delivery systems.

Once the appropriate patient is selected, he or she undergoes an intrathecal trial performed with single boluses, epidural continuous trials, or intrathecal continuous trials. Based on patients' response as measured by 50% reduction in pain, improved functional capability, or reduced side effects, the patient can proceed with an implant. Medications currently approved for intrathecal use are morphine, ziconotide, and baclofen. **Table 3** lists the various combinations of intrathecal medications.[14]

Table 2	
Patient selection for intrathecal drug-delivery systems	
Relative Indications	**Relative Contraindications**
Inability to tolerate oral medications	Anticoagulation therapy
Fear of side effects or addiction	Leukopenia <2 × 10^9/L Neutropenia <1000 μL Thrombocytopenia <20 × 10^3/μL
Receiving aggressive chemotherapy regimens with high toxicity profile	Active infections or methicillin-resistant *Staphylococcus aureus*
Pain refractory	Spinal cord tumors
Visceral tumors that affects other forms of absorption of medications	Body size not sufficient to accept pump bulk
Pathologic fractures or diffuse bone metastasis	
Neuropathic pain states due to surgery, chemotherapy, or radiation	
Minimum life expectancy >3 mo	
Pelvic tumors or tumors with high rate of metastatic spread to bone[14]	

Table 3
Lists the cancer pain best practices algorithm

	Nociceptive	Mixed Pain	Neuropathic Pain
First line	Morphine or hydromorphone	Morphine/ hydromorphone with bupivacaine	Bupivacaine
Second line	First-line drugs or fentanyl/sufentanil with bupivacaine and clonidine	First-line drugs or fentanyl/sufentanil with bupivacaine and clonidine	First-line drugs or fentanyl/sufentanil with bupivacaine
Third line	Second-line drugs with either baclofen or other lipophilic or hydrophilic opioid	—	—
Fourth line	Second-line drugs with anesthetic, antineuropathic medication, and NMDA antagonist	—	—

Abbreviation: NMDA, *N*-methyl-D-aspartate.

INTERVENTIONAL TREATMENT FOR CANCER PAIN

Various nociceptive pathways can be blocked by using local anesthetics in the nervous system to alleviate cancer pain on a temporary or long-term basis, allowing them to undergo treatment that might be needed to alleviate the cancer. An example concerns a patient with mesothelioma and metastatic disease to the rib cage. He required a series of 8 radiation treatments to suppress the expansion of his tumor. Unfortunately he was unable to lie still for 45 minutes to undergo these treatments. The patient therefore underwent intercostal blockade with 0.5% marcaine 45 minutes before radiation therapy, which provided pain relief to undergo the radiation treatment required. Neurolytic blockade can also assist the oncologist and radiation oncologist to facilitate cancer treatment. Another example is anesthetizing the lumbar plexus and its roots for patients undergoing treatment of sacral malignancies caused by direct invasion of bladder or rectal cancer, to facilitate temporary pain relief while undergoing treatment. There have also been case reports of physicians inserting lumbosacral plexus catheters for continuous infusions of anesthetic for palliative care (**Figs. 6** and **7**).[15]

Neurolysis and Chemotactic Agents

Neurolysis with chemotaxic agents has also been described over the years to be effective in treating refractory cancer pain for periods of time, but in certain anatomic regions there is risk of motor deficit or paralysis if there is too much diffusion of medication. Radiofrequency ablation is another option for destroying or denaturing nerves. Pancreatic and abdominal cancers are extremely painful, as shown in **Fig. 1**. If pancreatic cancer is diagnosed early enough, some patients will undergo surgical resection. However, those who have advancing stages of pancreatic cancer will suffer from direct invasion into the celiac plexus. There are multiple ways of blocking the celiac plexus, but these techniques carry risk owing to the close proximity of the aorta. Even if blockade is obtained for short-term relief, performing neurolytic blockade with phenol has been associated with spinal cord infarction and paralysis. Therefore, other approaches to the pancreas include lesser and greater splanchnic nerve supply

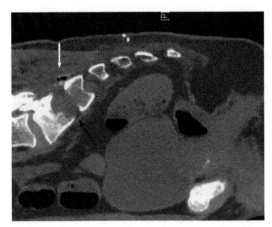

Fig. 6. A patient with metastatic lung cancer to S1 with continuous pain. Dashed arrow indicates tumor. White arrow indicates catheter tip and continuous infusion of ropivacaine over tumor.

branches to the celiac plexus (**Fig. 8**). Various techniques have been described for blocking the splanchnic nerves. In the author's practice, patients receiving a greater than 50% reduction in pain after splanchnic nerve blocks are considered for radiofrequency lesioning. The splanchnic nerve blocks are performed under fluoroscopic guidance with a combination of 2 mL of 2% xylocaine, 3 mL of 0.5% marcaine, and 40 mg dexamethasone phosphate (**Figs. 9** and **10**). The patient is evaluated with a pain diagram for the first 24 hours and the efficacy of the procedure recorded via a follow-up call. The patient is then followed up after 1 week. Should the procedure be effective, the patient is considered as a candidate for rhizotomy.

SPLANCHNIC NERVE RHIZOTOMY FOR PANCREATIC PAIN RELIEF

Treating pain derived from pancreatic cancer can be extremely difficult. Pancreatic cancer is one of the most deadly, and is associated with a high degree of pain. Aside

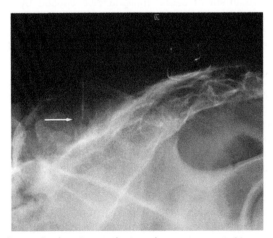

Fig. 7. Lateral radiograph showing catheter placement over S1 neuroforamen (*white arrow*). Personal files.

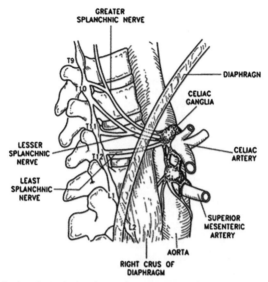

Fig. 8. Anatomy of splanchnic chain. (*From* Carachi R, Currie JM. New Tools in the treatment of motility disorders in children. Semin Pediatr Surg 2009;18:274–7; with permission.)

from medications, interventional techniques such as celiac plexus blocks and neurolysis have been associated with severe complications. An alternative is to use radiofrequency lesioning of the splanchnic nerves to provide a safe and longer-term treatment for the pancreatic pain.

Raj and colleagues[16] described rhizotomy as an effective technique for the treatment of pancreatic pain, with minimal side effects. The author uses a technique similar to that described by Gauci,[17] performed on an outpatient basis with local anesthetic. Sedation is not used for this procedure because it tends not to be painful with local anesthetic

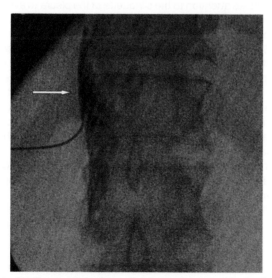

Fig. 9. Anteroposterior fluoroscopic view of splanchnic nerve block after 2 mL of Omnipaque, 180 mg/mL. White arrow indicates lateral dye spread.

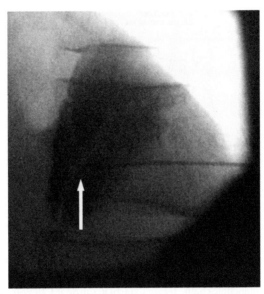

Fig. 10. Lateral fluoroscopic view of splanchnic nerve block after 2 mL of Omnipaque, 180 mg/mL. White arrow indicates needle of T12 anterior part of vertebral body.

and a blunt-needle technique. The procedure takes less than 15 minutes, so patient does not have to fast. Should patients have problems with anxiety or pain, lorazepam (Ativan) is prescribed if they do not already have it, with the recommendation that that they take their pain medications 30 minutes before the procedure.

- The patient is placed in a prone position on the fluoroscopy table, and the T11 and T12 vertebral body is identified. The image is then rotated obliquely so that the supra-articular process is under the anterior third of the superior vertebral body. One must pay close attention to the silhouette of the pleura to avoid pneumothorax.
- Under intermittent fluoroscopy, the skin is locally anesthetized with 1 to 2 mL of 2% lidocaine without epinephrine with a 25-gauge needle.
- A 3.5-inch 25 gauge spinal needle is advanced under intermittent fluoroscopy to anesthetize the deep muscle structures with lidocaine without epinephrine.
- A 16-gauge intravenous angiocatheter is guided under intermittent fluoroscopy in the direction of the anterior vertebral body of T12 with a slight superior tilt. The stylet is then removed. A 100- or 145-mm blunt radiofrequency cannula with a 10-mm active tip is then advanced under intermittent fluoroscopy until contact with vertebral body. Once the vertebral body is contacted, the fluoroscope is angled to a lateral position.
- With a lateral projection, the needle tip is advanced to the anterior one-third of the vertebral body. Confirmation is obtained with lateral and anteroposterior pictures (**Fig. 11**; lateral view only).
- Confirm position by stimulating at 50 Hz at 0.6 mV. In general, patients will feel no sensation at all but sometimes patients will complain of tightness in their stomach. Position is further confirmed with 2 Hz at a voltage of 3.0 mV to make sure there is no motor stimulation. If placement is not proper, one can contact the diaphragmatic nerves and discern stimulation of the diaphragm.
- Use of Omnipaque to demonstrate spread along the lateral vertebral bodies and avoidance of intravascular uptake may be beneficial.

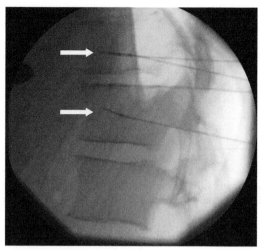

Fig. 11. Placement of radiofrequency needles for splanchnic lateral view. White arrows over the anterior third of T11 and T12 vertebral body.

- The splanchnic nerve is anesthetized with 3 mL of 2% xylocaine without epinephrine, and lesioning is carried out at 80°C for 75 seconds, after which the cannulas are rotated 180° and lesioning is repeated.
- This procedure is performed on both sides of the patient.
- The cannulas are removed and a sterile dressing is applied.

POSTOPERATIVE CARE

- The patient is monitored for 15 minutes to make sure vital signs are stable, and discharged home.
- Unlike with typical rhizotomy of the medial branch nerves, the author has not seen a postinjection flare. In general any soreness can be managed with patients' current pain medications. If they are sore at the injection site, ice is applied. Patients should experience about 6 to 9 months of pain relief, and the procedure may be repeated.

COMPLICATIONS AND MANAGEMENT

- Complications from the procedure consist of:
  1. Infection
  2. Bleeding
  3. Pneumothorax from improper placement
- To help minimize the risk of pneumothorax, use of blunt needles in addition to understanding of proper fluoroscopic guidance is necessary.

OUTCOMES AND FUTURE CONSIDERATIONS

The success rate of splanchnic nerve radiofrequency is sparse in the literature. Papadopoulos and colleagues[18] demonstrated in patients with malignant pain a significant improvement in quality of life and reduction in pain during the first 5 months after the procedure. Raj and colleagues[16] looked at 107 patients with both malignant and nonmalignant abdominal pain, and found that 40% of patients who had both splanchnic nerve blocks and radiofrequency lesioning had excellent results at

Table 4
Genetic markers and their association with pharmacologic metabolism

Genetic Marker	Pharmacologic Implications
CYP2C9, VKORC1	NSAID therapy, phenytoin, warfarin metabolism
CYP2C19	Diazepam, citalopram, sertraline
CYP2D6	Opioids, tapentadol, amphetamines, tramadol, duloxetine, fluoxetine, paroxetine, venlafaxine, cyclobenzaprine, bupropion
CYP3A4, CYP3A5	Buprenorphine, methadone, buprenorphine and naloxone, meperidine, fentanyl

6 months. Future research into utilization of splanchnic nerve rhizotomy for pancreatic pain should involve more prospective studies and look at bipolar radiofrequency lesioning to provide a bigger lesion and potentially longer duration of efficacy.

FUTURE PHARMACOLOGIC AND NONPHARMACOLOGIC THERAPIES
Genetic Testing

Over the past decade there has been increasing concern about the cost of health care. Often, inefficiency is due to using a trial-and-error approach to determine the appropriate medications, because of lack of evidence. Recent advances in pharmacogenetic testing have enabled physicians to obtain a drug-metabolism profile of their patients by obtaining a swab from the inside of the buccal mucosa. In opioid therapy one will examine the CYP450 system, primarily at the CYP2D6, CYP2C9, CYP2C19, CYP3A4, CYP3A5, and VKORC1. These genetic markers evaluate the patient's ability to metabolize certain drugs (**Table 4**). Test results assess a person's ability to metabolize medications. The analysis of the cytochrome P450 system is broken down into accelerated, broad/normal, compromised, and deficient. To interpret these grades one must know the outcomes of each grade (**Table 5**).

Case Example

A 58 year old female with metastatic pancreatic cancer to bone presents for treatment. She is unable to take nonsteroidal anti-inflammatory therapy because she is being treated with anticoagulants. Before starting treatment, genetic testing is obtained and reveals the following:

CYP2C9/VKORC1	Grade B normal/broad/extensive metabolizer
CYP2C19	Grade B normal/broad/extensive metabolizer
CYP2D6	Grade C compromised/intermediate metabolizer
CYP3A4	Grade B normal/broad/extensive metabolizer
COMT	Grade B normal/broad/extensive metabolizer
CYP1A2	Grade B normal/broad/extensive metabolizer

These results demonstrate that she is compromised to opioids or other medications that primarily use the CYP2D6 system to become active in the body. Therefore, normal dosages of a medication using this genetic marker to break down into an active metabolite might cause inadvertent overdose of adverse reactions if this test was not performed before initiating therapy. **Table 4** lists some of the medications that are metabolized by the CY2D6 as well as the other enzymes.

Table 5
List of enzymes and associated pharmacological metabolism

CYP2C19 Enzymes Metabolize	CYP2D6 Enzymes Metabolize	CYP2C9 Enzymes Metabolize
Tricyclics	AHDH	Hypoglycemics
Amitriptyline	Modafinil	Glipzide
Imipramine	Amphetamine	Glimepiride
SSRI's	Atomoxetine	Tolbutamide
Citalopram	Methyphenidate	Glyburide
Escitalopram	Psychotropics	Anticoagulants
Sertaline	Aripiprazole	S-warfarin
Anticonvulsant	Risperidone	Diuretic
Diazepam	Haloperidol	Torsemide
Oncology	Thioridazine	ARB's
Cyclophosphamide	Clozipine	Losartan
Proton Pump	Donepezil	Irbesartan
Omeprazole	Tricylcics	Statins
Lansoprazole	Nortriptyline	Fluvastatin
Pantoprazole	Clomipramine	Rosuvastatin
ETC.	Deipramine	NSAID's
Antiplatelet	SSRI's	Celecoxib
Clopidogrel	Fluoxetine	Diclofenac
Other	Paroxetine	Meloxicam
Proquanil	Sertaline	Naproxen
Atovaquone	Opioids	Ibuprofen
Melfinavir	Hydrocodone	Indomethacin
Tolbutamide	Codeine	Anticonvulsant
Carisoprodol	Tramadol	Valproic acid
	Beta blockers	Phenytoin
	Carvedilol	Other:
	Metoprolol	Sildenafil
	Timolol	
	Propanolol	
	Antiarrythmics	
	Flecainide	
	Propafenone	
	Quinadine	
	Mexilitine	
	Oncology	
	Tamoxifen	
	Doxorubicine	
	SNRI's	
	Duloxetine	
	Venlafaxine	

(continued on next page)

Table 5
(continued)

CYP3A4 Enzymes Metabolize		CYP1A2 Enzymes Metabolize	COMT Enzymes Metabolize
Psychotropics	Statins	Psychotropics	Catecholamines
Carbamazepine	Atorvastatin	Clomipramine	Epinephrine
Aripiprazole	Lovastatin	Imipramine	Norepinephrine
Quetiapine	Simvastatin	Fluvoxamine	Dopamine
Mirtazapine	Sex hormones	Antipsychotics	Parkinsons
Trazodone	Finasteride	Haloperidol	Carbidopa/
Sertraline	Estradiol	Clozipine	levodopa
Oncology	Progesterone	Olanzapine	Cardiac inotropic
Vincristine	Ethinylestradiol	Muscle relaxers	Dobutamine
Vinblastine	Testosterone	Cyclobenzaprine	Isoproterenol
Imatinib	HIV	Tizanidine	Methyldopa
Erlotinib	Amprenavir	Cardiovascular	Catechol estrogens
Doxorubicin	Efavirenz	Mexiletine	2-hydroxyestrodial
Cardiovascular	Atripla	Other	4-hydroxyestrodial
Amilodipine	Atazanavir	Theophylline	
Diltiazem	Ritonavir	Caffeine	
Felodipine	Opioids	Zolmitriptan	
Nifedipine	Buprenorphine	Acetaminophen	
Verapamil	Fentanyl		
Antiarrythmic	Methadone		
Amiodarone	Oxycodone		
Other	Tranquilizers		
Tacrolimus	Alprazolam		
Cyclosporine	Midazolam		
Hydrocortisone	Sedative		
Dexamethasone	Zolpidem		
Donepezil	Eszoplidone		
Erythromycin			
Clarithromycin			

TRANSCRANIAL MAGNETIC STIMULATION

A nonpharmacologic technique that is proving interesting in the management of pain is transcranial magnetic stimulation. This treatment is based on enhancing the descending inhibitory pathways through magnetic stimulation of the prefrontal cortex. Studies have demonstrated that repetitive transcranial magnetic stimulation of the prefrontal cortex can enhance production of serotonin and norepinephrine. This method has obtained approval from the Food and Drug Administration for major depression refractory to oral medication. Transcranial magnetic stimulation consists of repetitive stimulation over the prefrontal cortex at an intensity of 120% of motor threshold. Repetitive impulses are provided to the patient at a rate of more than 5 seconds with a 25-second rest. The sessions take 37.5 minutes to complete and are performed daily for a total of 30 treatments. Studies evaluating functional magnetic resonance imaging (MRI) have demonstrated in patients without pain that one treatment of transcranial magnetic stimulation can increase the thermal threshold in almost 13% of patients treated. This finding correlates with those of functional MRI demonstrating increased activity in the right superior frontal gyrus and insula, and anterior and posterior cingulate gyri. Increased superior frontal activity was significantly associated with decreased pain-intensity ratings.[19] Various clinical trials studying the effects of transcranial magnetic stimulation on fibromyalgia and other areas of pain are currently under way.

SUMMARY

Although the diagnosis of cancer has been stereotyped as a disease to end all, pain treatment in cancer is showing hopeful prospects. A strong background in anatomy and physiology is the foundation on which to approach pain in a patient with cancer, with multiple options accessible. Using new medications geared at enhancing the descending inhibitory pathways in combination with classic pharmacologic treatment can improve a patient's quality of life and reduce side effects. Interventional therapy to inhibit various peripheral structures improves a patient's quality of life. Clinicians must look not only at the disease but also how it is affecting the patient. Reducing pain has been reported to enhance the quality of life of patients with cancer and has been associated with longer survival rates. Being diligent to always reassess treatment is the answer to effectively managing complicated cases of cancer pain. It is hoped that this article will give the reader pause for thought as to how patients suffering from pain can be helped, rather than being merely instructive. Pain is always changing and, therefore, an astute physician will know how to address the treatment at any time by understanding how pain works.

REFERENCES

1. Marcus DA. Epidemiology of cancer pain. Current Pain Headache Rep Aug 2011; 15(4):231–4.
2. Simone C. Cancer patient attitudes toward analgesic usage and pain intervention. Clin J Pain 2012;28(2):157–62.
3. Medical Services Commission. Palliative care for the patient with incurable cancer or advanced disease. Part 2. Pain and symptom management. Victoria (Canada): British Columbia Medical Services Commission; 2011. p. 44.
4. Moulin DE. Opioid treatment for cancer pain and chronic noncancer pain. In: Merskey H, Loeser JD, Dubner R, editors. The paths of pain 1975-2005. Seattle (WA): IASP Press; 2005. p. 469–82.

5. Yaksh TL. Opioid analgesia: the last 30 years. In: Merskey H, Loeser JD, Dubner R, editors. The paths of pain 1975-2005. Seattle (WA): IASP Press; 2005. p. 209–28.
6. Fields HL, Heinricher MM. Anatomy and physiology of a nocioceptive modulatory system. Philos Trans R Soc Lond B Biol Sci 1985;308(1136):361–74.
7. Millan MJ. Descending control of pain. Prog Neurobiol 2002;66:355–474.
8. Burgess SE, Gardell LR, Ossipov MH, et al. Time dependent descending facilitation from the rostral ventromedial medulla maintains, but does not initiate, neuropathic pain. J Neurosci 2002;22:5129–36.
9. Sang CN. NMDA-receptor antagonists in neuropathic pain: experimental methods of clinical trials. J Pain Symptom Manage 2000;19(Suppl 1):S21–5.
10. Hemmings H, Egan T. Pharmacology and physiology for anesthesia: foundations and clinical application. Chapter 14. 2013. p. 235–52.
11. Dray A. Pharmacology of inflammatory pain. In: Merskey H, Loeser JD, Dubner R, editors. The paths of pain 1975-2005. Seattle (WA): IASP Press; p. 177–90.
12. Campbell FA, Tramer MR, Carroll D, et al. Are cannabinoids an effective and safe treatment option in the management of pain? A quality systematic review. BMJ 2001;323:13–6.
13. Johnson JR, Burnell-Nugent M, Lossignol D, et al. Multicenter, double-blind, randomized, placebo-controlled, parallel group study of the efficacy, safety, and tolerability of THC: CBD extract and THC extracts in patients with intractable cancer related pain. J Pain Symptom Manage 2010;39:169–79.
14. Stearns L, Boortz-Marx R, Du Pen S, et al. Intrathecal drug delivery for management of cancer pain: a multidisciplinary consensus of best clinical practices. J Support Oncol 2005;3(6):399–408.
15. Zaporowska-Stachowiak I, Kotlinska-Lemieszek A, Kowalski G, et al. Lumbar paravertebral blockade as intractable management method in palliative care. Onco Targets Ther 2013;6:1187–96.
16. Raj PP, Sahinler B, Lowe M. Radiofrequency lesioning of the splanchnic nerves. Pain Pract 2002;2(3):241–7.
17. Gauci CA. Sympathetic nervous system radiofrequency and pulsed radiofrequency. In: Manual of RF techniques. Meggen (Switzerland): Flivo Press SA; 2004. p. 95–100.
18. Papadopoulos D, Kostopanagiotou G, Batistaki C. Bilateral thoracic splanchnic nerve radiofrequency thermocoagulation for the management of end stage pancreatic abdominal cancer pain. Pain Physician 2013;16:125–33.
19. Martin L, Borckardt J, Reeves S, et al. A pilot functional MRI study of the effects of prefrontal rTMS on pain perception. Pain Med 2011;14:999–1009.

Side Effects of Commonly Prescribed Analgesic Medications

Gregory T. Carter, MD, MS[a,b,]*, Vicky Duong, BS, PharmD(c)[c],
Stanley Ho, BS, PharmD(c)[c], Kathryn C. Ngo, BS, PharmD(c)[c],
Christopher L. Greer, BPharm[a,c], Douglas L. Weeks, PhD[a,c]

KEYWORDS

- Analgesics • Side effects • Adverse drug events • Patient counseling • Chronic pain

KEY POINTS

- Analgesics, including opioids, steroidal and nonsteroidal anti-inflammatory drugs, aspirin, acetaminophen, antiepileptics, and serotonin-norepinephrine reuptake inhibitors are medications commonly used to treat many forms of pain.
- All of these medications may have significant adverse side effects.
- Adverse effects may occasionally be inseparable from desired effects. Side effects are often dose dependent and time dependent.
- It is critical that the prescribing practitioner and the dispensing pharmacist provide a thorough, understandable review of the potential side effects to all patients before these drugs are administered.
- Proper monitoring and follow-up during therapy are crucial.

INTRODUCTION

Pain is classified by duration as either acute or chronic, with chronic pain usually lasting longer than 3 months.[1,2] Chronic pain typically is associated with longer-term medication exposure, thus increasing the likelihood of adverse events. Complex regimens with multiple medications, particularly when there are several prescribers, often result in a lack of continuity of care and proper monitoring; this can also be associated with inadequate patient education. Many drugs have names that sound alike or look alike, and drug names are sometimes miswritten, misheard, and

[a] St. Luke's Rehabilitation Institute, 711 South Cowley Street, Spokane, WA 99202-1330, USA;
[b] University of Washington, School of Medicine, Seattle, WA 98195, USA; [c] Department of
Pharmacotherapy, Washington State University, Spokane, WA 99202-1330, USA
* Corresponding author. St. Luke's Rehabilitation Institute, 711 South Cowley Street, Spokane,
WA 99202-1330.
E-mail address: gtcarter@uw.edu

Phys Med Rehabil Clin N Am 25 (2014) 457–470
http://dx.doi.org/10.1016/j.pmr.2014.01.007
1047-9651/14/$ – see front matter © 2014 Elsevier Inc. All rights reserved.

Table 1
Major adverse effects of opioids

Classification	Drugs	Adverse Effects and Relative Risks
Phenanthrenes	Morphine	*Dermatologic:* Pruritus (≤80%) *Gastrointestinal:* Constipation (≥9%), nausea (oral, 7% and >10%; epidural or intrathecal, 15%–70%), vomiting (>10%) *Neurologic:* Dizziness (6%), headache (>10%), lightheadedness, somnolence (≥9%) *Renal:* Urinary retention (oral, <5%; epidural/intrathecal, 15%–70%)
	Codeine	*Cardiovascular:* Hypotension (1%–10%), tachycardia or bradycardia (1%–10%) *Dermatologic* (1%–10%): Pruritus (1%–10%), rash (1%–10%), urticaria (1%–10%) *Gastrointestinal:* Constipation (>10%), nausea (1%–10%), vomiting (1%–10%), anorexia (1%–10%), xerostomia (1%–10%) *Neurologic:* Drowsiness (>10%), dizziness (1%–10%), lightheadedness (1%–10%), sedated, somnolence *Renal:* Urinary retention *Respiratory:* Dyspnea (1%–10%) *Ophthalmic:* Blurred vision (1%–10%), visual disturbances
	Hydromorphone	*Dermatologic:* Flushing (extended-release, <2%), pruritus (extended-release, 1%–8%), sweating *Gastrointestinal:* Constipation (extended-release, 7%–31%), nausea (extended-release, 9%–28%), vomiting (extended-release, 6%–14%) *Neurologic:* Asthenia (extended-release, 1%–11%), dizziness (extended-release, 2%–11%), headache (extended-release, 5%–12%), lightheadedness, sedated (extended-release, <2%), somnolence (extended-release, 1%–15%)
	Oxycodone	*Dermatologic:* Pruritus (controlled-release, 13%; immediate-release, ≥3%), Sweating (controlled-release, 5%; immediate-release, <3%) *Gastrointestinal:* Abdominal pain (≤5%), constipation (controlled-release, 23%; immediate-release, ≥3%), nausea (controlled-release, 23%; immediate-release, ≥3%), vomiting (controlled-release, 12%; immediate-release, ≥3%), xerostomia (controlled-release, 6%; immediate-release, <3%) *Neurologic:* Asthenia (controlled-release, 6%; immediate-release, ≥3%), dizziness (controlled-release, 13%; immediate-release, ≥3%), headache (controlled-release, 7%; immediate-release, 23%; immediate-release, ≥3%), somnolence (controlled-release, 23%; immediate-release, ≥3%)

Levorphanol	*Cardiovascular:* Hypotension (1%–10%) *Dermatologic:* Pruritus (>10%) *Gastrointestinal:* Constipation (1%–10%), nausea (>10%), vomiting (1%–10%) *Psychiatric:* Altered mental status (1%–10%), disturbance in mood (1%–10%)
Hydrocodone[a]	*Dermatologic:* Pruritus, rash *Gastrointestinal:* Constipation, bowel obstruction, nausea, vomiting, pharyngeal dryness, xerostomia *Neurologic:* Confusion, dizziness, impaired cognition, lethargy, sedated, somnolence *Psychiatric:* Anxiety, dysphoric mood, euphoria, fear, mood swings *Renal:* Urinary retention, spasm of bladder, urethral spasm *Respiratory:* Depression, tight chest
Oxymorphone	*Cardiovascular:* Hypotension (<10%) *Dermatologic:* Pruritus (≤15.2%), sweating symptom (1% to <10%) *Gastrointestinal:* Abdominal pain (1% to <10%), constipation (4.1%–27.6%), nausea (2.9%–33.1%), vomiting (≤15.6%), xerostomia (1% to <10%) *Neurologic:* Confusion (≤10%), dizziness (≤17.8%), headache (2.9%–12.2%), somnolence (1.9%–19.1%) *Respiratory:* Dyspnea (1% to <10%), hypoxia (1% to <10%) *Other:* Fever (1%–14.2%)
Buprenorphine	*Dermatologic:* Application-site erythema (5%–10%), application-site irritation (3%–5%), application-site rash (6%–9%), pruritus, application site (4%–15%) *Gastrointestinal:* Constipation (14%), nausea (23%), vomiting (11%), xerostomia (≥5%) *Neurologic:* Dizziness (16%), headache (16%), somnolence (14%)—does have ceiling dose for analgesia. Not recommended above 30 mg total daily dose. Buprenorphine is associated with less QTc prolongation than methadone, but this can occur at higher doses
Butorphanol	*Gastrointestinal:* Nausea and vomiting (13%) *Neurologic:* Dizziness (19%–54%), insomnia (11%), sedated (30%–40%), somnolence (43%–88%) *Respiratory:* Nasal congestion (13%), long-term use of intranasal product (13%)

(continued on next page)

Table 1
(continued)

Classification	Drugs	Adverse Effects and Relative Risks
Phenylpiperidines	Fentanyl	*Dermatologic:* Application-site reaction (adults, ≥1%; pediatrics, 3%–10%), diaphoresis (adults: transdermal ≥10%, sublingual ≥1%; pediatrics: transdermal ≥1%), pruritus (transdermal, 3%–10%; sublingual, ≥1%) *Gastrointestinal:* Abdominal pain (transdermal, 3%–10%; sublingual, ≥1%), constipation (adults, ≥10%; pediatrics, 3%–10%), diarrhea (adults: transdermal 3%–10%, sublingual ≥1%; pediatrics: transdermal ≥1%), indigestion (transdermal, 3%–10%; sublingual, ≥1%), loss of appetite (transdermal, 3%–10%; sublingual, ≥1%), nausea (≥10%), vomiting (≥10%), xerostomia (adults: transdermal ≥10%, sublingual ≥1%; pediatrics: transdermal ≥1%) *Neurologic:* Asthenia (adults, ≥9.7%; pediatrics, 3%–10%), confusion (adults: transdermal ≥10%, sublingual ≥1%; pediatrics: transdermal ≥1%), dizziness (adults, 3%–10%; pediatrics, ≥1%), feeling nervous (3%–10%), headache (transdermal, 3%–10%; sublingual, ≥1%), insomnia (adults, ≥1%; pediatrics, 3%–10%), somnolence (adults, ≥9.5%; pediatrics, 3%–10%) *Psychiatric:* Anxiety (adults, 3%–10%; pediatrics, ≥1%), depression (adults: transdermal 3%–10%, sublingual ≥1%; pediatrics: transdermal ≥1%), euphoria (3%–10%), hallucinations (adults: transdermal 3%–10%, sublingual ≥1%; pediatrics: transdermal ≥1%) *Renal:* Urinary retention (adults: transdermal 3%–10%, sublingual <1%; pediatrics: transdermal ≥1%) *Respiratory:* Dyspnea (adults: transdermal 3%–10%, sublingual 10.4%; pediatrics: transdermal ≥1%), upper respiratory infection (3%–10%) *Other:* Fatigue (transdermal, 3%–10%; sublingual, ≥1%), influenza-like symptoms (3%–10%)
	Alfentanil	*Cardiovascular:* Bradyarrhythmia (14%), hypertension (18%), hypotension (10%), tachycardia (12%) *Gastrointestinal:* Nausea (28%), vomiting (18%)
	Sufentanil	*Cardiovascular:* Bradyarrhythmia (3%–9%), Hypotension (3%–9%) *Dermatologic:* Pruritus (25%) *Gastrointestinal:* Nausea (3%–9%), vomiting (3%–9%) *Musculoskeletal:* Muscle rigidity, chest wall (3%–9%) *Neurologic:* Somnolence (3%–9%)
	Meperidine[a]	*Dermatologic:* Sweating, pruritus, rash, urticaria *Gastrointestinal:* Abdominal cramps, anorexia, biliary spasm, constipation, nausea, paralytic ileus, sphincter of Oddi spasm, vomiting, xerostomia *Neurologic:* Agitation, confusion, delirium, disorientation, dizziness, lightheadedness, sedation *Neuromuscular and skeletal:* Muscle twitching, myoclonus, tremor, weakness *Ocular:* Visual disturbances

Other	Methadone[a]	*Cardiovascular:* Cardiac dysrhythmia, hypotension *Endocrine metabolic:* Diaphoresis *Gastrointestinal:* Constipation, nausea, vomiting *Neurologic:* Asthenia, dizziness, lightheadedness, sedated
	Tapentadol	*Gastrointestinal:* Constipation (8%–17%), nausea (21%–30%), vomiting (8%–18%) *Neurologic:* Dizziness (17%–24%), headache (extended-release tablets, 10%–15%), somnolence (12%–15%); avoid combining with SNRI or SSRI
	Tramadol	*Dermatologic:* Flushing (8%–16%), pruritus (3%–11.9%) *Gastrointestinal:* Constipation (9%–46%), nausea (15%–40%), vomiting (5%–17%), dyspepsia (1%–13) *Neurologic:* Dizziness (7%–28.2%), headache (3%–15.8%), insomnia (1%–10.9%), somnolence (4%–20.3%) *Neuromuscular and skeletal:* Weakness (4%–12%); avoid combining with SNRI or SSRI

Abbreviations: SNRI, serotonin–norepinephrine reuptake inhibitor; SSRI, selective serotonin reuptake inhibitor.

References:

1. Alfentanil [package insert]. Lake Forest, IL: HOSPIRA, Inc; 2004.
2. Butrans [package insert]. Stamford, CT: Purdue Pharma L.P.; 2012.
3. Cherny N, Ripamonti C, Pereira J, et al. Strategies to manage the adverse effects of oral morphine: an evidence-based report. J Clin Oncol 2001;19(4):2542–54.
4. Codeine [package insert]. Columbus, OH: Roxane Laboratories, Inc; 2013.
5. Demerol [package insert]. Lake Forest, IL: HOSPIRA, Inc; 2010.
6. Dilaudid [package insert]. Stamford, CT: Purdue Pharma L.P.; 2009.
7. Dolophine [package insert]. Columbus, OH: Roxane Laboratories Inc; 2013.
8. Duragesic [package insert]. Titusville, NJ: Janssen Pharmaceuticals, Inc; 2009.
9. Levorphanol [package insert]. Columbus, OH: Roxane Laboratories Inc; 2011.
10. Micromedex Healthcare Series [Internet database]. Greenwood Village (CO): Thomson Healthcare.
11. Pharmaceutical Press. Methyl salicylate. MARTINDALE—the complete drug reference. MICROMEDEX Healthcare Series. 2006. Available at: http://www-thomsonhc-com.offcampus.lib.washington.edu/hcs. Accessed September 20, 2013.
12. MS Contin [package insert]. Corona, CA: Watson Pharmaceuticals, Inc; 2009.
13. Norco [package insert]. Corona, CA: Watson Pharmaceuticals, Inc; 2007.
14. Nucynta [package insert]. Titusville, NJ: Janssen Pharmaceuticals, Inc; 2009.
15. Opana [package insert]. Chadds Ford, PA: Endo Pharmaceuticals, Inc; 2012.
16. Oxycontin [package insert]. Stamford, CT: Purdue Pharma L.P.; 2012.
17. Ryzolt [package insert]. Stamford, CT: Purdue Pharma L.P.; 2011.
18. Schug SA, Zech D, Grond S. Adverse effects of systemic opioid analgesics. Drug Saf 1992;7(3):200–13.
19. Stadol [package insert]. Columbus, OH: Roxane Laboratories Inc; 2009.
20. Subutex [package insert]. Richmond, VA: Reckitt Benckiser Pharmaceuticals, Inc; 2011.
21. Sufenta [package insert]. Lake Forest, IL: Akorn, Inc; 2008.

[a] Frequency of adverse effects not defined.

Table 2
Major adverse effects of nonsteroidal anti-inflammatory medication

	Oral NSAIDs
Cardiovascular	Edema (<9%), palpitation, hypertension. A recent meta-analysis looking at the cardiovascular effects of NSAIDs (including selective COX-2 inhibitors) shows that the risks are similar. Naproxen is associated with less cardiovascular risk than other NSAIDs[a]
Dermatologic	Rash (3%–9%), itching (<9%)
Central nervous system	Dizziness (3%–9%), headache (1%–3%), nervousness (1%–3%) Indomethacin: Headache (12%) Ketorolac: Headache (17%)
Endocrine and metabolic	Fluid retention (≤9%)
Gastrointestinal	Epigastric pain (3%–9%), heartburn (3%–9%), nausea (3%–9%), abdominal pain/cramps/distress (1%–3%), appetite decreased (1%–3%), constipation (1%–3%), diarrhea (1%–3%), dyspepsia (1%–3%), flatulence (1%–3%), vomiting (1%–3%), stomatitis
General	Dyspnea (3%–9%), thirst
Hepatic	Ketoprofen: Liver function test abnormality (<15%)
Otic	Tinnitus (3%–9%)
Renal	Ketorolac: Renal function abnormal
	Topical NSAIDs
Dermatologic	Dermatitis (11%), pruritus (4%), erythema (<1%), paresthesia (<1%), dryness (<1%), vesicles (<1%), irritation (<1%), papules (<1%), itching
	COX-2 Selective Inhibitor
Gastrointestinal	Abdominal pain (4%), diarrhea (5%), dyspepsia (8%), flatulence (2%), nausea (3%)
Cardiovascular	The selective action on COX-2 does reduce gastrointestinal side effects but dos not eliminate cardiovascular complications (see above for NSAIDs)[a]
Central, peripheral nervous system	Dizziness (2%), headache (15%); in higher doses may produce disorientation, particularly in elderly
Psychiatric	Insomnia (2%)
Respiratory	Pharyngitis (2%), rhinitis (2%), sinusitis (5%), upper respiratory infection (8%)
Dermatologic	Rash (2%)

Abbreviations: COX-2, cyclooxygenase-2; NSAID, nonsteroidal anti-inflammatory drug.

References:
1. Ibuprofen: Drug information. UpToDate. Available at: http://www.uptodateonline.com.
2. Indomethacin: Drug information. UpToDate. Available at: http://www.uptodateonline.com.
3. Ketorolac: Drug information. UpToDate. Available at: http://www.uptodateonline.com.
4. Ketoprofen: Drug information. UpToDate. Available at: http://www.uptodateonline.com.
5. Meloxicam: Drug information. UpToDate. Available at: http://www.uptodateonline.com.
6. Naproxen: Drug information. UpToDate. Available at: http://www.uptodateonline.com.
7. Naprosyn [package insert]. South San Francisco, CA: Genentech USA Inc; 2010.
8. Voltaren Gel [package insert]. Parsippany, NJ: Novartis Consumer Health Inc; 2013.
9. Celebrex [package insert]. New York, NY: Pfizer Inc; 2011.
[a] Coxib and traditional NSAID Trialists' (CNT) Collaboration. Vascular and upper gastrointestinal effects of nonsteroidal anti-inflammatory drugs: meta-analyses of individual participant data from randomised trials. Lancet 2013;382(9894):769–79.

misread. All of these factors contribute to the likelihood of adverse drug events (ADEs).[3,4] Counseling with patient communication is an important way to avoid medication errors, and to help patients understand the intended effects as well as the side effects of their drugs. Proper patient counseling by both physicians and pharmacists will help prevent ADEs. Studies have shown that appropriate medication counseling for patients can save money, unnecessary hospitalization, and possibly prevent harm

Table 3
Major adverse effects of acetaminophen

	Oral
Dermatologic	Rash
	Rare, serious: Stevens-Johnson syndrome, toxic epidermal necrolysis (TEN), acute generalized exanthematous pustulosis (AGEP)
Central nervous system	Dizziness, insomnia (1%–7%), headache (1%–10%)
Endocrine, metabolic	May increase chloride, uric acid, glucose
	May decrease sodium, bicarbonate, calcium
Hematologic	Anemia, blood dyscrasias (neutropenia, pancytopenia, leukopenia)
Hepatic	Bilirubin increased, alkaline phosphatase increased. For adults and children 12 y and older, the recommended maximum daily dose of acetaminophen 3000 mg in 24 h
Psychiatric	Agitation (>5%)
Renal	Ammonia increased, nephrotoxicity with chronic overdose, analgesic nephropathy
Gastrointestinal	Nausea (adults 34%, children >5%), vomiting (adults 15%, children >5%), constipation (>5%)
	Intravenous
Cardiovascular	Edema (peripheral), hypervolemia, hypo-/hypertension, tachycardia
Central nervous system	Headache (adults 10%, children >1%), insomnia (adults 7%, children >1%), anxiety, fatigue
Dermatologic	Pruritus (children >5%), rash
Endocrine, metabolic	Hypoalbuminemia, hypokalemia, hypomagnesemia, hypophosphatemia
Gastrointestinal	Constipation (children >5%), abdominal pain, diarrhea
Hematologic	Anemia
Hepatic	Transaminase increased
Local	Infusion-site pain
Neuromuscular, skeletal	Muscle spasms, pain in extremity, trismus
Ocular	Periorbital edema
Renal	Oliguria (children >1%)
Respiratory	Atelectasis (>5%), abnormal breath sounds, dyspnea, hypoxia, pleural effusion, pulmonary edema, stridor, wheezing

References:
   1. Kociancic T, Reed MD. Acetaminophen intoxication and length of treatment: how long is long enough? Pharmacotherapy 2003;23(8):1052–9.
   2. Rowden AK, Norvell J, Eldridge DL, et al. Acetaminophen poisoning. Clin Lab Med 2006;26(1): 49–65.

or even death in patients.[5] Patients' understanding of their medication regimen assists in the identification of drug-related problems. Early identification of drug-related problems has also been shown to be associated with a lower rate of preventable ADEs.[6]

GENDER CONSIDERATIONS

Women and men feel pain differently and respond to treatment differently.[7,8] Women report more severe and longer-lasting pain than men, and there are gender differences in pharmacokinetics. Notable reasons for these differences include the lower body weight in women. Women also have a higher percentage of body fat, which can also affect the volume of distribution.[7,8] Adults are often given the same dose of

Table 4 Major adverse effects of commonly used topical analgesics	
Capsaicin	Local: Redness (63%), burning sensation, pain (42%) Pruritus (2%–6%), papules (6%), edema (4%), dryness (2%), swelling (2%) Systemic: Hypertension (2%, transient) Nausea (5%), vomiting (3%) Nasopharyngitis (4%), sinusitis (3%), bronchitis (2%)
Lidocaine (cream, patch)	Localized: Redness, edema, itching, rash, paleness *Patch:* petechia, bruising, irritation, pain exacerbation Systemic: (if dose is large enough) Hypotension (3%), nausea (<1%) Bradycardia, methemoglobinemia Lightheadedness, nervousness, euphoria, confusion, dizziness, sensations of heat, cold or numbness, tremors, drowsiness Serious, but rare: cardiac arrest, cardiac dysrhythmia, respiratory depression
Lidocaine/ prilocaine (cream)	Localized: Paleness (37%), redness (30%), alterations in temperature sensations (7%), edema (6%), itching (2%), rash (<1%) Systemic: Unlikely to occur, owing to small doses Same as systemic adverse drug reactions listed above under lidocaine
Methyl salicylate, menthol, camphor	Localized: Irritation, burns, redness Systemic (in larger doses, frequent application): Salicylate toxicity (nausea, vomiting, respiratory distress, apnea, confusion, seizures, coma, pulmonary edema, hyperthermia, cardiovascular collapse, death)

References:
1. Rowden AK, Norvell J, Eldridge DL, et al. Effectiveness and safety of topical versus oral nonsteroidal anti-inflammatory drugs: a comprehensive review. Phys Sportsmed 2013;41(2):64–74.
2. Derry S, Moore RA, Rabbie R. Topical NSAIDs for chronic musculoskeletal pain in adults. Cochrane Database Syst Rev 2012;9:CD007400.

Table 5
Major adverse effects and relative risk of antiepileptics

Drugs	Adverse Effects and Relative Risk
Carbamazepine	*Cardiovascular:* Hypotension *Dermatologic:* Pruritus (8%), rash (7%) *Gastrointestinal:* Constipation (10%), nausea (29%), vomiting (18%), xerostomia (8%) *Neurologic:* Asthenia (8%), ataxia (15%), dizziness (44%), somnolence *Ophthalmic:* Blurred vision (6%), nystagmus
Phenytoin[a]	*Dermatologic:* Morbilliform eruption, rash (5%–10%) *Gastrointestinal:* Constipation, drug-induced gingival hyperplasia, nausea, vomiting *Neurologic:* Ataxia, coordination problem, nystagmus, slurred speech *Psychiatric:* Confusion, feeling nervous
Lamotrigine	*Dermatologic:* Rash (immediate-release, ≤10% [adult]; 14% [pediatric]) *Gastrointestinal:* Abdominal pain (immediate-release, 5%–10%), diarrhea (immediate-release, 6%–11%; extended-release, 5%), indigestion (immediate-release, 2%–7%), nausea (immediate-release, 7%–25%; extended-release, 7%), vomiting (immediate-release, 5%–20%; extended-release, 6%) *Neurologic:* Asthenia (immediate-release, 2%–8%; extended-release, 6%), ataxia (immediate-release, 2%–11%), coordination problem (immediate-release, 6%–7%; extended-release, 3%), dizziness (immediate-release, 7%–54%; extended-release, 14%), headache (immediate-release, 29%), insomnia (immediate-release, 5%–10%), somnolence (immediate-release, 9%–17%; extended-release, 5%), tremor (immediate-release, 4%–10%; extended-release, 6%), vertigo (immediate-release, 2%; extended-release, 3%) *Ophthalmic:* Blurred vision (immediate-release, 11%–25% [adults] and 4% [children]; extended-release, 3%), diplopia (immediate-release, 24%–49% [adults] and 5% [children]; extended-release, 5%) *Psychiatric:* Anxiety (immediate-release, 4%; extended-release, 3%), depression (immediate-release, 4%; extended-release, 3%) *Reproductive:* Dysmenorrhea (immediate-release, 5%–7%) *Respiratory:* Rhinitis (immediate-release, 7%–14%) *Other:* Pain (immediate-release, 5%)
Oxcarbazepine	*Gastrointestinal:* Abdominal pain (adult, ≤13%), indigestion (adult, ≤6%; pediatric, 2%), nausea (adult, 7%–29%; pediatric, 19%), vomiting (adult, 5%–36%; pediatric, 33%) *Neurologic:* Abnormal gait (adult, ≤17%; pediatric, 8%), ataxia (adult, 1%–31%; pediatric, 13%), dizziness (adult, 8%–49%; pediatric, 28%), headache (adult, 8%–32%; pediatric, 31%), impairment of balance (5%–7%), somnolence (adult, 5%–36%; pediatric, 31%–34.8%), tremor (adult, 1%–16%; pediatric, 6%) *Ophthalmic:* Abnormal vision (adult, 1%–14%; pediatric, 13%), diplopia (adult, 1%–40%; pediatric, 17%), nystagmus (adult, 2%–26%; pediatric, 9%) *Other:* Fatigue (adult, 3%–21%; pediatric, 13%)
Zonisamide[a]	*Dermatologic:* Pruritus *Gastrointestinal:* Loss of appetite (13%) *Neurologic:* Ataxia (6%), dizziness (13%), somnolence (17%), unable to concentrate (6%) *Ophthalmic:* Amblyopia *Psychiatric:* Agitation (9%), depression (6%) *Other:* Disturbance in speech (5%)

(continued on next page)

Table 5 (continued)	
Drugs	**Adverse Effects and Relative Risk**
Lacosamide	*Gastrointestinal:* Nausea (7%–17%) *Neurologic:* Dizziness (16%–53%), headache (11%–14%) *Ophthalmic:* Diplopia (6%–16%)
Rufinamide	*Cardiovascular:* Shortened QT interval (46%–65%) *Gastrointestinal:* Nausea (7%–12%), vomiting (5%–17%) *Neurologic:* Ataxia (4%–5.4%), dizziness (2.7%–19%), headache (16%–27%), somnolence (11%–24.3%) *Ophthalmic:* Blurred vision (6%), diplopia (4%–9%) *Other:* Fatigue (9%–16%)

References:
1. Carbamazepine [package insert]. East Hanover, NJ: Novartis, Inc; 2013.
2. Lacosamide [package insert]. Smyrna, GA: UCB, Inc; 2011.
3. Lamotrigine [package insert]. Kalamazoo, MI: Torrent Pharmaceuticals, Ltd; 2012.
4. Micromedex® Healthcare Series [Internet database]. Greenwood Village (CO): Thomson Healthcare.
5. Oxcarbazepine [package insert]. Rockville, MD. Supernus Pharmaceuticals, Inc; 2012.
6. Perucca P, Gilliam FG. Adverse effects of antiepileptic drugs. Lancet Neurol 2012;11(9): 792–802.
7. Pharmaceutical Press. MARTINDALE—the complete drug reference. MICROMEDEX Healthcare Series. 2006. http://www-thomsonhc-com.offcampus.lib.washington.edu/hcs. Accessed September 26, 2013.
8. Phenytoin [package insert]. New York, NY: Pfizer, Inc; 2011.
9. Rufinamide [package insert]. Woodcliff Lake, NJ: Eisai, Inc; 2011.
10. Zonisamide [package insert]. Teaneck, NJ: Eisai Inc; 2006.
[a] Frequency of adverse effects not defined.

drug regardless of body weight, so women tend to have higher serum concentrations of drugs. Other gender differences in bioavailability, metabolism, and renal elimination may also be involved in medication effects. Drug metabolism and distribution differ between women and men. The menstrual cycle can affect drug blood levels as a result of fluctuating body fluid mass, which can result in differing renal drug clearance in women caused by changes in glomerular filtration. These factors need to be taken into consideration during patient counseling.

Treating chronic pain can be seen as layered with available first-line, second-line, and third-line pharmacologic treatments. Historically many drugs used to treat chronic pain are considered adjuvant analgesics. These medications are, by definition, agents whose primary indication is not analgesia. For example, tricyclic antidepressants and antiepileptic drugs (AEDs) have been the mainstay in the treatment of neuropathic pain. Even today these drugs are still used primarily as pain medications, although neither is approved by the Food and Drug Administration (FDA) for this use. Newer drugs such as the serotonin-norepinephrine reuptake inhibitor duloxetine (Cymbalta) and the AED pregabalin (Lyrica) are approved by the FDA for analgesic use.[9,10]

Tables 1–7 review the common adverse side effects and the percentages associated with use of the particular drug classes. In general, side effects are fairly class specific.

Table 6
Major adverse effects and relative risks of SNRI medications

	Cymbalta
Cardiovascular	Palpitation (1%–2%)
Central nervous system	Headache (14%), somnolence (12%), fatigue (11%), dizziness (10%), insomnia (10%), agitation (5%), anxiety (3%), dream abnormal (2%)
Dermatologic	Hyperhidrosis (7%)
Endocrine and metabolic	Decreased libido (4%), hot flushes (3%), orgasm abnormality (3%)
Gastrointestinal	Nausea (25%), xerostomia (15%), constipation (10%), diarrhea (10%), decreased appetite (9%), abdominal pain (6%), vomiting (5%), dyspepsia (2%), weight loss (2%)
Genitourinary	Erectile dysfunction (5%), ejaculation delayed (3%), ejaculatory dysfunction (2%)
Hepatic	Alanine aminotransferase > 3× upper limit of normal
Miscellaneous	Influenza (3%)
Neuromuscular and skeletal	Muscle spasms (3%), tremor (3%), musculoskeletal pain (1%), paresthesia (1%), rigors (1%)
Ocular	Blurred vision (3%)
Respiratory	Nasopharyngitis (5%), cough (3%)
	Effexor
Cardiovascular	Vasodilation (2%–6%), hypertension (3% in patients receiving <100 mg/d, ≤13% in patients receiving >300 mg/d), palpitation (3%), tachycardia (2%), chest pain (2%), orthostatic hypotension (1%), edema
Central nervous system	Headache (25%–38%), somnolence (12%–26%), dizziness (11%–24%), insomnia (15%–24%), nervousness (6%–21%), anxiety (2%–11%), yawning (3%–8%), abnormal dreams (3%–7%), chills (2%–7%), agitation (2%–5%), confusion (2%), abnormal thinking (2%), depersonalization (1%), depression (1%–3%), fever, migraine, amnesia, hypoesthesia, vertigo
Dermatologic	Rash (3%), pruritus (1%), bruising
Endocrine and metabolic	Decreased libido (2%–8%), hypercholesterolemia (5%), increased triglycerides
Gastrointestinal	Nausea (21%–58%), xerostomia (12%–22%), anorexia (8%–17%), constipation (8%–15%), abdominal pain (8%), diarrhea (8%), vomiting (3%–8%), dyspepsia (5%–7%), weight loss (1%–6%), flatulence (3%–4%), taste perversion (2%), appetite increased, belching, weight gain
Genitourinary	Abnormal ejaculation/orgasm (2%–19%), impotence (6%), urinary frequency (3%), urination impaired (2%), urinary retention (1%), metrorrhagia, prostatic disorder, vaginitis
Miscellaneous	Diaphoresis (7%–19%), infection (6%), flu-like syndrome (2%), trauma (2%)
Neuromuscular and skeletal	Weakness (8%–19%), tremor (1%–10%), hypertonia (3%), paresthesia (3%), twitching (3%), arthralgia, neck pain, trismus
Ocular	Accommodation abnormal (6%–9%), abnormal or blurred vision (4%–6%), mydriasis (2%)
Otic	Tinnitus (2%)
Respiratory	Pharyngitis (7%), sinusitis (2%), bronchitis, cough increased, dyspnea

(continued on next page)

Table 6
(continued)

Pristiq	
Cardiovascular	Orthostatic hypotension (8%), syncope (<2%), tachycardia (<2%)
Central nervous system	Dizziness (10%–13%), insomnia (9%–12%), somnolence (≤9%), fatigue (7%), anxiety (3%–5%), abnormal dreams (2%–3%)
Dermatologic	Hyperhidrosis (10%–11%), Alopecia (<2%), angioedema (<2%), photosensitivity reaction (<2%), rash (<2%)
Endocrine and metabolic	Libido decreased (males 4%–5%), cholesterol (increased by ≥50 mg/dL and ≥261 mg/dL: 3%–4%), anorgasmia (females 1%; males ≤3%), prolactin increased (<2%), hot flushes (1%)
Gastrointestinal	Nausea (22%–26%), xerostomia (11%–17%), constipation (9%), appetite decreased (5%–8%), vomiting (≤4%), weight gain (<2%)
Genitourinary	Urinary retention (<2%)
Hepatic	Liver function tests abnormal (<2%)
Neuromuscular and skeletal	Tremor (≤3%), dystonia (<2%), stiffness (<2%), weakness (<2%)
Ocular	Blurred vision (3%–4%), mydriasis (2%)
Savella	
Cardiovascular	Orthostatic hypotension (5%), syncope (<5%), tachycardia (<5%)
Central nervous system	Dizziness (12%), insomnia (12%), somnolence (≤5%), fatigue (5%), anxiety (3%)
Dermatologic	Hyperhidrosis (10%–11%), Alopecia (<2%), angioedema (<2%), photosensitivity reaction (<2%), rash (<2%)
Endocrine and metabolic	Libido decreased (males 4%–5%), cholesterol (increased by ≥50 mg/dL and ≥261 mg/dL: 3%–4%), anorgasmia (females 1%; males ≤3%), prolactin increased (<2%), hot flushes (1%)
Gastrointestinal	Nausea (6% stop drug because of this), xerostomia (10%), constipation (10%), appetite decreased (8%–10%), vomiting (3%–5%), weight gain or loss (3%–5%)
Genitourinary	Urinary retention (<2%)
Hepatic	Liver function tests abnormal (<2%)
Neuromuscular and skeletal	Tremor (≤3%), dystonia (<2%), stiffness (<2%), weakness (<2%)
Ocular	Blurred vision (3%–4%), mydriasis (2%)

References:
Cymbalta:
1. Duloxetine: Drug information. UpToDate. Available at: http://www.uptodateonline.com.
2. Cymbalta [package insert]. Indianapolis, IN: Eli Lilly and Company; 2012.
Effexor:
3. Venlafaxine: Drug information. UpToDate. Available at: http://www.uptodateonline.com.
Serotonin syndrome or neuroleptic malignant syndrome (NMS)-like reactions may occur with SNRIs and SSRIs. The risk of this is dose dependent and is greatly increased by concomitant use of serotonergic drugs (including triptans) or drugs that impair the metabolism of serotonin; this includes monoamine oxidase inhibitors (MAOIs), antipsychotics, or other dopamine antagonists.
Signs of serotonin syndrome include mental status changes (eg, confusion, agitation, hallucinations), autonomic instability (eg, tachycardia, hyperthermia), neuromuscular changes (eg, hyperreflexia, incoordination) and gastrointestinal symptoms (eg, nausea, vomiting, diarrhea). In its most severe form serotonin syndrome may resemble neuroleptic malignant syndrome. Signs of this include hyperthermia and muscle rigidity.
4. Desvenlafaxine: Drug information. UpToDate. Available at: http://www.uptodateonline.com.
5. Pristiq [package insert]. Philadelphia, PA: Pfizer; 2013.
6. Available at: http://www.fda.gov/Safety/MedWatch/Safety.

Table 7
Major adverse effects and relative risks of oral steroids

	Prednisone, Prednisolone
Cardiovascular	Hypertension, congestive heart failure in susceptible patients Body fluid retention—prednisolone
Central nervous system	Headache
Dermatologic	Impaired wound healing, bruising, thin fragile skin Acne, ecchymosis, superinfection—prednisolone
Endocrine, metabolic	Body fluid retention, impaired glucose tolerance, increased appetite, weight gain, Cushing syndrome, adrenal suppression Children: growth suppression Lipid abnormalities—prednisolone
Gastrointestinal	Abdominal distention, pancreatitis
Immunologic	Immune suppression (prolonged use)
Musculoskeletal	Osteoporosis, tendon rupture, steroid myopathy
Ocular	Intraocular pressure increased, glaucoma
Psychiatric	Disturbance in mood, irritability, euphoria, other psychiatric reactions (frequency estimated to be 5%–6% in adults)
	Dexamethasone, Hydrocortisone
Cardiovascular	Hypertension
Dermatologic	Atrophic condition of skin, impaired wound healing
Endocrine, metabolic	Cushing syndrome Children: growth suppression
Immunologic	Immune suppression
Musculoskeletal	Osteoporosis
Ocular	Cataract (5%), raised intraocular pressure (25%)
Psychiatric	Depression, euphoria
Respiratory	Pulmonary tuberculosis
	Fludrocortisone, Methylprednisolone – Common
Cardiovascular	Edema
Dermatologic	Bruising, impaired wound healing, petechiae, rash, urticaria
Endocrine, metabolic	Abnormal electrolytes, hypokalemia, hyperglycemia, weight gain due to sodium and water retention Children: decreased body growth
Gastrointestinal	Abdominal distention, peptic ulcer disease
Musculoskeletal	Drug-induced myopathy, muscle weakness
Neurologic	Headache, vertigo
Renal	Glycosuria
Reproductive	Irregular periods

(continued on next page)

Table 7 (continued)	
Budesonide—Oral	
Cardiovascular	Edema (<7%)
	Chest pain, facial edema, tachycardia (<5%)
Central nervous system	Headache (21%), dizziness (<7%), mood swings (7%)
Dermatologic	Bruising (5%–15%), acne (<15%), hirsutism (5%), alopecia (<5%)
Gastrointestinal	Nausea (11%), diarrhea (10%)
Respiratory	Infection (11%), sinusitis (8%)
Miscellaneous	Fat redistribution (moon face, buffalo hump) (3%–11%)

References:
1. Budesonide: Drug information. UpToDate. Available at: http://www.uptodateonline.com.
2. Dexamethasone: Drug information. UpToDate. Available at: http://www.uptodateonline.com.
3. Fludrocortisone: Drug information. UpToDate. Available at: http://www.uptodateonline.com.
4. Hydrocortisone: Drug information. UpToDate. Available at: http://www.uptodateonline.com.
5. Methylprednisolone: Drug information. UpToDate. Available at: http://www.uptodateonline.com.
6. Micromedex Healthcare Series [Internet database]. Greenwood Village (CO): Thomson Healthcare. Updated periodically.
7. Prednisolone: Drug information. UpToDate. Available at: http://www.uptodateonline.com.
8. Prednisolone Summary of Product Characteristics, Cyprus: Chelonia Healthcare Limited. 2008. Available at: http://www.drugs.com/uk/pdf/leaflet/160279.pdf. Accessed September 26, 2013.
9. Prednisone: Drug information. UpToDate. Available at: http://www.uptodateonline.com.
[a] <1%: Venous thrombosis (life-threatening) for all.

REFERENCES

1. Jensen MP, Abresch RT, Carter GT, et al. Chronic pain in persons with neuromuscular disorders. Arch Phys Med Rehabil 2005;86(6):1155–63.
2. Molton I, Jensen MP, Ehde DM, et al. Coping with chronic pain among younger, middle-aged, and older adults living with neurologic injury and disease: a role for experiential wisdom. J Aging Health 2008;20:972–96.
3. Fu H, Price KL, Nilsson ME, et al. Identifying potential adverse events dose-response relationships via bayesian indirect and mixed treatment comparison models. J Biopharm Stat 2013;23(1):26–42.
4. Schnipper JL, Kirwin JL, Cotugno MC, et al. Role of pharmacist counseling in preventing adverse drug events after hospitalization. Arch Intern Med 2006;166(5):565–71.
5. Altavela JL, Jones MK, Ritter M. A prospective trial of a clinical pharmacy intervention in a primary care practice in a capitated payment system. J Manag Care Pharm 2008;14(9):831–43.
6. Ross S, Ryan C, Duncan EM, et al. Perceived causes of prescribing errors by junior doctors in hospital inpatients: a study from the PROTECT programme. BMJ Qual Saf 2013;22(2):97–102.
7. Kalthoff S, Winkler A, Freiberg N, et al. Gender matters: Estrogen receptor alpha (ERα) and histone deacetylase (HDAC) 1 and 2 control the gender-specific transcriptional regulation of human uridine diphosphate glucuronosyltransferases genes (UGT1A). J Hepatol 2013;59(4):797–804.
8. Wiesenfeld-Hallin Z. Sex differences in pain perception. Gend Med 2005;2(3):137–45.
9. Wielage R, Bansal M, Wilson K, et al. Cost-effectiveness of duloxetine in chronic low back pain: a Quebec societal perspective. Spine 2013;38(11):936–46.
10. Smith MT, Moore BJ. Pregabalin for the treatment of fibromyalgia. Expert Opin Pharmacother 2012;13(10):1527–33.

Special Article
Epidural Steroid Injections for Radicular Lumbosacral Pain: A Systematic Review

Epidural Steroid Injections for Radicular Lumbosacral Pain: A Systematic Review

Tatyana A. Shamliyan, MD, MS[a],*, J. Bart Staal, PhD[b],
David Goldmann, MD[a], Megan Sands-Lincoln, MPH, PhD[a]

KEYWORDS

- Epidural injection • Steroids • Lumbosacral radicular syndrome • Low back pain

KEY POINTS

- A systematic review of the literature suggests that off-label epidural steroid injections provide short-term but not long-term (>12 weeks) relief of leg pain and improvement in function in patients with benign lumbosacral radicular syndrome. The clinical importance of steroid benefits is small (<10 points improvement on a 100-point scale).
- Different steroids are similarly effective in reducing pain and disability in the short term but do not do so in a dose-responsive manner.
- Injection of steroids is no more effective than injection of local anesthetics alone.
- Postprocedural complications are uncommon, but the risk of contamination and serious infections is very high.
- Evidence is insufficient to posit an association between short-term effectiveness of steroid injections and differing patient characteristics.
- Based on high-quality evidence, routine use of off-label epidural steroid injections in adults with benign radicular lumbosacral pain is not recommended.

INTRODUCTION

The prevalence of acute and chronic low back pain in adults has increased more than 100% in the last decade and continues to increase dramatically in the aging population, affecting both men and women in all ethnic groups.[1] Low back pain contributes to

This work was supported by Elsevier Clinical Solutions, Evidence-Based Medicine Center. The authors have nothing to disclose. Drs T.A. Shamliyan, D. Goldmann, and M. Sands-Lincoln are Elsevier employees.
[a] Elsevier Clinical Solutions, Evidence-Based Medicine Center, Philadelphia, PA, USA;
[b] Scientific Institute for Quality of Healthcare (IQ Healthcare), Radboud University Nijmegen Medical Centre, Nijmegen, The Netherlands
* Corresponding author. Evidence-Based Medicine Center, Elsevier, 1600 John Fitzgerald Kennedy Boulevard, Philadelphia, PA 19103.
E-mail address: t.shamliyan@elsevier.com

lost productivity, disability, and substantial health care expenditures,[2] and is the leading determinant of years lived with disability.[3]

The goals of conservative treatment of chronic low back pain (pain persisting for >12 weeks)[4] are to decrease pain, improve function, reduce opioid use, and obviate spinal surgery.[5] Most available clinical guidelines do not recommend routine use of invasive treatments, including epidural steroid injections, for the management of chronic low back pain.[6]

However, many clinicians do not adhere to these guidelines.[7] The Office of Inspector General (OIG) of the United States Department of Health and Human Services concluded that more than 30% of epidural injections were inappropriate, and resulted in $45 million of improper Medicare payments, and an additional $23 million in improper facility payments.[8] Lack of adherence to guideline recommendations among generalist physicians may relate to difficulties in communicating to patients the benefits and harms of available treatments for low back pain.[9]

Many studies, including systematic reviews,[10–16] suffer from inconsistent methodology and provide conflicting conclusions and recommendations about the benefits and harms of epidural treatments, making clinical decisions even more difficult. Individual randomized studies[17–29] use various definitions of low back pain, evaluate different steroid administration routes and doses, and provide inconsistent measures of treatment success. Therefore, this article aims to provide a comprehensive overview of currently available reviews and primary epidemiologic studies to inform evidence-based clinical decision making in the treatment of benign chronic low back pain.

METHODS

The authors formulated the following clinical questions as the basis for this overview. (1) What are the short-term and the long-term efficacy and safety of epidural steroid injections in the treatment of chronic radicular lumbosacral pain in community-dwelling adults? (2) What patient characteristics may modify treatment benefits and harms?

The target population was defined as community-dwelling adults age 18 and older with benign radicular lumbosacral pain lasting more than 12 weeks.[4,30] Lumbosacral radicular syndrome was defined as radiculopathy, nerve root compromise, nerve root compression, disc herniation, radiculitis, nerve root pain, or nerve root entrapment.[31,32] This review relied on diagnostic methods provided by the authors of the original studies. It was determined whether the following factors modified the effects of treatment: patient age, gender, ethnicity, socioeconomic status, duration of pain, and prior response to analgesics; and comorbidities including obesity, osteoporosis, and history of spinal trauma, diabetes, or arterial hypertension.

Eligible interventions included off-label epidural steroid injections administered with or without fluoroscopic guidance. The effects of different routes of steroid administration (eg, caudal, transforaminal, or interlaminar) and different steroid formulations and doses (Appendix 1 Tables 1 and 2; available at www.pmr.theclinics.com) were examined as well as the frequency of injections if provided by the investigators. Comparators included placebo, epidural injection of anesthetics, and nonpharmacologic treatments including physical therapy or acupuncture/acupressure.

Outcomes included pain, global symptom relief, functional improvement and reduction in disability, patient perception of improvement, return to work, use of opioid and nonopioid analgesia, need for surgery, and quality of life. Outcomes at both short-term and long-term (>12 weeks) follow-up were examined. Minimum clinically important improvement in outcomes was defined as a greater than 50% reduction in pain or disability scores.[32,33]

Also examined were the adverse effects of treatment related to epidural technique (eg, dural puncture, hematoma or infections) and those related to the pharmacologic effects of the injected drugs (eg, weight gain, fluid retention, hyperglycemia or hypertension).

Study Inclusion Criteria

Guidelines, systematic reviews, and randomized controlled clinical trials (RCTs) in English, and large observational cohorts to assess treatment safety, were examined.[34,35] Harms were defined as the totality of all possible adverse consequences of an intervention. Investigators sometimes defined harmful effects as unrelated to steroid treatments. Harms were analyzed regardless of how investigators related them to treatments.[36]

Study Exclusion Criteria

Studies of pregnant women and patients with recent trauma, tumors, or cauda equina syndrome were excluded, as were studies of children and nursing home residents, studies of surgical treatments, and studies that did not examine the effect of epidural steroid injections on eligible patient outcomes.

The authors relied on the study design used for indexing of the references in bibliographic databases (Appendix 2; available at www.pmr.theclincs.com). However, clinical reviews that did not meet systematic review definitions were excluded regardless of indexing.

Search Strategy

In accordance with a protocol developed a priori (registration number CRD42014007011),[37] all relevant articles published in English up to January 10, 2014, in PubMed, Embase, Science Direct, and the Cochrane Library (see Appendix 2 for the exact search strings) were identified. To identify unpublished data, a search was made of the trial registry clinicaltrials.gov. The bibliographies of identified articles were scanned, and study investigators were contacted for additional publications. A separate search for relevant cost-effectiveness studies was conducted.

Two authors performed initial eligibility determination for the studies, and all co-authors contributed to resolving differences. Information was abstracted about study population, interventions, comparators, and outcomes. Minimum datasets (eg, number of the subjects in treatment groups and events) were abstracted to estimate absolute risk difference, relative risk, and number needed to treat for categorical variables.[38] Means and standard deviations of continuous variables were abstracted to calculate standardized mean differences, odds ratios, and numbers needed to treat, assuming a 25% control group rate of improvement in pain or function.[38] Two co-authors cross-checked abstracted data with the texts of the original articles.

Quality Assessment of the Studies

This overview used the Assessment of Multiple Systematic Reviews (AMSTAR) scale for systematic reviews,[39] the Appraisal of Guidelines for Research and Evaluation (AGREE II) scale for clinical guidelines,[40] the Cochrane risk of bias tool for randomized trials,[41] and the risk of bias tool for nonrandomized studies from the Agency for Healthcare Research and Quality.[42] A low risk of bias was assumed when RCTs met all the risk of bias criteria, a medium risk of bias if at least 1 of the risk-of-bias criteria was not met, and a high risk of bias if 2 or more risk-of-bias criteria were not met.[43] An unknown risk of bias was assigned for the studies with poorly reported risk-of-bias criteria.

Synthesis of Evidence

An overview of the reviews was conducted following the framework of the Cochrane collaboration.[38] Although no meta-analysis was performed, the authors calculated absolute risk difference, number needed to treat, and the number of attributable events per 1000 treated based on data from the published randomized trials, using Meta-Analyst software[44] and STATA[45] software. Statistical significance was evaluated at a 95% confidence level. Correction coefficients for zero events were used as a default option in both software programs, and intention to treat was used for evidence synthesis. Superiority of drugs under comparison was hypothesized.[46] This review relied on pooling criteria and heterogeneity statistics from published meta-analyses, and assessed reporting bias following the recommendations of the Agency for Healthcare Research and Quality.[47]

To examine the role of patient characteristics, a search was undertaken for subgroup analyses by patient demographics, pain type, prior treatment response, and comorbidities in systematic reviews and randomized trials, including significant interaction effects.[38]

Quality Assessment of the Body of Evidence

The authors assigned quality of evidence ratings as high, moderate, low, or very low, according to risk of bias in the body of evidence, directness of comparisons,[48] precision and consistency in treatment effects, and the evidence of reporting bias, using GRADE methodology.[49–52]

Treatment effect estimates were defined as precise when pooled estimates had reasonably narrow 95% confidence intervals and pooled sample size was greater than 300.[53] Justification of the sample size was not included in grading of the evidence, nor were post hoc statistical power analyses conducted.

In assessing the quality of evidence in all studies, the authors looked for a dose-response association, the strength of association, and evidence of any reporting bias. The strength of the association was evaluated, defining a priori a large effect when the relative risk was greater than 2 and a very large effect when the relative risk was greater than 5.[38] A small treatment effect was construed when the relative risk was significant but less than 2. For standardized continuous measures of pain and function, the magnitude of the effect was defined as small, moderate, and large, corresponding to standardized mean differences in standard deviation units of 0 to 0.5, 0.5 to 0.8, and greater than 0.8, respectively.[54]

A high quality of evidence was assigned to well-designed RCTs with consistent findings. The quality of evidence was downgraded to moderate if at least 1 of 4 strength-of-evidence criteria was not met; for example, moderate quality of evidence was assigned if there was a medium risk of bias in the body of evidence or if the results were not consistent or precise. The quality of evidence was downgraded to low if 2 or more criteria were not met.

A low quality of evidence was assigned to nonrandomized studies, and upgraded for the rating if there was a strong or dose-response association. Evidence was defined as insufficient when no studies provided valid information about treatment effects. This approach was applied regardless of whether the results were statistically significant.

Strength of Recommendations

Strength of the recommendations was assigned based on overall quality of evidence, balances between benefits and harms, and cost, using GRADE methodology.[50,55,56]

RESULTS

A total of 344 references were retrieved, which included 79 references for this review (**Fig. 1**). Eighteen systematic reviews were identified that synthesized data from 65 RCTs (Appendix 1 Table 3). Eleven publications of RCTs that were omitted from the reviews or published after the reviews were identified (Appendix 1 Table 4). Excluded studies are referenced in Appendix 2 to assure transparency in studies selection. There was evidence of reporting bias, because only 3 of 7 eligible studies registered

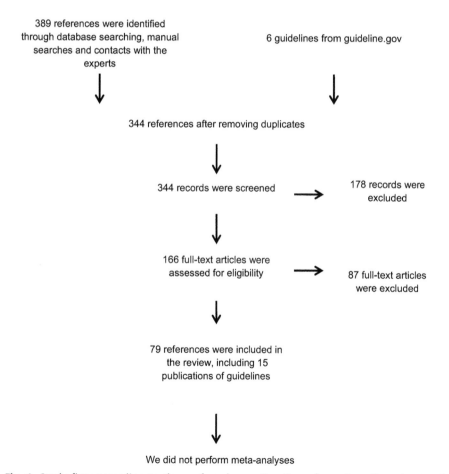

Fig. 1. Study flow according to the preferred reporting items for systematic reviews and meta-analyses. (*From* Liberati A, Altman DG, Tetzlaff J, et al. The PRISMA statement for reporting systematic reviews and meta-analyses of studies that evaluate health care interventions: explanation and elaboration. J Clin Epidemiol 2009;62(10):e1–34.)

in clinicaltrials.gov had been published. The reporting quality of the primary studies was generally poor, with unclear allocation concealment and incomplete reporting of treatment-effect means with variance that precluded comprehensive meta-analyses of data pertaining to all primary and secondary outcomes.

Benefits of Epidural Steroids

No consistent evidence was found for clinically important sustained benefits from epidural steroids in adults with radicular lumbosacral pain. Primary studies and systematic reviews did not necessarily relate outcomes to exact duration of symptoms or to a success from prior treatments.

Systematic reviews provided conflicting conclusions. The high-quality systematic review by members of the Cochrane Collaboration did not distinguish among interlaminar, caudal, or transforaminal epidural injection techniques for lumbosacral radicular syndrome, and found no clinically important benefits with use of epidural steroids (see Appendix 1 Table 3).[14,57]

By contrast, the reviews authored by members of the American Society of Interventional Pain Physicians (ASIPP) included results from both RCTs and observational studies stratified by injection techniques and type of spinal disorders, and concluded that there is good evidence of short-term and long-term pain reduction and improvement in function with epidural steroids (see Appendix 1 Table 3).[11,15,16,58] These reviews categorized results from individual studies as positive, negative, or statistically insignificant, but failed to address the clinical importance of these categories and did not provide rates of clinically significant improvements in pain and disability, number needed to treat, or attributable events for clinical decision making. The primary studies and the reviews reported multiple outcomes at different short-term and long-term time points without considering statistical multiple hypothesis testing.

The reviews conducted by evidence-based practice centers concluded that there are short-term but not long-term benefits with epidural steroids in patients with sciatica (see Appendix 1 Table 3).[31,32,59–63] The authors of one recent high-quality review[31,32] converted continuous measurements of pain and disability to common scales from 0 (no pain or disability) to 100 (worst possible pain or disability), and reported weighted means of short-term pain reduction of 6% and disability of 3%. These small statistically significant effects have questionable clinical importance.

Injection Technique

No single specific injection technique improved back pain. A statistically significant short-term reduction in leg pain was reported with caudal injection, but not with interlaminar or transforaminal approaches.[32] A statistically significant reduction in long-term leg pain was reported with transforaminal injection, but not with caudal or interlaminar approaches.[32] A statistically significant reduction in short-term disability was reported with caudal injection, but not with interlaminar or transforaminal approaches.[32]

Steroid Dose

Systematic reviews found no evidence to suggest that a series of epidural injections was any more effective than a single injection (see Appendix 1 Table 3).[13] Individual RCTs found no evidence of improvement in steroid benefits with increasing dose (see Appendix 1 Table 4).[64,65]

Comparative Effectiveness of Epidural Steroids

Individual RCTs found no consistent evidence of superior efficacy of one steroid over the others (see Appendix 1 Table 4).[66,67] Moreover, injection of anesthetic alone resulted in reduction in pain and disability similar to that derived from a combination of steroids with anesthetic (see Appendix 1 Table 4).[23,24,68]

Epidural Steroid Safety

Harms associated with epidural steroid injections were rarely reported in individual RCTs and systematic reviews (Appendix 1 Table 5). One large observational study of more than 10,000 epidural injections reported that crude rates of selected postsurgical complications were rare (see Appendix 1 Table 5).[69] Other reviews reported a rate of dural puncture frequency between 2% and 5%, and rare cases of postdural puncture syndrome.[16] One recent systematic review analyzed reports from the Centers for Disease Control and Prevention and the Food and Drug Administration as well as all published evidence of contaminated epidural steroid injections, and concluded that these substantial harms outweighed any short-term benefits.[70] Several case series published during the last decade reported that development of abscesses after epidural steroids sometimes resulted in paraplegia and death.[71] Primary studies including RCTs and observational studies did not measure all well-known steroid-related adverse effects (Appendix 1 Table 6).

Cost-Effectiveness

Conclusions about cost-effectiveness of epidural steroid injections are inconsistent.[72,73] A recent analysis concluded that caudal epidural steroid injections are cost-effective when compared with combined conservative and invasive treatments.[2]

Quality of the Evidence

High-quality evidence suggests that epidural steroid injections provide short-term but not long-term leg-pain relief and improvement in function for patients with lumbosacral radicular syndrome when compared with placebo (**Fig. 2**). The clinical importance of these small changes in pain and disability is questionable. High-quality evidence also suggests that caudal corticosteroid injections are better than placebo in reducing leg pain at short-term but not long-term follow-up (Appendix 1 Table 7, **Tables 1–4**). Low-quality evidence suggests that caudal corticosteroid injections result in short-term improvement in disability. Very low-quality evidence suggests that transforaminal corticosteroid injections are better than placebo in reducing leg pain at long-term follow-up, with no improvement in disability (see Appendix 1 Table 7, **Tables 1–4**). Low-quality evidence supports similar effectiveness of different steroids on pain and disability.[66,67] Low-quality evidence finds no dose-response association between steroid doses and improvement in outcomes.[64,65]

Moderate-quality evidence suggests that epidural steroids are not better than anesthetics in improving pain or disability or in reducing the need for surgery (**Fig. 3**). High-quality evidence indicates that short-term postprocedural complications are uncommon but that the risks of contamination and serious infections are very high (see Appendix 1 Table 5, **Table 4**).

Evidence of an association between patient characteristics and steroid effects was insufficient.

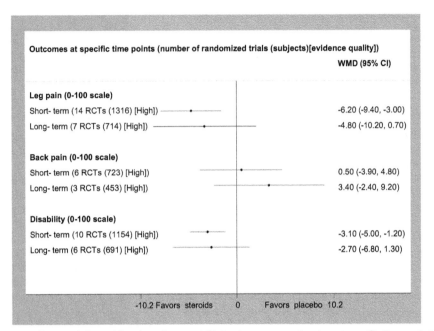

Fig. 2. Efficacy of the epidural corticosteroid injections versus placebo at specific time points in adults with sciatica (results from systematic review). Short term: less than 12 weeks. Long term: 12 weeks or more. CI, confidence interval; RCT, randomized controlled trial; WMD, weighted mean difference. (*Data from* Pinto RZ, Maher CG, Ferreira ML, et al. Epidural corticosteroid injections in the management of sciatica: a systematic review and meta-analysis. Ann Intern Med 2012;157(12):865–77.)

DISCUSSION

This review found no evidence of sustained, clinically important improvement in back pain or disability, and no reduction in need for surgery or opioid use after epidural steroid injections in adults with chronic low back pain. Current evidence suggests that epidural steroid injections provide some short-term improvement in radicular lumbosacral pain and disability. This conclusion is based on statistically significant differences that are likely not clinically significant in most treated patients. These results are consistent with recommendations in most published guidelines on the treatment of radicular low back pain. Most of these guidelines do not mention epidural steroids or recommend them (Appendix 1 Table 8). Those that do comment on the uneven quality of evidence relating to the 3 injection techniques (caudal, interlaminar, and transforaminal approaches), and provide different recommendations for symptoms of differing etiology including disc herniation and/or radiculitis, discogenic pain without disc herniation, and spinal stenosis. Guidelines from the ASIPP[11,74–76] provide a stronger recommendation in favor of epidural steroid use; however, the guideline development process did not require transparent peer review by all societies concerned with treatment of adults with radicular lumbosacral pain. The British Pain Society[77] guideline recommends that only patients with severe radicular pain lasting more than 2 weeks should be referred to a specialist who can consider magnetic resonance imaging–guided steroid injections or surgery.

The North America Spine Society[78] guideline recommends fluoroscopy-guided epidural steroid injections for short-term symptom relief in patients with neurogenic

Table 1
Effects of epidural corticosteroid injections on pain (results from systematic reviews)

Outcome	Type of Pain[a]	Effect Measure (95% CI) NNT	OR[b] (95% CI)	No. of RCTs (Subjects) Quality of Evidence	Comments
Intervention: Epidural Corticosteroid Injection vs Placebo (All Techniques Combined)					
Outcome: Back pain at short-term follow-up[32]	Sciatica[c]	WMD 0.5 (−3.9 to 4.8); NNT = NS	OR 0.8–1.2 (NS)	6 RCTs (723) High	No difference
Outcome: Back pain at long-term follow-up[32]	Sciatica	WMD 3.4 (−2.4 to 9.2); NNT = NS	OR 1.1 (NS)	3 RCTs (453) High	No difference
Outcome: Leg pain at short-term follow-up[32]	Sciatica	WMD −6.2 (−9.4 to −3.0); NNT = 10	OR 0.5 (0.4; 0.8)	14 RCTs (1316) High	Favors epidural corticosteroid injection
Outcome: Leg pain at long-term follow-up[32]	Sciatica	WMD −4.8 (−10.2 to 0.7); NNT = NS	OR 0.6 (0.3; 1.0)	7 RCTs (714) High	No difference
Intervention: Epidural Caudal Corticosteroid Injection vs Placebo					
Outcome: Leg pain at short-term follow-up	Sciatica	SMD −0.32 (−0.61; −0.04); NNT = 11	OR 0.6 (0.3; 0.9)	2 RCTs (192) High	Favors epidural corticosteroid injection
Outcome: Leg pain at long-term follow-up[32]	Sciatica	SMD −0.30 (−0.58; −0.01); NNT = 12	OR 0.6 (0.3; 1.0)	2 RCTs (187) Moderate	No difference
Intervention: Epidural Interlaminar Corticosteroid Injection vs Placebo					
Outcome: Leg pain at short-term follow-up[32]	Sciatica	SMD −0.40 (−0.80; 0.00); NNT = 9	OR 0.5 (0.2; 1.0)	6 RCTs (613) Moderate	No difference
Outcome: Leg pain at long-term follow-up[32]	Sciatica	SMD −0.16 (−0.71; 0.39); NNT = 20	OR 0.7 (0.3; 2.0)	2 RCTs (298) High	No difference

(continued on next page)

Table 1
(continued)

Outcome	Type of Pain[a]	Effect Measure (95% CI) NNT	OR[b] (95% CI)	No. of RCTs (Subjects) Quality of Evidence	Comments
Intervention: Epidural Transforaminal Corticosteroid Injection vs Placebo					
Outcome: Leg pain at short-term follow-up[32]	Sciatica	SMD −0.24 (−0.52; 0.05); NNT = 14	OR 0.6 (0.4; 1.1)	3 RCTs (270) Moderate	No difference
Outcome: Leg pain at long-term follow-up[32]	Sciatica	SMD −0.93 (−1.52; −0.33); NNT = 5	OR 0.2 (0.1; 0.6)	1 RCT (48) Very low	Favors epidural transforaminal corticosteroid injection
Intervention: Epidural Corticosteroid Injections (All Techniques Combined) vs Control					
Outcome: Any pain at 12 mo[59]	Low back pain	SMD −0.12 (−0.27; 0.04); NNT = 27	0.8 (0.6; 1.1)	9 RCTs (683) Moderate	No difference

Abbreviations: CI, confidence interval; NNT, number needed to treat; NS, not statistically significant; OR, odds ratio; RCT, randomized controlled trial; SMD, standardized mean difference; WMD, weighted mean difference.
[a] In this table and hereafter, patient subpopulations were defined according to the definitions provided in the studies.
[b] In this table and hereafter, ORs were calculated based on WMD.
[c] Radiculopathy, nerve root compromise, nerve root compression, lumbosacral radicular syndrome, disc herniation, radiculitis, nerve root pain, and nerve root entrapment.

Table 2
Effects of epidural corticosteroid injections on disability (results from systematic reviews)

Outcomes	Type of Pain	Effect Measure (95% CI) NNT	OR (95% CI)	No of RCTs (Subjects) Quality of Evidence	Comments
Intervention: Epidural Corticosteroid Injection vs Placebo (All Techniques Combined)					
Outcome: Disability at short-term at follow-up[32]	Sciatica[a]	WMD −3.1 (−5.0 to −1.2); NNT = 16	OR 0.7 (0.5; 0.9)	10 RCTs (1154) High	Favors epidural corticosteroid injection
Outcome: Disability at long-term at follow-up[32]	Sciatica	WMD −2.7 (−6.8 to 1.3); NNT = NS	OR 0.7 (0.4; 1.1)	6 RCTs (691) High	No difference
Intervention: Epidural Caudal Corticosteroid Injection vs Placebo					
Outcome: Disability at short-term at follow-up[32]	Sciatica	SMD −0.31 (−0.60; −0.03); NNT = 11	OR 0.6 (0.3; 0.9)	2 RCTs (192) Low	Favors epidural caudal corticosteroid injection
Intervention: Epidural Interlaminar Corticosteroid Injection vs Placebo					
Outcome: Disability at short-term at follow-up[32]	Sciatica	SMD −0.19 (−0.39; 0.02); NNT = 17	OR 0.7 (0.5; 1.0)	3 RCTs (383) Low	No difference
Intervention: Epidural Transforaminal Corticosteroid Injection vs Placebo					
Outcome: Disability at short-term at follow-up[32]	Sciatica	SMD −0.12 (−0.39; 0.16); NNT = NS	OR 0.8 (0.5; 1.3)	2 RCTs (205) Low	No difference
Intervention: Epidural Corticosteroid Injections (All Techniques Combined) vs Control					
Outcome: Disability at 12 mo[59]	Low back pain	SMD 0.09 (−0.35; 0.54); NNT = NS	1.2 (0.5; 2.6)	9 RCTs (843) Moderate	No difference

[a] Radiculopathy, nerve root compromise, nerve root compression, lumbosacral radicular syndrome, disc herniation, radiculitis, nerve root pain, and nerve root entrapment.

Table 3
Effects of various techniques of epidural corticosteroid injections on need for surgery (results from systematic reviews)

Comparisons	Type of Pain	ARD (95% CI) NNT	Relative Risk (95% CI)	No. of RCTs (Subjects) Evidence Quality	Comments
Caudal steroids vs control[59]	Low back pain	0.00 (−0.07; 0.07) NNT = NS	0.8 (0.4; 1.7)	4 RCTs (323) Moderate	No differences
Interlaminar steroids vs control[59]	Low back pain	0.01 (−0.05; 0.07) NNT = NS	1.1 (0.8; 1.4)	7 RCTs (682) Moderate	
Transforaminal steroids vs control[59]	Low back pain	0.00 (−0.08; 0.07) NNT = NS	1.1 (0.7; 1.5)	7 RCTs (456) Moderate	
Epidural steroids vs control[59]	Low back pain	0.00 (−0.03; 0.04) NNT = NS	1.0 (0.9; 1.3)	18 RCTs (1497) Moderate	

claudication or radiculopathy. The American College of Physicians and the American Pain Society[4,60] concluded that epidural steroids are potential treatment options in cases of prolapsed lumbar disc with persistent radicular symptoms not responding to noninvasive therapy.

Individualized treatment recommendations in the guidelines are largely based on expert opinion, as no well-designed RCTs demonstrate sustained clinically important benefits from epidural steroids for specific patient populations. For informing individualized treatment decisions, the evidence is insufficient in clarifying differences in steroid effects by patient characteristics including demographics, causes of back pain, and comorbidities. Evidence is also insufficient to conclude that epidural steroids have any salutary effect on patients' quality of life.

Limitations of this work include the fact that the authors relied on published evidence and did not contact principal investigators for additional information about study methodology and unreported outcomes. Treatment effects from published randomized controlled trials and one meta-analysis were recalculated. Suboptimal quality of reporting in primary studies precluded comprehensive meta-analysis of all examined outcomes.

Implications for Future Research

Future research should combine patient-level data from all published and unpublished randomized trials, categorize treatment effect by clinical importance, and provide the number needed to treat to explore clinically meaningful improvement in patient subpopulations by demographics, prior treatment response, spinal pathology, and comorbidities. Patient registries would provide additional insight into long-term safety and in to the association between quality of care rendered by health care providers and meaningful patient outcomes.

Implications for Clinical Practice

In concordance with some current guidelines, clinicians perform epidural injections in increasing numbers of patients.[79,80] Patient preferences for choosing invasive treatments for low back pain remain unclear. Based on this analysis, the authors conclude

Table 4
Harms of epidural corticosteroid injections

Harm Definitions	Incidence of Harms	Relative Incidence Rate	Studies	Evidence Quality	Comments
Intra- and short-term postsurgical complications	No differences	No differences	5 RCTs (429)[22–25,27,28,65,66,68]	Low	No difference
Serious adverse effects from contaminated epidural steroids injections	>14,000 patients were exposed to contaminated steroids, >337 developed meningitis, and 25 died of aspergillosis	Substantial increase in risk of serious harms associated with epidural steroids injections	Systematic review, 43 references to the CDC and FDA reports and observational studies[16,70]	High	Epidural steroid injections were associated with substantial risk of infectious contaminations and patient harms
Epidural abscess	Death and paraplegia were reported in patients with abscesses after epidural steroid injections	No control	11 noncontrolled case series and case reports[71]	Very low	Multiple cases of abscesses after epidural steroid injections were published in the last several decades

Abbreviations: CDC, Centers for Disease Control and Prevention; FDA, Food and Drug Administration.

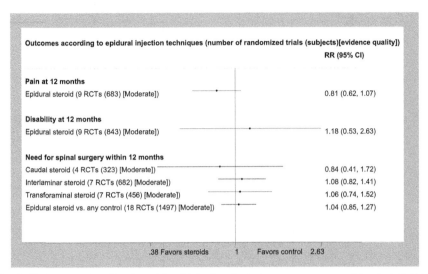

Fig. 3. Outcomes according to epidural injection techniques versus any epidural control injections in adults with chronic low back pain (results from systematic review). RR, relative risk. (*Data from* Choi HJ, Hahn S, Kim CH, et al. Epidural steroid injection therapy for low back pain: a meta-analysis. Int J Technol Assess Health Care 2013;29(3):244–53.)

that the evidence does not support routine use of epidural steroid injections for chronic radicular lumbosacral pain. Patients should be informed that benefit from steroid injection is likely to be short-lived and may carry the risk of contamination. If chosen for treatment, epidural injections should be administered in specialized centers by trained physicians, prioritizing patient safety and taking all precautions to eliminate the risk of contamination.[81,82] However, whenever possible, guideline-recommended conservative treatment options should be offered first in adults with chronic low back pain.[4,30,33]

REFERENCES

1. Freburger JK, Holmes GM, Agans RP, et al. The rising prevalence of chronic low back pain. Arch Intern Med 2009;169(3):251–8.
2. Manchikanti L, Benyamin RM, Falco FJ, et al. Recommendations of the Medicare Payment Advisory Commission (MEDPAC) on the health care delivery system: the impact on interventional pain management in 2014 and beyond. Pain Physician 2013;16(5):419–40.
3. Vos T, Flaxman AD, Naghavi M, et al. Years lived with disability (YLDs) for 1160 sequelae of 289 diseases and injuries 1990-2010: a systematic analysis for the Global Burden of Disease Study 2010. Lancet 2012;380(9859):2163–96.
4. Chou R, Qaseem A, Snow V, et al. Diagnosis and treatment of low back pain: a joint clinical practice guideline from the American College of Physicians and the American Pain Society. Ann Intern Med 2007;147(7):478–91.
5. Dagenais S, Haldeman S. Evidence-based management of low back pain. In: Dagenais S, Haldeman S, editors. Evidence-based management of low back pain. St Louis (MO): Mosby; 2012. p. 1–12.
6. Dagenais S, Tricco AC, Haldeman S. Synthesis of recommendations for the assessment and management of low back pain from recent clinical practice guidelines. Spine J 2010;10(6):514–29.

7. Mafi JN, McCarthy EP, Davis RB, et al. Worsening trends in the management and treatment of back pain. JAMA Intern Med 2013;173(17):1573–81.
8. Levinson DR. Inappropriate Medicare payments for transforaminal epidural injection services. US Department of Health and Human Services Office of Inspector General; 2010. OEI-05-09-00030. Available at: http://oig.hhs.gov/oei/reports/oei-05-09-00030.pdf. Accessed January 22, 2014.
9. Williams CM, Maher CG, Hancock MJ, et al. Low back pain and best practice care: a survey of general practice physicians. Arch Intern Med 2010;170(3):271–7.
10. Koes BW, Scholten RJ, Mens JM, et al. Efficacy of epidural steroid injections for low-back pain and sciatica: a systematic review of randomized clinical trials. Pain 1995;63(3):279–88.
11. Boswell MV, Trescot AM, Datta S, et al. Interventional techniques: evidence-based practice guidelines in the management of chronic spinal pain. Pain Physician 2007;10(1):7–111.
12. Luijsterburg PA, Verhagen AP, Ostelo RW, et al. Effectiveness of conservative treatments for the lumbosacral radicular syndrome: a systematic review. Eur Spine J 2007;16(7):881–99.
13. Novak S, Nemeth WC. The basis for recommending repeating epidural steroid injections for radicular low back pain: a literature review. Arch Phys Med Rehabil 2008;89(3):543–52.
14. Staal JB, De Bie R, De Vet HC, et al. Injection therapy for subacute and chronic low-back pain. Cochrane Database Syst Rev 2008;(3):CD001824.
15. Manchikanti L, Buenaventura RM, Manchikanti KN, et al. Effectiveness of therapeutic lumbar transforaminal epidural steroid injections in managing lumbar spinal pain. Pain Physician 2012;15(3):E199–245.
16. Parr AT, Manchikanti L, Hameed H, et al. Caudal epidural injections in the management of chronic low back pain: a systematic appraisal of the literature. Pain Physician 2012;15(3):159–98.
17. Vad VB, Bhat AL, Lutz GE, et al. Transforaminal epidural steroid injections in lumbosacral radiculopathy: a prospective randomized study. Spine 2002;27(1):11–6.
18. Valat JP, Giraudeau B, Rozenberg S, et al. Epidural corticosteroid injections for sciatica: a randomised, double blind, controlled clinical trial. Ann Rheum Dis 2003;62(7):639–43.
19. Buttermann GR. Treatment of lumbar disc herniation: epidural steroid injection compared with discectomy. A prospective, randomized study. J Bone Joint Surg Am 2004;86-A(4):670–9.
20. Arden NK, Price C, Reading I, et al. A multicentre randomized controlled trial of epidural corticosteroid injections for sciatica: the WEST study. Rheumatology (Oxford) 2005;44(11):1399–406.
21. Manchikanti L, Cash KA, McManus CD, et al. Preliminary results of a randomized, equivalence trial of fluoroscopic caudal epidural injections in managing chronic low back pain: part 1–Discogenic pain without disc herniation or radiculitis. Pain Physician 2008;11(6):785–800.
22. Manchikanti L, Cash KA, McManus CD, et al. Preliminary results of a randomized, double-blind, controlled trial of fluoroscopic lumbar interlaminar epidural injections in managing chronic lumbar discogenic pain without disc herniation or radiculitis. Pain Physician 2010;13(4):E279–92.
23. Manchikanti L, Cash KA, McManus CD, et al. One-year results of a randomized, double-blind, active controlled trial of fluoroscopic caudal epidural injections

with or without steroids in managing chronic discogenic low back pain without disc herniation or radiculitis. Pain Physician 2011;14(1):25–36.

24. Manchikanti L, Cash KA, McManus CD, et al. Lumbar interlaminar epidural injections in central spinal stenosis: preliminary results of a randomized, double-blind, active control trial. Pain Physician 2012;15(1):51–63.

25. Manchikanti L, Cash KA, McManus CD, et al. Fluoroscopic lumbar interlaminar epidural injections in managing chronic lumbar axial or discogenic pain. J Pain Res 2012;5:301–11.

26. Manchikanti L, Singh V, Cash KA, et al. Effect of fluoroscopically guided caudal epidural steroid or local anesthetic injections in the treatment of lumbar disc herniation and radiculitis: a randomized, controlled, double blind trial with a two-year follow-up. Pain Physician 2012;15(4):273–86.

27. Manchikantis L, Cash KA, McManus CD, et al. Results of 2-year follow-up of a randomized, double-blind, controlled trial of fluoroscopic caudal epidural injections in central spinal stenosis. Pain Physician 2012;15(5):371–84.

28. Manchikanti L, Cash KA, McManus CD, et al. A randomized, double-blind, active-controlled trial of fluoroscopic lumbar interlaminar epidural injections in chronic axial or discogenic low back pain: results of 2-year follow-up. Pain Physician 2013;16(5):E491–504.

29. Manchikanti L, Cash KA, Pampati V, et al. A randomized, double-blind, active control trial of fluoroscopic cervical interlaminar epidural injections in chronic pain of cervical disc herniation: results of a 2-year follow-up. Pain Physician 2013;16(5):465–78.

30. Chou R, Atlas SJ, Stanos SP, et al. Nonsurgical interventional therapies for low back pain: a review of the evidence for an American pain society clinical practice guideline. Spine 2009;34(10):1078–93.

31. Pinto RZ, Maher CG, Ferreira ML. Review: epidural corticosteroids reduce short-but not long-term leg pain and disability in sciatica. Ann Intern Med 2013;158(10):JC7.

32. Pinto RZ, Maher CG, Ferreira ML, et al. Epidural corticosteroid injections in the management of sciatica: a systematic review and meta-analysis. Ann Intern Med 2012;157(12):865–77.

33. Chou R, Huffman LH. Medications for acute and chronic low back pain: a review of the evidence for an American Pain Society/American College of Physicians clinical practice guideline. Ann Intern Med 2007;147(7):505–14.

34. Norris S, Atkins D, Bruening W, et al. Selecting observational studies for comparing medical interventions. In: Agency for Healthcare Research and Quality. Methods Guide for Comparative Effectiveness Reviews [posted June 2010]. Rockville, MD. Available at: http://www.effectivehealthcare.ahrq.gov/ehc/products/196/454/MethodsGuideNorris_06042010.pdf.

35. Norris SL, Atkins D, Bruening W, et al. Observational studies in systematic [corrected] reviews of comparative effectiveness: AHRQ and the Effective Health Care Program. J Clin Epidemiol 2011;64(11):1178–86.

36. Chou R, Aronson N, Atkins D, et al. AHRQ series paper 4: assessing harms when comparing medical interventions: AHRQ and the effective health-care program. J Clin Epidemiol 2010;63(5):502–12.

37. Liberati A, Altman DG, Tetzlaff J, et al. The PRISMA statement for reporting systematic reviews and meta-analyses of studies that evaluate health care interventions: explanation and elaboration. J Clin Epidemiol 2009;62(10):e1–34.

38. Higgins J, Green S, editors. Cochrane handbook for systematic reviews of interventions. Version 5.1.0. London: The Cochrane Collaboration; 2011. Cochrane book series.

39. Shea BJ, Hamel C, Wells GA, et al. AMSTAR is a reliable and valid measurement tool to assess the methodological quality of systematic reviews. J Clin Epidemiol 2009;62(10):1013–20.

40. Collaboration A. Development and validation of an international appraisal instrument for assessing the quality of clinical practice guidelines: the AGREE project. Qual Saf Health Care 2003;12(1):18–23.

41. Higgins JP, Altman DG, Gotzsche PC, et al. The Cochrane Collaboration's tool for assessing risk of bias in randomised trials. BMJ 2011;343:d5928.

42. Viswanathan M, Berkman ND, Dryden DM, et al. Assessing Risk of Bias and Confounding in Observational Studies of Interventions or Exposures: Further Development of the RTI Item Bank. Methods Research Report. (Prepared by RTI–UNC Evidence-based Practice Center under Contract No. 290-2007-10056-I). AHRQ Publication No. 13-EHC106-EF. Rockville, MD: Agency for Healthcare Research and Quality; August 2013. Available at: www.effective healthcare.ahrq.gov/reports/final.cfm.

43. Viswanathan M, Ansari MT, Berkman ND, et al. Assessing the risk of bias of individual studies in systematic reviews of health care interventions. Agency for Healthcare Research and Quality Methods Guide for Comparative Effectiveness Reviews. AHRQ Publication No. 12-EHC047-EF; March, 2012. Available at: www.effectivehealthcare.ahrq.gov/.

44. Wallace BC, Schmid CH, Lau J, et al. Meta-Analyst: software for meta-analysis of binary, continuous and diagnostic data. BMC Med Res Methodol 2009;9:80.

45. Egger M, Smith GD, Altman DG. Systematic reviews in health care: meta-analysis in context. 2nd edition. London: BMJ Books; 2001.

46. Treadwell JR, Uhl S, Tipton K, et al. Assessing equivalence and noninferiority. J Clin Epidemiol 2012;65(11):1144–9.

47. Balshem H, Ansari M, Norris S, et al. Finding grey literature evidence and assessing for outcome and analysis reporting biases when comparing medical interventions: AHRQ and the Effective Health Care Program. AHRQ and the Effective Health Care Program Methods Guide for Comparative Effectiveness Reviews. (Prepared by the Oregon Health and Science University and the University of Ottawa Evidence-based Practice Centers under Contract Nos. 290-2007-10057-I and 290-2007-10059-I) (AHRQ Publication No. 13(14)-EHC096-EF). Rockville (MD): Agency for Healthcare Research and Quality; November, 2013. Available at: www.effectivehealthcare.ahrq.gov/reports/final.cfm.

48. Guyatt GH, Oxman AD, Kunz R, et al. GRADE guidelines: 8. Rating the quality of evidence–indirectness. J Clin Epidemiol 2011;64(12):1303–10.

49. Balshem H, Helfand M, Schunemann HJ, et al. GRADE guidelines: 3. Rating the quality of evidence. J Clin Epidemiol 2011;64(4):401–6.

50. Canfield SE, Dahm P. Rating the quality of evidence and the strength of recommendations using GRADE. World J Urol 2011;29(3):311–7.

51. Guyatt GH, Oxman AD, Santesso N, et al. GRADE guidelines 12. Preparing summary of findings tables-binary outcomes. J Clin Epidemiol 2013;66(2):158–72.

52. Guyatt GH, Oxman AD, Schunemann HJ. GRADE guidelines-an introduction to the 10th-13th articles in the series. J Clin Epidemiol 2013;66(2):121–3.

53. Guyatt GH, Oxman AD, Kunz R, et al. GRADE guidelines 6. Rating the quality of evidence–imprecision. J Clin Epidemiol 2011;64(12):1283–93.

54. Cohen J. Statistical power analysis for the behavioral sciences. 2nd edition. Hillsdale (NJ): Lawrence Erlbaum Associates; 1988.

55. Baker A, Young K, Potter J, et al. A review of grading systems for evidence-based guidelines produced by medical specialties. Clin Med 2010;10(4):358–63.

56. Djulbegovic B, Trikalinos TA, Roback J, et al. Impact of quality of evidence on the strength of recommendations: an empirical study. BMC Health Serv Res 2009;9:120.

57. Staal JB, De Bie RA, De Vet HC, et al. Injection therapy for subacute and chronic low back pain: an updated Cochrane review. Spine 2009;34(1):49–59.

58. Benyamin RM, Manchikanti L, Parr AT, et al. The effectiveness of lumbar interlaminar epidural injections in managing chronic low back and lower extremity pain. Pain Physician 2012;15(4):E363–404.

59. Choi HJ, Hahn S, Kim CH, et al. Epidural steroid injection therapy for low back pain: a meta-analysis. Int J Technol Assess Health Care 2013;29(3): 244–53.

60. Chou R, Atlas SJ, Stanos SP, et al. Interventional therapies, surgery, and interdisciplinary rehabilitation for low back pain. Spine 2009;34(10):1066–77.

61. Quraishi NA. Transforaminal injection of corticosteroids for lumbar radiculopathy: systematic review and meta-analysis. Eur Spine J 2012;21(2):214–9.

62. Rabinovitch DL, Peliowski A, Furlan AD. Influence of lumbar epidural injection volume on pain relief for radicular leg pain and/or low back pain. Spine J 2009;9(6):509–17.

63. Roberts ST, Willick SE, Rho ME, et al. Efficacy of lumbosacral transforaminal epidural steroid injections: a systematic review. PM R 2009;1(7):657–68.

64. Kang SS, Hwang BM, Son HJ, et al. The dosages of corticosteroid in transforaminal epidural steroid injections for lumbar radicular pain due to a herniated disc. Pain Physician 2011;14(4):361–70.

65. Owlia MB, Salimzadeh A, Alishiri G, et al. Comparison of two doses of corticosteroid in epidural steroid injection for lumbar radicular pain. Singapore Med J 2007;48(3):241–5.

66. Datta R, Upadhyay KK. A randomized clinical trial of three different steroid agents for treatment of low backache through the caudal route. Med J Armed Forces India 2011;67(1):25–33.

67. Huda N, Bansal P, Gupta SM, et al. The efficacy of epidural depomethylprednisolone and triamcinolone acetate in relieving the symptoms of lumbar canal stenosis: a comparative study. J Clin Diagn Res 2010;4(4):2842–7.

68. Manchikanti L, Singh V, Cash KA, et al. The role of fluoroscopic interlaminar epidural injections in managing chronic pain of lumbar disc herniation or radiculitis: a randomized, double-blind trial. Pain Pract 2013;13(7):547–58.

69. Manchikanti L, Malla Y, Wargo BW, et al. A prospective evaluation of complications of 10,000 fluoroscopically directed epidural injections. Pain Physician 2012;15(2):131–40.

70. Epstein N. The risks of epidural and transforaminal steroid injections in the Spine: commentary and a comprehensive review of the literature. Surg Neurol Int 2013;4(Suppl 2):S74–93.

71. Molloy RE, Benzon HT. Chapter 40. Interlaminar epidural steroid injections for lumbosacral radiculopathy. In: Benson HT, Raja SN, Molloy RE, et al, editors. Essentials of pain medicine and regional anesthesia (2nd edition). Philadelphia: Elsevier Inc; 2005. p. 331–40.

72. Lewis R, Williams N, Matar H, et al. The clinical effectiveness and cost-effectiveness of management strategies for sciatica: systematic review and economic model. Health Technol Assess 2011;15(39):1–578.

73. Price C, Arden N, Coglan L, et al. Cost-effectiveness and safety of epidural steroids in the management of sciatica. Health Technol Assess 2005;9(33): 1–58, iii.

74. Manchikanti L, Falco FJ, Singh V, et al. An update of comprehensive evidence-based guidelines for interventional techniques in chronic spinal pain. Part I: introduction and general considerations. Pain Physician 2013;16(Suppl 2): S1–48.
75. Manchikanti L, Abdi S, Atluri S, et al. An update of comprehensive evidence-based guidelines for interventional techniques in chronic spinal pain. Part II: guidance and recommendations. Pain Physician 2013;16(Suppl 2):S49–283.
76. Manchikanti L, Boswell MV, Singh V, et al. Comprehensive evidence-based guidelines for interventional techniques in the management of chronic spinal pain. Pain Physician 2009;12(4):699–802.
77. Lee J, Gupta S, Price C, et al. Low back and radicular pain: a pathway for care developed by the British Pain Society. Br J Anaesth 2013;111(1):112–20.
78. North American Spine Society. Diagnosis and treatment of degenerative lumbar spinal stenosis. NASS Evidence-Based Clinical Guidelines Committee; 2011. Available at: www.spine.org/Documents/ResearchClinicalCare/Guidelines/LumbarStenosis.pdf.
79. Manchikanti L, Boswell MV, Giordano J. Evidence-based interventional pain management: principles, problems, potential and applications. Pain Physician 2007;10(2):329–56.
80. Stout A. Epidural steroid injections for low back pain. Phys Med Rehabil Clin N Am 2010;21(4):825–34.
81. Goertz M, Bonsell J, Bonte B, et al. Adult acute and subacute low back pain. Institute for Clinical Systems Improvement. Available at: https://www.icsi.org/_asset/bjvqrj/LBP.pdf. Accessed November, 2012.
82. Helm S, Glaser S, Falco F, et al. A medical-legal review regarding the standard of care for epidural injections, with particular reference to a closed case. Pain Physician 2010;13(2):145–50.

Index

Note: Page numbers of article titles are in **boldface** type.

A

Acetaminophen
    in discogenic low back pain management, 310
    side effects of, 462
Acupuncture
    in discogenic low back pain management, 311
    in MPS management, 364
Adhesive capsulitis
    in HSP differential diagnosis, 417
Alfentanil
    side effects of, 460
Analgesia/analgesics
    side effects of, **457–470**. *See also specific drugs, e.g.,* Morphine
        gender effects on, 464, 466
        introduction, 457, 463–464
        phenanthrenes, 458–459
        phenylpiperidines, 460–461
        topical analgesics, 464
Antidepressant(s)
    tricyclic
        in MPS management, 362
Antiepileptic agents
    side effects of, 465–466
Axonopathy
    in CTS diagnosis, 234–235

B

Back pain
    low
        discogenic, **305–317**. *See also* Discogenic low back pain
Benzodiazepines
    in MPS management, 361–362
Biacuplasty
    in discogenic low back pain management, 312–313
Botulinum toxin
    in HSP management, 427
    in MPS management, 366–368
Brachial plexus nerve injury
    in HSP differential diagnosis, 415–416

Phys Med Rehabil Clin N Am 25 (2014) 491–504
http://dx.doi.org/10.1016/S1047-9651(14)00028-X
1047-9651/14/$ – see front matter © 2014 Elsevier Inc. All rights reserved.

Moving?

Make sure your subscription moves with you!

To notify us of your new address, find your **Clinics Account Number** (located on your mailing label above your name), and contact customer service at:

Email: **journalscustomerservice-usa@elsevier.com**

800-654-2452 (subscribers in the U.S. & Canada)
314-447-8871 (subscribers outside of the U.S. & Canada)

Fax number: **314-447-8029**

Elsevier Health Sciences Division
Subscription Customer Service
3251 Riverport Lane
Maryland Heights, MO 63043

*To ensure uninterrupted delivery of your subscription, please notify us at least 4 weeks in advance of move.

Printed and bound by CPI Group (UK) Ltd, Croydon, CR0 4YY

03/10/2024

01040497-0008